THE CANCER PREVENTION DIET

THE CANCER PREVENTION DIET

Michio Kushi's Nutritional Blueprint for the Prevention and Relief of Disease

By MICHIO KUSHI
with ALEX JACK

ST. MARTIN'S PRESS
NEW YORK

Note to the reader:

It is advisable for the reader to seek the guidance of a
physician and appropriate nutritionist before implementing
the approach to health suggested by this book. It is
essential that any reader who has any reason to suspect
cancer or illness, contact a physician promptly. Neither
this nor any other book should be used as a substitute for
professional medical care or treatment.

Library of Congress Cataloging in Publication Data

Kushi, Michio.
    The cancer-prevention diet.

    Bibliography: p.
    Includes index.
    1. Cancer——Diet therapy——Recipes. 2. Cancer——
Nutritional aspects. 3. Cancer——Prevention.
4. Macrobiotic diet——Recipes. I. Jack, Alex, 1945–
II. Title.
RC271.D52K87 1983   616.99'40654   83–3023
ISBN 0–312–11837–6

Design by Mina Greenstein

10 9 8 7 6 5 4 3

Contents

Part III RECIPES AND MENUS

Preface

Life moves in a spiral, and each generation faces in slightly different form the obstacles and challenges of the past. In his 1849 book, *Cancerous and Cancroid Growths*, British physician John Hughes Bennett proposed a nutritional approach to preventing malignancy. "It seems to be a prudent step to diminish all those dietetic substances easily converted into fat, including not only oily matters themselves but starch and sugar. . . . These are points which, although at present unknown, will, I trust, erelong be investigated and understood," the onetime president of the Royal Medical Society continued, "and then we shall begin to have glimpses of what ought to constitute a sure and certain guide to the constitutional treatment of numerous diseases of nutrition, and, among the rest, of cancer."

Only in the last decade has modern medicine begun to investigate systematically a daily diet high in fat, refined flour, and sugar and its relationship to cancer, heart disease, and other degenerative illnesses. The exact mechanism of tumor formation at the cellular level is still imperfectly understood. However, in the last several years, most of the major American, Canadian, and European medical associations have recommended that, pending further research, the general public adopt a Prudent Diet low in saturated and unsaturated fat, cholesterol, and refined carbohydrates and high in whole grains, vegetables, and fresh fruit.

Virology, genetics, and immunology have commanded most of the attention and grants in cancer research until now. However, after a century of neglect, nutrition, the perennial stepchild of modern medicine, is finally gaining recognition as a potential Cinderella science in this effort. There is reason to believe that the slipper of dietary common sense, in combination with other lifestyle and environmental factors, will eventually be found to fit the relevant epidemiological, laboratory, and clinical data. If this holistic approach wins widespread acceptance, the chapter on cancer, one of the most sorrowful in human history, will have a happy ending.

Even though most of the Prudent Diets advanced during the last decade are moving in the right direction, some are more prudent than others. A few are based on the nutritional requirements of experimental animals that may not always be appropriate for humans. Others are derived from computer analyses programmed by people themselves suffering the same diseases that they hope to eliminate. However, perhaps the weakest link between dietary guidelines and their implementation is the lack of adequate recipes and menus. How does an ordinary person, family, school cafeteria, or hospital kitchen translate general proposals to lower fat and increase fiber into daily meals? The nation's food writers and cooking columnists have moved to fill this vacuum by publishing various menu plans to help protect against cancer. Basically they call for consuming a little less of everything that people already are eating and suspect are not particularly good for them. The menus do not reflect the fundamental change in the quality of food selection, preparation, or cooking that is needed if cancer, heart disease, and other degenerative illnesses are truly to be eliminated.

The approach to health presented in this book has evolved naturally in both East and West. We call it the Cancer-Prevention Diet because it has protected most of the human family from cancer and related diseases for more than a hundred generations. During the last two decades, hundreds of thousands of people around the world have successfully adopted this way of eating, under the name macrobiotics, and found that it not only protects them from serious disease but also is delicious and satisfying. This includes hundreds of people from all walks of life who have relieved already existing cancers with the recipes and menus developed by Aveline Kushi and introduced in this volume.

Over the centuries, many individuals, communities, and cultures have contributed to the approach presented in this book. The authors would especially like to express their deep appreciation and gratitude to the late Yukikazu Sakurazawa (George Ohsawa) and his wife Lima, who have inspired modern macrobiotics, and to the few remaining traditional societies that have kept alive the intuitive culinary wisdom of the past.

Also, we are thankful to the many practitioners down through the ages, both Eastern and Western, traditional healers and medical doctors, therapists and researchers, who have devoted their lives to studying diet and disease. We appreciate all current medical, educational, and governmental efforts, as well as individual initiatives, to improve personal, family, and public health. We wish to work together with all organizations and people concerned with the problem of cancer and modern society. We hope that this book serves as a contribution to this common goal and we welcome any comments or suggestions on cooperation in the future.

Natural foods and holistic healing practices are gradually entering the mainstream of American society. This book also represents the unfolding experience and insight of thousands of contemporary macrobiotic health and dietary counselors, teachers, cooks, organic farmers and gardeners, natural foods store personnel, authors and artists who are actively involved in transforming world health through a return to whole foods and a more natural way of life.

New directions in medicine are also emerging as we prepare for the century ahead. We are grateful to the many doctors, nurses, nutritionists, public health educators, medical journalists, and cancer patients and their families who have participated since 1977 in the East West Foundation's annual conference on a nutritional approach to cancer and other degenerative diseases, and related activities. These include Robert S. Mendelsohn, M.D., author, syndicated columnist, and former chairman of the Medical Licensure Committee for the State of Illinois; Nicholas Mottern, a congressional staff member, who contributed to the U.S. Senate Select Committee on Nutrition and Human Need's report *Dietary Goals for the United States;* Drs. Edward Kass and Frank Sacks of Harvard Medical School; Marilyn Light, president of the American Hypoglycemia Foundation; Marian Tompson, founder of the La Leche League; and William Castelli, M.D., director of the Framingham Heart Study.

Participants also included Stephen Appelbaum, Ph.D., of the Menninger Foundation; Jonathan Lieff, M.D., of the Shattuck Hospital, Boston; Frederic Ettner, M.D., of the American International

Hospital, Zion, Illinois; Norman Ralston, D.V.M., from Dallas; Marc Van Cauwenberghe, M.D., from Ghent, Belgium; Keith Block, M.D., from Evanston, Illinois; Christiane Northrup, M.D., from Portland, Maine; Peter Klein, M.D., from Rockville, Maryland; Kristen Schmidt, R.N., from Cincinnati; Chandrasekhar Thakkur, M.D., from Bombay; Hideo Ohmori of the Japan C.I. Foundation; Shizuko Yamamoto, director of the East West Center in New York; William Dufty, author of *Sugar Blues;* Gloria Swanson, film star, author, and inspirational example of a healthy way of life; the late Jean Kohler, professor of music at Ball State University, and his wife Mary Alice, authors of *Healing Miracles from Macrobiotics;* and Peter Barry Chowka, medical journalist and commentator.

Useful assistance in preparing this book has been provided by our families and friends. We would especially like to thank Aveline Kushi for developing the recipes and menus and Lawrence Kushi, a doctoral student at the Harvard School of Public Health, for looking over some of the medical sections. Understanding, literary support, and gentle encouragement were also given by Esther Jack, Homer Jack, Lucy Williams, Jonathan Williams, Sherman Goldman, Ann Purvis, Tom Monte, Karin Stephan, David Brisson, Eric Zutrau, and Frank Salvati.

Research was conducted at the Boston Public Library, the Brookline Public Library, and the Countway Library of Medicine of Harvard University. We are fortunate to have these resources in the Boston area. At the back of this book, we include our own reference section. Please turn to the glossary to look up any medical terms and food items that may be unfamiliar.

Various other colleagues deserve mention for their ongoing work in presenting information on cancer and diet to the public through classes, workshops, seminars, and other books and magazine articles. These include Bill Tara, Carolyn Heindenry, and Olivia Oredsen of the Kushi Institute and Kushi Foundation; Edward Esko, author and editor of several other publications on cancer and diet; Steve Minkin of the *East West Journal;* and Gary Smith of the East West Foundation. We are grateful to them and their staffs for advice and encouragement, as well as the many friends at macrobiotic educational centers in this country and abroad who are working to create a healthy and peaceful world.

In seeing this book into final form, we wish to thank Flo Nakamura and Anna Picchioni for secretarial help. We are especially grateful to Julia Coopersmith, our literary representative, and Ashton Applewhite, our editor at St. Martin's. Their prudent editorial guidelines, enthusiasm, and gracious help all along the way are deeply appreciated. We also wish to thank Tom Dunne, Pamela Dorman, Ina Shapiro, Mab Gray, and Margaret Willard at St. Martin's for their contributions to the publication of this volume.

Society as a whole is on the threshold of a breakthrough in its application of diet to the prevention and relief of illness. We hope that this book contributes to modern humanity's understanding of cancer and to the future health and happiness of generations without end.

MICHIO KUSHI
ALEX JACK

Brookline, Massachusetts
February 16, 1982

THE CANCER
PREVENTION
DIET

PART I

Preventing Cancer Naturally

1.

Cancer, Diet, and Macrobiotics

When I first came to America nearly thirty-five years ago, the expected cancer rate was about one out of eight people. Today this rate has risen to 30 percent of the population, or nearly one out of every three people, according to the American Cancer Society. In 1983 more than 440,000 Americans will die of the disease, and another 855,000 new cases will be detected. Another 400,000 cases of usually non-fatal skin cancer will also arise this year. If this increase continues at the present rate, by the end of the century, 50 percent of the population then living will develop cancer during their lifetime, and thirty to thirty-five years from now virtually everyone will have the disease at some time before their death.

Recently I was reading a copy of *Time* magazine and happened to glance at the obituary column. I noticed that almost everyone on the list that week had died of cancer. They included Stefan Cardinal Wyszynski, the Roman Catholic prelate of Poland; Soong Ch'ing-ling, the widow of Sun Yat Sen and a high official of the People's Republic of China; Charles Yost, a former U.S. ambassador to the United Nations; and Mary Lou Williams, the black jazz composer. Clearly cancer is one of the great levelers of the modern age. It strikes the high and the low, rich and poor, male and female, young and old, black and white, Westerner and Oriental, capitalist and communist, saint and sinner. There is hardly a family today untouched.

Other chronic and degenerative illnesses are also on the rise. Thirty years ago the rate of mental illness in America was one out of twenty. It has now more than doubled to over one out of ten. Forty-two million people in this country have cardiovascular disorders, 37-million have high blood pressure, 35-million have allergies, 14- to 28-million suffer from alcoholism, tens of millions abuse drugs, 13-million have birth defects, 11-million are diabetic, 5-million are mentally retarded, 2-million have epilepsy, about 1-million have Parkinson's disease, and one-half-million have multiple sclerosis.

One of the most dramatic increases in recent decades has been in the rise of sexual disorders. In 1982 the British Medical Association, for example, reported that new cases of venereal disease in Great Britain had risen 1,700 percent since 1957. In both Europe and North America, herpes and other sexually transmitted diseases (STD) have assumed epidemic proportions. In addition, infertility is on the increase. Since the 1920's, the average sperm count in American males has dropped by 39 percent according to medical tests, and one recent study of otherwise healthy college males showed that 23 percent were functionally sterile. Moreover, about 800,000 American women, many of childbearing age, currently have their ovaries or uteruses surgically removed each year because of cancer or the fear of cancer.

A host of new diseases has developed to further challenge medical science and national health. Toxic shock syndrome, Legionnaire's disease, and Kaposi's sarcoma, to mention a few, have affected thousands of people, and millions of others are afraid of developing these disorders. Meanwhile, old illnesses are coming back in more virulent form. New varieties of pneumonia and other infectious diseases have been reported for which there is no medical relief on the horizon. A 1982 Tufts University Medical School study found that 75 percent of the population sampled now carries a significant level of antibiotic-resistant bacteria in their digestive system. Even the simple common cold, despite a much publicized medical campaign begun twenty years ago under President Kennedy, remains largely immune to effective treatment. In fact, few major sicknesses, if any, can really be cured by modern methods. In some cases pain and other discomfort can be relieved and the symptoms temporarily diminished or controlled, but, fundamentally, illness cannot be cured and sooner or later reappears.

Given these and many other trends, we can see that modern civilization as a whole is on the verge of self-destruction as a result of deep-seated chronic biological degeneration. This includes the United States, Canada, the Soviet Union, Eastern and Western Europe, Japan, Australia, China, and many other parts of Asia, Africa, and Latin America. The threat of possible extinction from degenerative disease and the inability of humanity in the future to reproduce itself is just as real as the danger posed by the accumulation of nuclear weapons. And, like the arms race, the time left to us to reverse this direction is very short. By the time the present generation grows to adulthood, we may be witnessing the complete decline of our recently developed modern way of life. The final collapse may come within the next thirty or, at the most, forty years.

The cancer problem, however, offers us the chance to seriously rethink our present understanding of health and sickness. It provides the opportunity to reexamine the basic premises of our way of life and work together as members of a common planetary family to build one healthy, peaceful world.

CANCER IN THE ANCIENT WORLD

The history of cancer goes back 2,500 years to ancient Greece where Hippocrates first identified and described the illness. In Greek the word *karkinos,* from which our word cancer comes, originally meant crab. The Father of Western medicine evidently chose the image because of the disease's crablike spread through the body. Though known and classified since ancient times, cancer was an extremely rare illness. Through most of recorded history it has affected only a tiny fraction of the world's population. For instance, cancer is not mentioned in the Bible, nor is it included in the Yellow Emperor's Classic of Internal Medicine, the ancient medical book of China. In most traditional societies, cancer was completely unknown. However, about the time of the Industrial Revolution, beginning in the seventeenth century, cancer gradually began to emerge in the West. In the 1830's Stanislas Tanchou, a French scientist who pioneered in the field of vital statistics, tabulated the mortality rates around Paris and reported that cancer deaths comprised about two percent of the total. At the beginning of the twentieth century, the cancer rate in the United States had reached about four percent. As recently as a generation ago, many forms of cancer common today were rare.

"In 1919, during my junior year at Washington University, a patient with cancer of the lung was admitted to the Barnes Hospital," Alton Oschner, M.D. recalls of his medical training in an article in *American Scientist.* "As was usual, the patient died. Dr. George

Dock, our Professor of Medicine, who was not only an eminent clinician and scientist but also an excellent pathologist, insisted upon the two senior classes witnessing the autopsy, and he stressed that the condition was so rare he thought we might never see another case as long as we lived." Dr. Oschner adds that he saw his next case of lung cancer in 1936, seventeen years later.

As modern civilization spread across the world, a legion of explorers, medical doctors, missionaries, and other travelers marveled at the almost complete absence of degenerative disease in native societies. In 1908 W. Roger Williams, a Fellow of the Royal College of Surgeons, chronicled the absence of cancer in overseas territories of the British Empire in his book, *The Natural History of Cancer*. In the 1920's Sir Robert McCarrison, Director of Nutritional Research in India, wrote about his discovery of the remote Hunza culture where disease was virtually unknown and people lived to an exceedingly old age. In the 1930's, Japanese educator George Ohsawa began his study of indigenous cultures culminating in his book, *Cancer and the Philosophy of the Far East*. Dental surgeon Weston Price performed fieldwork among the Indians of North America, the Eskimo, the Polynesians, and the Australian Aborigines and reported no trace of cancer in his 1945 publication, *Nutrition and Physical Degeneration*.

These four medical detectives and others tried to explain why traditional peoples living in the tropics, polar regions, islands, and other cultures removed from modern civilization remained immune to cancer, heart disease, and even tooth decay. After careful observation and research, including laboratory testing in some cases, they each independently concluded that cancer was a disease of overnutrition caused by intake of sugar, white flour, and other refined foods, as well as excess protein and fat. When these items were introduced into primitive societies, cancer and other degenerative diseases followed close behind.

A few professional cancer researchers drew the obvious conclusions from reports such as these, as well as from epidemiological studies comparing diets and incidence of disease among different populations. In the July 1927 medical journal, *Cancer*, William Howard Hay, M.D. conjectured:

Think back over the years of cancer research, of the millions spent, the time consumed, the pains expended . . . and where are we today? Is it not time to take stock of our basic conception of cancer to see if there is not something radically wrong with this, to account for the years of utter and complete failure to date? . . . Cancer has been consistently on the increase. . . . Is it possible that the cause of cancer lies in our departure from natural foods? It would surely look so to any man from Mars, but we have lived so long on processed foods deficient in vitamines and tissue salts that we are in a state of unbalanced nutrition almost from birth. . . . We have come to regard our [refined] foods as the hallmark of civilization, when it is a fact that these very foods set the stage for every sort of ill, including cancer.

THE STAFF OF LIFE

All civilizations prior to ours recognized the primacy of food and agriculture and enshrined dietary concerns in their household economies, religions, and literature and art. Cooked whole grains, in particular, have constituted humanity's staple food for thousands of years, and, until fairly recently, were eaten as the staple food throughout the world. For example, rice and millet were principal foods in the Orient; wheat, oats, and rye in Europe; buckwheat in Russia and Central Asia; sorghum in Africa; barley in the Middle East; and corn in the Americas. In fact, the English word for food is *meal*, or ground grain, while in Japanese, the term used for meal is *gohan*, which means cooked rice.*

In the ancient world, nutritional therapy formed the core of medical understanding and practice. Hippocrates' writings, for example, are permeated with dietary considerations, and he frequently emphasizes the importance of wheat and barley, the two principal grains of the Hellenistic world. "I know too that the body is affected differently by bread according to the manner in which it is prepared," he explains in *Tradition in Medicine*. "It differs according as it is made

*The Old English word *meat* also originally meant daily food, staple fare: oats, barley, rye, wheat, and the edible part of nuts and fruits. Later the word took on four connotations: 1) green meat or grains and vegetables, 2) baked meat or bread (cf. *Hamlet*, "The Funerall Bakt-meats/ Did coldly furnish forth the Marriage Tables"), 3) sweetmeats or pastries, and 4) butcher's meat (also known as red-, dark-, horse-, and hard-meat). Later, when the generic words for staple food in the Bible were translated into the vernacular, confusion about the original meaning of the concept *meat* arose. In the King James Version, it refers to staple food as this passage from Genesis makes clear: "Behold, I have given you every herb bearing seed, which is upon the face of all the earth, and every tree, in the which is the fruit of a tree yielding seed; to you it shall be for meat."

from pure flour or meal with bran, whether it is prepared from win-
nowed or unwinnowed wheat, whether it is mixed with much water
or little, whether well mixed or poorly mixed, overbaked or under-
baked, and countless other points besides. The same is true of the
preparation of barley meal. The influence of each process is considerable and each has a totally different effect from another. How can
anyone who has not considered such matters and come to understand
them, possibly know anything of the diseases that afflict mankind?
Each one of the substances of a man's diet acts upon his body and
changes it in some way and upon these changes his whole life
depends. . . ."

The matter of food became so important to the founder of Western medicine that he coined another new word, *diaita*, to refer to a
way of life. From this Greek word our modern word *diet* comes.
Today its meaning has narrowed to signify weight loss or restricted
regimen, but the proper meaning is a mode of living of which food
selection and preparation is the main factor.

In treating serious illnesses in the fifth century B.C., Hippocrates
stressed the importance of using dietary methods. In *The Book on
Nutriment* he declares, "Let food be thy medicine and medicine thy
food." The Hippocratic Oath, still taken by modern medical doctors,
states, in part: "I will apply dietetic measures for the benefit of the
sick according to my ability and judgment; I will keep them from
harm and injustice. I will neither give a deadly drug to anybody if
asked for it, nor will I make a suggestion to this effect. . . . I will not
use the knife. . . ." His favorite remedy was cooked whole-grain barley cereal. He hailed this broth as "smooth, consistent, soothing; slippery and fairly soft; thirst-quenching and easily got rid of; doesn't
produce constipation or rumbling or swell up the stomach." He described various ways the barley meal could be modified for different
illnesses and supplemented dietary adjustments with simple, safe
compresses made of grains, vegetables, and herbs, which could be
prepared in the home. In the case of cancer, he warned against surgery: "If treated the patients die quickly; but if not treated, they hold
out for a long time."

CANCER IN MEDIEVAL TIMES

Hippocrates' careful attention to diet and environment won widespread renown. His conviction that disease had a natural rather than
a supernatural origin represented a break with the past and set the

direction for the medicine of the future. Until the seventeenth century, his natural healing methods and those of Galen, the second-century Roman physician, were widely practiced in the European and Arab worlds. In the Middle Ages, Maimonides, the famous Jewish physician, formulated a similar dietary philosophy and cautioned against eating "any kind of meal so completely sifted that not a trace of bran remains in it."

The *Divine Comedy* alludes to the origin of cancer. The key passage comes in a discussion between Dante and Virgil, his guide through the Inferno and Purgatory, on the necessity of heeding Nature's teaching and following "her laws, her fruits, her seasons." Dante characterizes the approach to life which ignores or scorns Nature as "a canker to every conscience" and throughout the early fourteenth-century epic extols the harmonious souls who followed a simple diet during their lifetime. For example, from the Bible he singles out Daniel for refusing the meat of the Babylonian king's table, and he locates the followers of Hippocrates atop the summit of the Earthly Paradise. As late as Shakespeare's day, the sixteenth century, Sir Thomas Elyot's *The Castle of Health*, a popular guide to home remedies, catalogued the effects of different foods upon the human body and recommended the consumption of cereal grains, principally rye and barley, to relieve serious illnesses.

Food selection and proper cooking also served as the cornerstone for preventing and relieving illness in the Far East. In the Yellow Emperor's Classic of Internal Medicine, Ch'i Po (the Hippocrates of the Orient) recommended that a broth of brown rice be eaten for ten days to cure cases of chronic disease. The Caraka Samhita, India's chief medical text dating to the first century A.D., equated the rise of illness in Hindu society with deterioration in diet. Other works warned against a departure from simple, whole foods, which then as now tended to be neglected by the rich and upper classes of society. For example, during the Song Dynasty, nearly a thousand years ago, a Chinese philosopher named Yang Fang complained that the children and grandchildren of officials "will be unwilling to eat vegetables and will look on greens and broth as coarse fare, finding beans, wheat, and millet meager and tasteless, and insisting on the best polished rice, and the finest roasts to satisfy their greedy appetites, with the products of the water and the land and the confections of human artifice set out before them neatly in ornamentally carved dishes and trays."

Further east, in 1714 Ekiken Kaibara, a Japanese physician and

Confucian scholar, completed *Yojokun,* a book on health and longevity describing the wisdom of adopting a brown-rice diet and disapproving of all symptomatic treatments for disease, including surgery.

THE RISE OF MODERN SCIENCE AND MEDICINE

Despite the calls for dietary common sense by Yang Fang, Maimonides, Sir Thomas Elyot, Ekiken Kaibara, and others, the spice trade generated by the Crusades and the discovery of the New World transformed traditional patterns of eating in East and West and ushered in the scientific age. With the overthrow of Hippocrates, Galen, Aristotle, and Ptolemy in the seventeenth and eighteenth centuries, the philosophy of natural healing, which had prevailed for two thousand years, declined, and Descartes' view of the world as a machine laid the conceptual groundwork for modern science and medicine. The doctrine of humors, which animated medicine in ancient Greece, the Middle Ages, and the Renaissance, quickly faded. Under this system, human constitutions and conditions, body organs, and different foods were classified according to varying combinations of Earth, Air, Water, and Fire, and an imbalance in these energies and their respective humors was believed to give rise to disease, including cancer. With the invention of the microscope and lifting of Church sanctions against dissection of the human body, a new view developed that saw illness as a manifestation of a chemical change in the body's tissues, usually localized in a particular organ. Treatment, according to this perspective, could also be chemical, directed to the diseased organ.

In the first laboratory experiment with cancerous tissue, Jean Astruc, a physician to eighteenth-century French and Polish monarchs, incinerated a piece of a human breast tumor and a piece of beefsteak in a retort and found they tasted the same. He concluded that cancerous growth had no more salty or bitter taste than ordinary cow's meat, the staple diet of royalty, and that the traditional humoral theories, which connected cancer with foods containing excess bile salts or acid, were wrong. On the basis of this test, future cancer researchers tended to dismiss the dietary hypothesis, which, in actuality, it had confirmed.

In other developments, Lavoisier laid the foundation for empirical study of respiration, oxidation, and caloric measurement. In France and England, the first hospitals devoted exclusively to cancer opened. In America, Dr. Benjamin Rush's treatment of yellow fever with calomel in 1793 ushered in the modern era of medical intervention and massive purging, bloodletting, blistering, and use of caustic dyes to root out disease. The eminent signer of the Declaration of Independence blamed Hippocrates for relying too much on the patient's own recuperative powers and held that "the work [of healing] must be taken out of nature's hand."

With the spread of the Industrial Revolution, traditional agriculture and food technology changed. By the early nineteenth century, steam-driven mills replaced water- and windmills, and nearly all aspects of breadmaking were mechanized and out of human hands. Tuberculosis, stomach ailments, and cancer increased as refined flour became widely available. A few eloquent health reformers warned against the declining use of whole grains. They include Reverend Sylvester Graham, popularizer of the whole-wheat Graham bread and Graham cracker; Mary Gove Nichols, leader of the Boston Ladies Physiological Society; and Ellen Harmon White, a founder of the Seventh Day Adventists, who championed unbolted flour and helped introduce soyfoods to this continent. However, these prophetic voices were ultimately lost in the analytical din of the nineteenth century as the engine of industrial society forged full steam ahead.

European society witnessed continued quantification and specialization in medical science and the rise of metabolic theory. The German scientist Liebig classified nourishment into protein, carbohydrate, and fat. The Austrian biologist Virchow developed cellular pathology and, as a scientific model, likened the cells of the body to citizens of a republic. In his view, disease represented a civil conflict among cells brought about by the intervention of outside forces. In the field of cancer, the Russian researcher Novinsky performed the first transplants of tumors in laboratory animals. In Vienna, Billroth introduced surgical removal of cancerous inner organs. In the Far East, Japanese medical students avidly turned to Western medicine following contact with Portuguese, Spanish, and Dutch surgeons. By 1868, under the Meiji rulers, Japan officially adopted the German medical system and prepared to assume its role in the technological forefront of the modern world. In China, government edicts outlawed the teaching and practice of traditional medicine as it had existed for thousands of years.

CANCER TREATMENT IN THE TWENTIETH CENTURY

With the rise of the petrochemical industry in the United States and Western Europe in the early part of the twentieth century, surgery and pharmacology consolidated their triumph over other approaches to medicine. The spread of chemical agriculture and factory farming revolutionized patterns of food consumption in the industrialized world. Nutrition became relegated to the back bunson burner as genetics, biochemistry, and radiation techniques dominated medical research.

Despite the general neglect of dietary concerns, a host of international population studies emerged during the middle part of the century linking cancer with high fat intake, refined carbohydrates, chemical additives, and other nutritional variables. Building on the earlier reports of the colonial medical doctors and anthropologists, epidemiologists concluded that cultures and subcultures eating a traditional diet of whole grains, cooked vegetables, and fresh seasonal fruit remained largely cancer-free.

One of the clearest warnings was sounded by Frederick L. Hoffman, LL.D., cancer specialist and consulting statistician for the Prudential Life Insurance Company. In his 1937 volume, *Cancer and Diet,* he stated:

> I have come to the essential conclusion that there has been a decided increase in the cancer death rate and progressively so during the last century ending with 1930. From this I reflect that the profound changes in dietary habits and nutritional condition of the population taking place during the intervening years have been world wide and due to the rapid and almost universal introduction of modified food products, conserved or preserved, refrigerated or sterilized, colored or modified, aside from positive adulteration by the addition of injurious mineral substances close to being of a poisonous nature. To a diminishing extent food is being consumed in its natural state, at least by urban populations everywhere, and to a lesser degree also among persons in rural communities.

In the 1940's and 1950's, laboratory studies on mice and other animals began to confirm these findings. Also, several European countries experienced a significant drop in cancer mortality rates during World Wars I and II when meat, dairy food, and eggs became scarce and local populations were forced to survive on brown bread, oats and barley meal, and home-grown produce.

Following World War II, frozen and enriched foods became more widely available, many tropical and subtropical foods such as oranges, grapefruits, and pineapples found their way to the daily breakfast table, and soft drinks, ice cream, candy bars, pizza, hamburgers, french fries, potato chips, and other fast foods became a way of life. As cancer rates climbed, the medical profession stepped up its technological arsenal. In 1971 President Nixon formally declared war on the disease and commissioned the National Cancer Institute to eradicate it. However, this mobilization largely excluded dietary means.

In 2,500 years, since cancer was first described in ancient Greece, medicine had come full circle. In *Epidemics*, Book I, Hippocrates cited factors for the physician to consider in making diagnoses and recommending treatment. At the head of the list comes "what food is given to him [the patient] and who gives it," followed by conditions of the climate and local environment, the patient's customs, mode of life, pursuits, age, speech, mannerisms, silences, thoughts, sleeping patterns, and dreams. Last on the list is physical symptoms. The priorities of modern medicine were just reversed. In 1973, according to a Harvard School of Public Health study, only four percent of the nation's medical schools had an independent course in nutrition.

A RETURN TO WHOLE FOODS

In nature, just as day follows night and valleys turn into mountains, societies regenerate after a long period of decay. In the modern world, the turning point came in the 1960's and 1970's when awareness of the deficiencies of the contemporary way of life and eating generated the natural foods and holistic health movements. Vegetarian and health foods had long been available, but their quality was often low and they appealed only to a tiny market. Suddenly, the postwar generation, which had become active in integrating Southern lunch counters and preserving the ricefields of Vietnam from destruction by bombs and chemical reagents, became conscious of the food they ate, and organized Food Days to consider the impact of modern agriculture on world hunger, energy conservation, and the quality of the environment.

By 1976 the concern for healthy food echoed through the halls of

Congress. In its historic report, *Dietary Goals for the United States*, the Senate Select Committee on Nutrition and Human Needs listed cancer as one of the six major degenerative diseases associated with improper nutrition. The report sent shock waves through the American food industry and medical profession. The cattle- and hog-growers' associations, the poultry and egg producers, and the refined salt institute condemned the report.

However, at the highest national level, the door had been opened for a return to healthy food. Within the next five years, dozens of medical and scientific associations corroborated the link between diet and degenerative disease. In his 1979 report, *Healthy People: Health Promotion and Disease Prevention*, the U.S. Surgeon General stated, "People should consume . . . less saturated fat and cholesterol . . . less red meat . . . more complex carbohydrates such as whole grains, cereals, fruits and vegetables." The American Heart Association, the American Diabetes Association, the American Society for Clinical Nutrition, and the U.S. Department of Agriculture issued similar statements. In 1981 a panel of the American Association for the Advancement of Science reported on the social impact of a change to a whole-grain diet. The scientists declared that changes in our eating habits could have significant beneficial effects on everything from land, water, fuel, and mineral use to the cost of living, unemployment, and the balance of international trade as well as reduce coronary heart disease by 88 percent and cancer by 50 percent.

In 1982 the National Academy of Sciences issued a 472-page report, *Diet, Nutrition, and Cancer*, calling upon the general public to reduce substantially consumption of foods high in saturated and unsaturated fat and increase daily intake of whole grains, vegetables, and fruit. The panel reviewed hundreds of current medical studies associating long-term eating patterns with the development of most common cancers, including those of the colon, stomach, breast, lung, esophagus, ovary, and prostate. The thirteen-member scientific committee suggested that diet could be responsible for 30 to 40 percent of cancers in men and 60 percent in women.

If followed up by the general public and the medical profession, *Diet, Nutrition, and Cancer* promises to end the second-class status of nutritional research in this country and abroad. The National Academy of Science's dietary guidelines are similar in direction to the Cancer-Prevention Diet that the East West Foundation, the *East*

West Journal, and other macrobiotic organizations have advanced during the past decade.

In addition, medical researchers at Harvard Medical School, Harvard School of Public Health, and affiliated hospitals in Boston, Massachusetts have conducted studies and reported on the protective health benefits of the macrobiotic dietary approach, particularly in lowering cholesterol and high blood pressure. These studies have been published in the *American Journal of Epidemiology,* the *New England Journal of Medicine, Journal of the American Medical Association,* and *Atherosclerosis.* For the past two years, the Lemuel Shattuck Hospital, a state-sponsored facility in Boston, has offered macrobiotic meals to its doctors and staff and is now offering lectures in Oriental medicine and philosophy. In 1982 researchers at the hospital from Tufts University Medical School conducted a double-blind study on a ward of psychiatric patients to measure the effects of a change to a macrobiotic diet.

At another institutional level, in Chesapeake, Virginia, the Tidewater Detention Center is initiating a macrobiotic dietary program designed to improve the health of its juvenile offenders. A preliminary experiment in which sugar was removed from the diet resulted in 45 percent less infractions and instances of aggressive behavior among inmates. Macrobiotic food is also available to prisoners in Lisbon, Portugal, and some who have taken advantage of this opportunity have undergone a change in consciousness and health, won early release, and gone on to useful, active lives. Several other prisons, institutions for exceptional children, and medical schools in the United States are in the process of initiating macrobiotic programs. Hundreds of thousands of people now following the Cancer-Prevention Diet are free of worry from cancer, heart disease, and other degenerative illnesses. Thousands of others who began the diet when they were ill have relieved their sicknesses and resumed healthy, meaningful lives.

The purpose of this book is to introduce the Cancer-Prevention Diet to many more people. This includes those who want to protect themselves and their families from cancer and those who already have cancer or precancerous conditions and are seeking an alternative or adjunct to surgery, radiation, or chemotherapy. In addition, we hope this book will help doctors and scientists better understand the origin and development of the disease as well as introduce simple and safe methods for its relief. To this end, we shall present a scientific model to account for the often confusing test results that many cancer researchers obtain as well as a comprehensive theory that can relate one cancer to another and locate the illness within the overall spectrum of health and disease.

THE MACROBIOTIC APPROACH

It is important to understand that macrobiotics is not just a diet in the modern sense of the term, but a way of life encompassing all dimensions of living. From such diverse phenomena as the size and shape of distant galaxies to the movements of subatomic particles, from the periodic rise and fall of civilizations to the patterns of our own individual lives, macrobiotic philosophy offers a unifying principle to understand the order of the universe as a whole.

Translated literally, *macro* is the Greek word for "great" or "long" and *bios* is the word for "life." Macrobiotics means the way of life according to the greatest or longest possible view. The earliest recorded usage of the term is found in the writings of Hippocrates. In the essay *Airs, Waters, and Places*, the Father of Western medicine introduces the word to describe a group of young men who are healthy and relatively long-lived. Other classical writers, including Herodotus, Aristotle, Galen, and Lucian, also used the term, and the concept came to signify living in harmony with nature, eating a simple balanced diet, and living to an active old age. In the popular imagination, macrobiotics became particularly associated with the Ethiopians of Africa, who were said to live 120 years or more, the Biblical patriarchs, and the Chinese sages. In *Pantagruel and Gargantua,* the sixteenth-century French humanist Rabelais mentions a fabulous Isle of the Macreons where his adventurers meet a sage named Macrobius who guides them along their way. In 1797 the German physician and philosopher Christoph W. Hufeland, M.D. wrote an influential book on diet and health entitled *Macrobiotics or The Art of Prolonging Life*.

In the Near and Far East, the macrobiotic spirit also guided and shaped civilization. Dietary common sense and principles of natural healing underlie the Bible, the I Ching, the Tao Te Ching, the Bhagavad Gita, the Kojiki, the Koran, and many other scriptures and epics. Down through the centuries, as we have seen, cultural movements surfaced in Asia to extol the benefits of the traditional way of eating and caution against increasingly artificial ways.

In the late nineteenth and early twentieth centuries, macrobiotics experienced a revival originating in Japan. Two educators, Sagen Ishitsuka, M.D. and Yukikazu Sakurazawa, cured themselves of serious illnesses by changing from the modern refined diet then sweeping Japan to a simple diet of brown rice, miso soup, sea vegetables, and other traditional foods. After restoring their health, they went on to integrate traditional Oriental medicine and philosophy with Vedanta, original Jewish and Christian teachings, and holistic perspectives in modern science and medicine. When Sakurazawa came to Paris in the 1920's, he adopted George Ohsawa as his pen name and called his teachings *macrobiotics*.

Thus macrobiotics today is a unique synthesis of Eastern and Western influences. It is the way of life according to the largest possible view, the infinite order of the universe. The practice of macrobiotics is the understanding and practical application of this order to our lifestyle, including the selection, preparation, and manner of eating of our daily food, as well as the orientation of consciousness. Macrobiotics does not offer a single diet for everyone but a dietary principle that takes into account differing climatic and geographical considerations, varying ages, sexes, and levels of activity, and ever-changing personal needs. Macrobiotics also embraces the variety and richness of all the world's cultures and heritages.

Broadly speaking, dietary practice according to macrobiotics is the way of eating that flourished from before the time of Homer to the Renaissance. It is the diet that Buddha ate under the tree of enlightenment and that Jesus shared with his disciples at the Last Supper. It is the diet that helped Moses free his people from bondage and that sustained the Pilgrims upon their arrival in the New World. Most of all macrobiotics is the way of life followed by ordinary people throughout history: farmers, shepherds, fishermen, merchants, traders, artisans, scribes, monks, bards. From the earliest campfires in the Ice Age to the latest space launches in the Atomic Age, countless mothers, fathers, daughters, sons, babies, and grandparents have shared nourishing food together and saved the seeds to plant the following spring.

To the eye of Heaven, our era is but a day. The spread of cancer and the proliferation of nuclear weapons are only passing shadows in humanity's prolonged adolescence. One day future generations will look back at the cult of modern civilization and regard its unnatural food and artificial way of life as a fad that flared up and extinguished itself in the relatively short span of four-hundred years. Under many names and forms, macrobiotics will continue as long as human life continues to exist, as its most fundamental and intuitive wisdom. It offers a key to restoring our health, a vision for regenerating the world, and a compass for charting our endless voyage toward freedom and enduring peace.

2.

Cancer and Modern Civilization

Over the last thirty-five years, modern medical science has mounted a tremendous campaign to solve the problems of cancer and other degenerative illnesses. To date, however, this large-scale effort has produced no lasting, comprehensive solutions.

In the field of cancer research, for example, modern medicine has pioneered such techniques as surgery, radiation therapy, laser therapy, chemotherapy, hormone therapy, and others. But these treatments are, at best, successful only in achieving temporary relief of symptoms. In the majority of cases they fail to prevent the disease from recurring, as they do not address the root cause or origin of the problem.

We believe that this biological decline is not irreversible, but that to prevent such a catastrophe from occurring we must begin to approach such problems as cancer with a new orientation. Specifically, we must begin to seek out the most basic causes and to implement the most basic solutions rather than continue the present approach of treating each problem separately in terms of its symptoms alone. The problem of degenerative disease affects us all in one way or another in all domains of modern life. Therefore, the responsibility of finding and implementing solutions should not be left only to those within the medical and scientific communities. We believe that the recovery of global health will emerge only through a cooperative effort involving people at all levels of society.

The epidemic of degenerative disease, the decline of traditional human values, and the decomposition of society itself are all clear indications that something is deeply wrong with the modern orientation of life. At present, we tend to value the development of civilization in terms of our advancing material prosperity. At the same time, we tend to undervalue the development of human consciousness, intuition, and spiritual development. But this viewpoint is out of proportion with the very nature of existence. The world of matter itself is a small, fragmental, and almost infinitesimal manifestation when compared to the vast currents of moving space and energy which envelop it and out of which it has come into physical existence.

Not only is the material world infinitesimally small by comparison, but also, as modern quantum physics has demonstrated, the more we analyze and take it apart, the more we discover that it actually has no concrete substance. The search for an ultimate unit of matter, which began with Democritus' assumption that reality could be divided into atoms and space, has ended in the twentieth century with the discovery that subatomic particles are nothing but charged matrixes of moving energy. Einstein's formulation that $E = MC^2$ signifies that matter is not solid material at all but ultimately waves of energy or vibration.

However, our limited senses easily delude us into believing that things have a fixed or unchanging quality, in spite of the fact that all of the cells, tissues, skin, and organs that comprise the human body are continuously changing. The red blood cells in the bloodstream live about 120 days. In order to maintain a relatively constant number of these cells, an astounding 200-million new cells are created every minute, while an equal number of old cells are continuously destroyed. The entire body regenerates itself about every seven years. As a result, what we think of as today's "self" is very different from yesterday's "self" and tomorrow's "self." This is obvious to parents who have watched their children grow. However, our development does not stop when we reach physical maturity: Our consciousness and judgment also change and develop during the entire period of life.

ENLARGING OUR PERSPECTIVE

In reality, there is nothing static, fixed, or permanent. Yet modern people frequently adopt an unchanging and inflexible attitude and, as a result, experience repeated frustration and disappointment when faced with the ephemerality of life. Today's culture which overemphasizes competition and material acquisition is based primarily on consumer values, and the successful production of consumer goods depends largely on mass marketing. In order to succeed, a product must stimulate or gratify our physical senses. Of itself, sensory satisfaction is not necessarily destructive; everyone is entitled to satisfy their basic senses. However, trouble arises when sensory gratification becomes a society's driving motive. This causes a society to degenerate, since the realm of the senses is extremely limited in comparison to our comprehensive native capacities, including emotion, intellect, imagination, understanding, compassion, insight, aspiration, and inspiration.

In the past, most people appreciated the simple, natural taste and texture of brown bread, brown rice, and other whole natural foods. Now, in order to stimulate the senses, whole-wheat bread has been replaced by soft, often sugary white bread, while brown rice is usually refined and polished into nutritionally deficient white rice.

At the same time, a food industry has developed to enhance sensory appeal by adding artificial colorings, flavorings, and texture agents to our daily foods. Over the last fifty years, this trend has extended to many items necessary for daily living, including clothing, cosmetics, housing materials, furniture, sleeping materials, and kitchenwares. As many people have discovered, however, the application of technology to the production of synthetic consumer goods often results in lower quality, poorer service, less material satisfaction, and is ultimately hazardous to our health. All in all, we have created a totally artificial way of life and have moved further and further from our origins in the natural world. By orienting our way of life against nature, we are separating ourselves from our evolutionary environment and threatening to weaken and destroy ourselves as a species that is naturally evolving on this planet.

Cancer is only one result of this total orientation. However, instead of considering the larger environmental, social, and dietary causes of cancer, most research up to now has been oriented in the opposite direction, viewing the disease mainly as an isolated cellular disorder. Most therapies focus only on removing or destroying the cancerous tumor while ignoring the overall bodily conditions that caused it to develop.

Cancer originates long before the formation of a malignant growth, and is rooted in the quality of the external factors that we select and consume in our day-to-day life. When a cancerous symptom is finally discovered, however, this external origin is overlooked, and the disease is considered to be cured as long as the symptom or tumor has been removed or destroyed. But because the cause has not been changed, the cancer will often return, in either the same form or some other form and location. This is usually met by another round of treatment that again ignores the cause. This type of approach represents an often futile attempt to control the disease by suppressing its symptoms.

In order to control cancer, we need to see beyond the immediate symptoms and consider larger factors such as the patient's overall blood quality, the types of food that have contributed to create that blood quality, and the mentality and way of life that have led the patient to consume those particular foods. It is also important to see beyond the individual patient and into the realm of society at large. Factors such as the trends of the food industry, the quality of modern agriculture, and our increasingly unnatural and sedentary way of life also apply.

OVERCOMING DUALISM

The modern way of thinking, which has culminated in this dead end, can be described as dualistic. It usually regards cancer as an aberration caused by certain factors (such as viruses, abnormal genes, or carcinogenic substances) that are viewed as "enemies." To cure the cancer, these "enemies" must be removed, sought out and destroyed, or bombarded by chemicals and radiation. A recent cover story on cancer in *Newsweek* illustrates the pervasiveness of this military way of thinking.

The invasion begins: deep in the bone marrow, a ragged-edged cell divides. Four days later the pair becomes four. The arithmetic is simple, the results devastating. Doubling again and again, the abnormal white-blood cells leach through the marrow, pour into the bloodstream and then spread to other tissues. . . . The counterattack is chemical warfare. Shot into the victim's bloodstream, an array of complex molecules takes on the malignant cells, each chemical fighting a specialized part of the battle. Vincristine interrupts the growth process and paralyzes some of the cells in mid-division. A drug called 6-MP sneaks inside other cells, stopping them from making the DNA they need to reproduce. Methotrexate acts like a Trojan horse: shaped like a vitamin that the voracious cancer cell needs, it is quickly gobbled up. But once inside, the molecule proves as indigestible as a pebble and the cell chokes and dies. Under the chemical onslaught, the tumor cells falter, stop and then retreat, leaving millions of their dead behind.

Our modern understanding of life, health and sickness, war and peace, and the nature of humanity is one sided. Dualistic thinking divides good from bad, friend from enemy, and health from illness, seeing the one as completely desirable and the other as totally undesirable. This divisive mode of thought actually underlies all of modern society, including education and religion, politics and economics, science and industry, communications and the arts. As long as our basic point of view is dualistic, it is impossible to cure fundamentally any sickness, whether diabetes, emphysema, leprosy, arthritis, mental illness, or even the common cold. The current mode of attack stems from our ignorance of the true nature of life and health. In a profound sense, while the riddle of cancer is testing our modern medical understanding, it is also challenging modern civilization itself.

For the past thirty years, I have been seriously studying this larger problem with many people. The first conclusion my associates and I reached was: If cancer is to be cured, it must first be understood. If it is to be understood, dualism must be outgrown in favor of a unified perspective. From this more holistic perspective, we can see that no enemy or conflict really exists. On the contrary, all factors proceed in a very harmonious manner, coexisting and supporting each other.

THE BENEFICIAL NATURE OF DISEASE

In our experience, cancer is only the final stage in a sequence of events in an illness through which individuals in the modern world tend to pass because we fail to appreciate the beneficial nature of disease symptoms. A healthy system can deal with a limited amount of excess nutrients or toxic materials taken in the form of daily food. This imbalance can be naturally eliminated through daily activity, sweat, urination, or other means. However, if we overconsume or increase the amount of toxins over a long period of time, the body begins to fall back upon more serious measures for elimination: fever, skin disease, and other superficial symptoms. Such sickness is a natural adjustment, the result of the wisdom of the body trying to keep us in natural balance.

Many people, however, are alarmed by those symptoms and think there is something unnatural or undesirable about them. So they try to suppress or control those natural manifestations with pills, cough syrups, or other medications, which separate them from the natural workings of their own bodies. If minor ailments are treated in this symptomatic way with no adjustment in what we consume, the excess held in the body eventually begins to accumulate in the form of fatty-acid deposits and chronically troublesome mucus, and manifests in vaginal discharges, ovarian cysts, kidney stones, or other troublesome conditions. In this state the body is still able at least to localize the excess and toxins that we continue to take in. By gathering the unwanted material in local areas, the rest of the body is maintained in a relatively clean and functioning condition. That process of localization is part of our natural healing power, saving us from total breakdown. But the modern view looks on those localizations as dangerous enemies to be destroyed and removed. Its attitude is comparable to the behavior of the inhabitants of a city troubled by too much waste. Instead of investigating the source of waste, the city dwellers blame the sanitation department for the accumulation of garbage in designated locations and decide to do away with the sanitation department.

As long as we continue to take in excessive nutrients, chemicals, and other factors that serve no purpose in the body, they must continue to accumulate somewhere in order to continue our normal living functions. If we don't allow them to accumulate in limited areas and form tumors, they will spread throughout the body, resulting in a total collapse of our vital functions and death by toxemia. Cancer is only the terminal stage of a long process. Cancer is the body's healthy attempt to isolate toxins ingested and accumulated through years of eating the modern unnatural diet and living in an artificial environment. Cancer is the body's last drastic effort to prolong life, even a few more months or years.

Cancer is not the result of some alien factor over which we have no control. Rather it is simply the product of our own daily behavior, including our thinking, lifestyle, and daily way of eating. We must go beyond looking at cancer at the cellular level and realize that our cells are constantly changing in quality, being nourished and rejuvenated as a result of nourishment and energy coming into them. Whatever is in the nucleus of a cell is nothing but the end result of what originally came in from the outside and formed the cell components. If the cell is abnormal, something coming in is abnormal, such as the blood, lymph, or vibrational energy including electromagnetic waves from the environment.

The cell is only the terminal of a long organic process and cannot be isolated from its surroundings and other body functions. Instead of focusing on the cell, we need to change the blood, lymph, and environmental conditions that have created malignant cells. Instead of treating isolated organs in the body, we need to treat the source of nourishment and other factors going into those organs and change the character of those organs. The proper place to perform cancer surgery is not in the operating room after the disease has run its course, but in the kitchen and in other areas of daily life before it has developed. By removing certain foods from the pantry and refrigerator, replacing them with the proper quality and variety of foods, and applying proper cooking methods, together with correcting environmental conditions and our daily way of life, we can ensure that cancer and other degenerative illnesses do not arise.

3.

Preventing Cancer Naturally

In considering two people living in the same environment, we often find that one develops cancer while the other does not. This difference must be the result of each person's own unique way of behavior, including thinking, lifestyle, and way of eating. When we bring these simple factors into a less extreme, more manageable balance, the symptoms of illness no longer appear. Accordingly, the following practices are beneficial in restoring balance to our lives:

SELF-REFLECTION

Sickness is an indication that our way of life is not in harmony with the environment. Therefore, to establish genuine health, we must rethink our basic outlook on life. In one sense, sickness results largely from thinking that life's main purpose is to give us sensory satisfaction, emotional comfort, or material prosperity. This more limited view places our happiness above that of those around us. Our daily life becomes competitive, aggressive, and demanding on the one hand or withdrawn, suspicious, and defensive on the other. In either case, we continually take in more than we are able to give out.

A more natural, harmonious balance can only be established by overcoming egocentric views and adopting a more universal attitude. As a first step, we can begin to offer our love and care to our parents, family, friends, and to all members of society, even extending our love and sympathy to those who have hurt us in some way or whom we think of as our enemies. By taking responsibility for all aspects of our lives, we begin to see that failure and illness contribute to our overall development as much as success and well-being. In reality, difficulties and obstacles challenge us to develop our intuition, compassion, and understanding. By appreciating the gift of life in all of its manifestations, we increase the universe's faith in us and life becomes an endlessly amusing and joyful adventure. If we have cancer, for example, we accept what it has to teach us about ourselves. We never lament over our fate and blame it on an accident, karma, evil spirits, or an indifferent cosmos. We look for the source of our problems within ourselves, and when we make a mistake we learn from it and gratefully move on.

Self-reflection involves using our higher consciousness to observe, review, examine, and judge our thoughts and behavior as well as contemplate the larger order of nature or what we might call the law of God. The more we reflect upon ourselves and the eternal order of change, the more refined and universal our awareness becomes. We begin to remember our origin, foresee our destiny, and understand what we came to accomplish upon this earth. As our consciousness develops, our life manifests the spirit of endless giving just as the universe itself expands infinitely. Our motto becomes, "One grain, ten thousand grains." For each seed planted in the soil, the earth returns many thousand seeds. By endlessly distributing our knowledge and insight, our understanding deepens and we become one with the eternal order of creation.

Self-reflection may take many forms, including a short period each day in quiet meditation or prayer. Questions we might ask and areas we might seek guidance in include the following:

1. Did I eat today in harmony with my environment?
2. Did I think of my parents, relatives, teachers, and elders with love and respect?
3. Did I happily greet everyone today and express an interest in their life?
4. Did I contemplate the sky, the trees, and the flowers and marvel at the wonders of nature?
5. Did I thank everyone and appreciate everything I experienced today?
6. Did I perform my tasks faithfully and thereby contribute to a more peaceful world?

RESPECT FOR THE NATURAL ENVIRONMENT

The relation between humanity and nature is like that between the embryo and the placenta. The placenta nourishes, supports, and sustains the developing embryo. It would be bizarre if the embryo were to seek to destroy this protecting organism. Likewise, it is simply a matter of common sense that we should strive to preserve the integrity of the natural environment upon which we depend for life itself. Over the last century, however, we have steadily contaminated our soil, water, and air and destroyed many of the plant and animal species on which our fragile ecology rests. Our daily way of life has also become more unnatural, relying heavily on synthetic fabrics and materials, and exposing us continually to great quantities of artificial electromagnetic radiation. These actually weaken our natural ability to resist disease.

A NATURALLY BALANCED DIET

The trillions of cells that make up the human body are created and nourished by the bloodstream. New blood cells are constantly being manufactured from the nutrients provided by our daily foods. If we eat improperly, the quality of our blood and cells, including our brain cells and quality of thinking, begins to deteriorate. Cancer, a disease characterized by the abnormal multiplication of cells, is largely the result of improper eating over a long period.

For restoring a sound, healthy blood and cell quality, the following dietary principles are recommended:

Harmony with the Evolutionary Order

Nature is continually transforming one species into another. A great food chain extends from bacteria and enzymes to sea invertebrates and vertebrates, amphibians, reptiles, birds, mammals, apes, and human beings. Complementary to this line of animal evolution is a line of plant development ranging from bacteria and enzymes to sea moss and sea vegetables, primitive land vegetables, ancient vegetables, modern vegetables, fruits and nuts, and cereal grains. Whole grains evolved parallel with human beings and therefore should form the major portion of our diet. The remainder of our food should be selected from among more remote evolutionary varieties of plants and may include land and sea vegetables, fresh fruit, seeds and nuts, and soup containing fermented enzymes and bacteria representing the most primordial form of life.

In traditional cancer-free societies, this way of eating is reflected in the natural development of infants and children. After conception, the human embryo develops from a single-celled fertilized egg into a multicellular infant and is nourished entirely on its mother's blood, analogous to the ancient ocean in which biological life began. At birth, mother's milk is the principal food, and as children began to stand, whole grains become their staple fare.

The exact proportion of plant food to animal food, with the latter being eaten primarily as a dietary supplement, also reflects our ancestors' understanding of nature's delicate balance. The ratio approximated seven parts vegetable food to about one part animal food. Modern views of geological and biological evolution have also found approximately the similar proportion in the evolutionary period of water life, roughly 2.8 billion years, compared to the period of land life, approximately 0.4 billion years. The structure of the human teeth offers another biological clue to humanity's natural way of eating. The thirty-two teeth include twenty molars and premolars for grinding grains, legumes, and seeds; eight incisors for cutting vegetables; and four canines for tearing animal and sea food. Expressed as a ratio of teeth designed for plant use and for animal use, the figure once again is seven to one. If animal food is eaten, it is ideally selected from among species most distant from human beings in the evolutionary order, especially fish and primitive sea life such as shrimp and oysters.

The modern notion that primitive hunting societies lived chiefly on mastadon, deer, birds, and other game has recently been shown by scientists to be exaggerated. Paleolithic cultures hunted mostly for undomesticated cereals and wild grasses and foraged for plants, berries, and roots. Animal life was taken only when necessary and consumed in small amounts. *The New York Times* science section reported on May 15, 1979 in a lengthy article on the early human diet:

Recent investigations into the dietary habits of prehistoric peoples and their primate predecessors suggest that heavy meat-eating by modern affluent societies may be exceeding the biological capacities evolution built into the human body. The result may be a host of diet-related health problems, such as diabetes, obesity, high blood pressure, coronary heart disease, and some cancers.

The studies challenge the notion that human beings evolved as aggressive hunting animals who depended primarily upon meat for survival. The new view—coming from findings in such fields as archaeology, anthropology, primatology, and comparative anatomy—instead portrays early humans and their forebears more as herbivores than carnivores. According to these studies, the prehistoric table for at least the last million and a-half years was probably set with three times more plant than animal foods, the reverse of what the average American currently eats.

Harmony with Universal Dietary Tradition

According to calulations based on U.S. Department of Agriculture surveys, from 1910 to 1976, the per capita consumption of wheat fell 48 percent, corn 85 percent, rye 78 percent, barley 66 percent, buckwheat 98 percent, beans and legumes 46 percent, fresh vegetables 23 percent, and fresh fruit 33 percent. Over this same period, beef intake rose 72 percent, poultry 194 percent, cheese 322 percent, canned vegetables 320 percent, frozen vegetables 1,650 percent, processed fruit 556 percent, ice cream 852 percent, yogurt 300 percent, corn syrup 761 percent, and soft drinks 2,638 percent. Since 1940, when per capita intake of chemical additives and preservatives was first recorded, the amount of artificial food colors added to the diet has climbed 995 percent.

U.S. per capita cereal products consumption, 1910-1970.

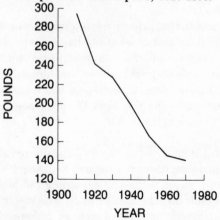

Source: USDA/ERS, 1975.

Per capita consumption of meat, poultry and fish, 1910-1970.

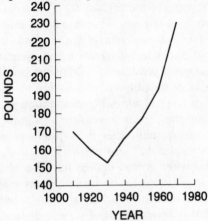

Source: USDA/ERS, 1975.

Despite the spread of refined and synthetic foods around the world, cooked whole grains, beans, and vegetables continue to be the principal foods in many cultures today. For example, corn tortillas and black beans are the staple foods in Central America, rice and soybean products are eaten throughout Southeast Asia, and whole and cracked wheat and chickpeas are staples in the Middle East. These regions have the lowest cancer rates in the world. For instance, a recent international study comparing the rate of cancer mortality in males in forty-four countries found the least cancer in El Salvador (23 deaths per 100,000 population), Thailand (25), and Egypt (42). In comparison, European nations registered the highest incidence: Luxembourg (212), Scotland (204), Czechoslovakia (200), Finland (192), Belgium (187), England (185), the Netherlands (183), France (178), and Denmark (163). Those countries in the upper range also included the United States (156), Australia (154), Canada (153), and Japan (140).

Harmony with the Ecological Order

It is advisable to base our diet primarily on foods produced in the same general area in which we live. For example, a traditional people like the Eskimo base their diet mostly on animal products, and this is appropriate in a polar climate. However, in India and other more tropical regions, a diet based almost entirely on grains and other vegetable foods is more conducive to health. When we begin to eat foods that have been imported from regions with different climatic conditions, however, we lose our natural immunity to diseases in our own local environment and a condition of chronic imbalance results. In recent decades, advances in refrigeration, transportation, and other technology have made it possible for millions of people in temperate zones to consume large quantities of pineapples, bananas, grapefruits, avocados, and other tropical and subtropical products. Similarly, people in southern latitudes are now consuming significant amounts of milk, cheese, ice cream, and other dairy products and frozen foods that were originally eaten in more northerly or arctic regions. Since 1948, for example, when frozen orange juice became available, the intake of frozen citrus drinks in the United States soared 11,600 percent. The violation of ecological eating habits contributes to biological degeneration and the development of serious disease.

Harmony with the Changing Seasons

A habit like eating ice cream in a heated apartment while snow is falling outside is obviously not in harmony with the seasonal order, nor is charcoal broiling steaks in the heat of summer. It is better to adjust naturally the selection and preparation of daily foods to harmonize with the changing seasons. For example, in colder weather we can apply longer cooking times, while minimizing the intake of raw salad or fruit. In the summer, lightly cooked dishes are more appropriate while the intake of animal food and heavily cooked items can be minimized.

Harmony with Individual Differences

Personal differences need to be considered in the selection and preparation of our daily foods, with variations according to age, sex, type of activity, occupation, original physiological constitution, present condition of health, and other factors. As individuals we are constantly developing physically, mentally, and spiritually, and our day-to-day eating naturally changes to reflect this growth. The following nutritional considerations are recommended to help us select a balanced diet:

1. Water—It is preferable to use clean natural water for cooking and drinking. Spring or well water is recommended for regular use.

It is best to avoid chemically treated municipal water or distilled water.

2. Carbohydrates—It is advisable to eat carbohydrates primarily in the form of polysaccharide glucose, such as that found in cereal grains, vegetables, and beans, while minimizing or avoiding the intake of monosaccharide or disaccharide sugars, such as those in fruit, honey, dairy foods, refined sugar, and other sweeteners.

3. Protein—Protein from such vegetable sources as whole grains and bean products is more easily assimilated by the body than protein from animal sources. When we examine the dietary patterns of people living in Hunza in Pakistan and Vilcabamba in Ecuador, who are noted for their health, vitality, and longevity, we find that they rely primarily on vegetable sources for protein. In a study recently published by *National Geographic,* the average daily caloric intake of a group of men in Hunza was found to be 1,923 calories, with 50 grams of protein, 35 grams of fat, and 354 grams of carbohydrate. In Vilcabamba, the average daily caloric intake was found to be 1,200 calories, with 35 to 38 grams of protein, 12 to 19 grams of fat, and 200 to 260 grams of carbohydrate. In both cases, protein was obtained principally from vegetable sources. Cancer, it should be noted, is virtually unknown in both these regions. In comparison, the average American consumes 3,300 calories per day, with 100 grams of protein, 157 grams of fat, and 380 grams of carbohydrate.

4. Fat—It is better to avoid the hard, saturated fats found in most types of meat and dairy products as well as the polyunsaturated fats found in margarine and hydrogenated cooking oils. Fat currently makes up about 40 percent of the modern diet and in medical studies is the nutrient most associated with degenerative illnesses, including heart disease and cancer. Whole grains, beans, nuts and seeds contain fat in the ideal proportions for daily consumption. For cooking purposes, high-quality unrefined sesame or corn oil is recommended for regular use.

5. Salt—It is better to rely primarily on natural sea salt, which contains a variety of trace minerals, and to avoid refined table salt, which is almost 100 percent sodium chloride.

6. Vitamins—Vitamins exist naturally in whole foods and should be consumed as a part of the food together with other nutrients. Vitamin pills and other nutritional supplements became popular in recent decades to offset the deficiencies caused by modern food refining. However, when taken as a supplement to our regular food, vitamins produce a chaotic effect on our body's metabolism. In its

report *Diet, Nutrition, and Cancer,* the National Academy of Sciences warned that some vitamins were toxic in high doses and advised that it was preferable to focus on whole foods rather than individual nutrients when planning our diet.

In a temperate, four-season climate, an optimum daily diet that will help protect against cancer and other serious illnesses consists of about 50 to 60 percent whole cereal grains, 5 to 10 percent soup (especially soups made with a fermented vegetable base and sea-based minerals), 25 to 30 percent vegetables prepared in a variety of styles, and 5 to 10 percent beans and sea vegetables. Supplementary foods for occasional use include locally grown fruits, preferably cooked; fish and other seafood; and a variety of seeds and nuts. (A complete description of the Cancer-Prevention Diet is presented in Chapter 5.)

AN ACTIVE DAILY LIFE

For many of us, modern life offers fewer physical and mental challenges than did life in the past. As a result, functions such as the active generation of caloric and electromagnetic energy, the circulation of blood and lymph, and the activity of the digestive, nervous, and reproductive systems often stagnate. However, a physically and mentally active life is essential for good health. The people living in Hunza and Vilcabamba remain active well into their eighties, nineties, and hundreds. Their cultures have no concept of retirement, and their elders continue to farm, garden, teach, and walk long distances until the very end of their days. In contrast, modern life has become sedentary, soft, and comfortable. After age fifty-five or sixty-five many people decline and die from lack of meaningful work or recreation. Regular physical and mental exercise, throughout life, will contribute to overall health and happiness.

4.

Diet and the Development of Cancer

To understand how cancer develops, use the analogy of a tree. A tree's structure is opposite to that of the human body. For example, the leaves of a tree have a more open structure and a green color, while the cells of the human body, which correspond to the leaves of a tree, have a more closed structure and are nourished by blood, which is red in color. A tree's sustenance comes from the nutrients absorbed through the external roots. The roots of the human body lie deep in the intestines in the region where nutrients are absorbed into the blood and lymph and then distributed to all of the body's cells. If the quality of nourishment is chronically poor in the soil or in the food that is consumed, the leaves of the tree or the cells of the body eventually lose their normal functional ability and begin to deteriorate. This condition results from the repeated intake of poor nutrients and does not arise suddenly. While it is developing, many other symptoms might arise in other parts of the tree trunk and branches or in the body.

Cancer develops over a period of time out of a chronically precancerous state. In my estimation, as many as 80 to 90 percent of Americans, Europeans, Japanese, and other modern people have some type of precancerous condition. The repeated overconsumption of excessive dietary factors causes a variety of adjustment mechanisms in the body which progressively develop toward cancer. Since the body at all times seeks balance with the surrounding environment, the normal process is for this excess to be eliminated or stored when it exceeds the body's capacity for elimination. Eventually, the overaccumulation will be stored in the form of excessive layers of fat, cholesterol, and the formation of cysts and tumors. Let us consider the gradual stages in this process, particularly in their relation to the appearance of cancer.

NORMAL DISCHARGE

Normal elimination occurs through the processes of urination, bowel movement, respiration (exhaling carbon dioxide), and perspiration, in which excessive chemical compounds are broken down into simple compounds and ultimately into carbon dioxide and water for discharge from the body. Discharge also occurs through physical, mental, and emotional activity. Mental discharge occurs in the form of wave vibrations, while emotions such as anger indicate that a great amount of excess is being eliminated.

Women have several additional means through which excess is naturally discharged. These include menstruation, childbirth, and lactation. Women have a distinct advantage over men in more efficiently discharging excess and thereby maintaining a cleaner condition. They tend to adjust more harmoniously with their environment and usually live longer than men. To compensate for this disadvantage, men usually go out into society and expend energy through additional physical, mental, and social activities. All of these processes take place continually throughout life. If we take in only a moderate amount of excess, they will proceed smoothly. However, if the quantity of excess is large, these natural processes are not capable of discharging it, and various abnormal processes begin.

ABNORMAL DISCHARGE

Today practically everyone eats and drinks excessively, which often triggers a variety of abnormal discharge mechanisms in the body such as diarrhea, excessive sweating, overly frequent bowel movements, or excessive urination. Habits like scratching the head, tapping the feet, and frequent blinking of the eyes also represent abnormal discharges of imbalanced energy, as do strong emotions such as fear, anger, and anxiety. Periodically, excess is discharged through more acute or violent symptoms such as a fever, coughing, sneezing, shouting, screaming, trembling, and shivering, as well as wild thoughts and behavior.

CHRONIC DISCHARGE

Chronic discharges are the next stage in this process and often take the form of skin diseases. These are common in cases where the kidneys have lost their ability to properly cleanse the bloodstream. For example, freckles, dark spots, and similar skin markings indicate the chronic discharge of sugar and other refined carbohydrates, while white patches indicate the discharge of milk, cottage cheese, or other dairy products.

Hard, dry skin arises after the bloodstream fills with fat and oil, eventually causing blockage of the pores, hair follicles, and sweat glands. When these blockages prevent the flow of liquid toward the surface, the skin becomes dry. Many people believe that this condition results from a lack of oil, when in fact it is caused by the intake of too much fat and oil.

Skin cancers are more serious forms of skin disease. However, skin disorders are usually not very serious, since in most cases the discharge of toxins toward the surface of the body permits the internal organs and tissues to continue functioning smoothly. However, if our eating continues to be excessive and we cannot eliminate effectively, the body will start to accumulate this excess in other locations.

ACCUMULATION

If we continue to eat poorly, we eventually exhaust the body's ability to discharge. This can be serious if an underlying layer of fat has developed under the skin which prevents discharge toward the surface of the body. Such a condition is caused by the repeated overconsumption of milk, cheese, eggs, meat, and other fatty, oily, or greasy foods. When this stage has been reached, internal deposits of mucus or fat begin to form, initially in areas that have some direct access to the outside and in the following regions:

Sinuses

The sinuses are a frequent site of mucous accumulation, and symptoms such as allergies, hay fever, and blocked sinuses often result. Hay fever and sneezing arise when dust or pollen stimulate the discharge of this excess, while calcified stones often form deep within the sinuses. Thick, heavy deposits of mucus in the sinuses diminish our mental clarity and alertness.

Inner Ear

The accumulation of mucus and fat in the inner ear interferes with the smooth functioning of the inner-ear mechanism and can lead to frequent pain, impaired hearing, and even deafness.

Lungs

Various forms of excess often accumulate in the lungs. Aside from the obvious symptoms of coughing and chest congestion, mucus often fills the alveoli or air sacs and breathing becomes more difficult. Occasionally, a coat of mucus in the bronchi can be loosened and discharged by coughing, but once the sacs are surrounded, it becomes more firmly lodged and can remain there for years. Then, if air pollutants or cigarette smoke enter the lungs, their heavier components are attracted to and remain in this sticky environment. In severe cases, these deposits can trigger the development of lung cancer. However, the underlying cause of this condition is the accumulation of sticky fat and mucus in the alveoli and in the blood and capillaries surrounding them.

Breasts

The accumulation of excess in this region often results in a hardening of the breasts and the formation of cysts. Excess usually accumulates here in the form of mucus and deposits of fatty acid, both of which take the form of a sticky or heavy liquid. These deposits develop into cysts in the same way that water solidifies into ice, a process that is accelerated by the intake of ice cream, cold milk, soft drinks, orange juice, and other foods that produce a cooling or freezing effect. Women who have breastfed are less likely to develop breast cysts or cancer since this reduces excess accumulation in this region.

Intestines

In many cases, excess will begin accumulating in the lower part of the body as mucus and fat deposits coating the intestinal wall. This will often cause the intestines to expand or become less flexible, resulting in a bulging abdomen. A large number of people in the United States have this problem. Young people are often very stylish and attractive. However, after the age of thirty, and particularly between the ages of thirty-five and forty, a large number of Americans lose their youthful appearance and become overweight.

Kidneys

Deposits of fat and mucus may also accumulate in the kidneys. Problems arise when these elements clog the fine network of cells in the interior of these organs, causing them to accumulate water and become chronically swollen. Since elimination is hampered, fluid that cannot be discharged is often deposited in the legs, producing periodic swelling and weakness. If someone with this condition consumes a large quantity of foods that produce a chilling effect, the deposited fat and mucus will often crystallize into kidney stones.

Reproductive Organs

In men, the prostate gland is a frequent site of accumulation. As a result of continued consumption of excess or imbalanced food, the prostate often becomes enlarged and hard fat deposits or cysts often form within and around it. This is one of the principal causes of impotence. In women, excess may also accumulate within and around the sexual organs leading to the formation of ovarian cysts, dermoid tumors, or the blockage of the Fallopian tubes. In some cases, mucus or fat in the ovaries or Fallopian tubes prevents the passage of the egg and sperm, resulting in an inability to conceive. Chronic vaginal discharge is one indication of accumulation in the reproductive region.

Although the symptoms that affect these inner organs may seem unrelated, they all stem from the same underlying cause. However, modern medicine often does not view them as related. For example, a person with hearing trouble or cataracts is often referred to an ear or eye specialist. However, cataracts are a symptom of a variety of related problems, such as mucous accumulation in the breasts, kidneys, and sexual organs.

STORAGE

In this stage, excess in various forms is stored within and around the deeper, vital organs, including the heart and the liver. In the case of the circulatory system, excess often accumulates around and inside the heart as well as within the heart tissues. Accumulation may also occur both in and around the arteries. These fatty deposits, including cholesterol accumulation, reduce the heart's ability to function properly and hamper the smooth passage of blood through the arteries. The end result is often a heart attack. The major causes of this problem are foods containing large amounts of hard, saturated fat. Many nutritionists and medical doctors are now aware of the relationship between the intake of saturated fats and cholesterol and cardiovascular disease, but they often overlook the effects of sugar and dairy products, both of which contribute greatly to the development of these illnesses.

Within the body, the proteins, carbohydrates, and fats that we consume often change into each other, depending on the amount of each consumed as well as the body's needs at a particular time. If we consume more of these than we need, the excess is normally discharged. However, the quantity of excess often exceeds the body's capacity to discharge it. When this happens, the excess is stored in the liver in the form of carbohydrate, in the muscles in the form of protein, or throughout the body in the form of fatty acids.

DEGENERATION OF THE BLOOD
AND LYMPH

If the bloodstream is filled with fat and mucus, excess will begin to accumulate, as we have seen, in the organs. Since the lungs and kidneys are usually affected first, their functions of filtering and cleansing the blood become less efficient. The situation leads to further deterioration of the blood quality and also affects the lymphatic system. Operations such as tonsillectomies also contribute to the deterioration of the lymphatic system since they reduce the ability of this system to cleanse itself. Such operations eventually lead to frequent swelling and lymph-gland inflammation, producing a chronic deterioration of the quality of the blood, particularly the red- and white-blood cells.

TUMORS

When the red blood cells begin to lose their capacity to change into normal body cells, an organism cannot long survive. Poorly functioning intestines can also contribute to the degeneration of blood quality, since the qualities of blood cells and plasma originate largely in the small intestine. In many cases, the villi of the small intestine are coated with fat and mucus, and the condition in the intestines is often acidic. A naturally healthy bloodstream will not be created in this type of environment.

Therefore, in order to prevent immediate collapse, the body localizes toxins at this stage in the form of a tumor. A tumor may be likened to a storage depot for the collection of degenerative cells from the bloodstream. As long as improper nourishment is taken in, the body will continue to isolate abnormal excess and toxins in specific areas, resulting in the continual growth of the cancer. When a particular location can no longer absorb toxic excess, the body must search for another place to localize it, and so the cancer spreads. This process continues until the cancer metastasizes throughout the body and the person eventually dies.

In summary, we may conclude that symptoms like dry skin, skin discharges, hardening of the breasts, prostate trouble, vaginal discharge, and ovarian cysts all represent potentially precancerous conditions. However, they need not develop toward cancer if we change our daily way of eating.

5.

The Macrobiotic Cancer-Prevention Diet

The following dietary recommendations have been formulated with universal human dietary traditions from both East and West in mind and have been further refined over several decades as a result of contemporary macrobiotic experience, which has relieved cancer, radiation sickness, and other modern physical and psychological disorders. When applied very carefully, these guidelines create a stabilized state of overall physiological balance. They may therefore be followed not only for the prevention of cancer, but also for the prevention of most other illnesses as well. This approach may be followed by persons already in generally good health. For those people who already have cancer or a serious precancerous condition, adjustments need to be made depending on the specific case, and, it is advisable to do so under the supervision of a qualified macrobiotics counselor or medical professional. These special adjustments are considered in full detail for each individual form of cancer in Part II of this book. People without a major health problem can follow the general Cancer-Prevention Diet outlined below.

WHOLE GRAINS

Approximately 50 to 60 percent of our daily food should consist by volume of cooked whole-cereal grains. These include brown rice, whole wheat, millet, oats, barley, corn, rye, and buckwheat, and they can be prepared according to a variety of cooking styles. When preparing brown rice, it is best to use a pressure-cooker made of stainless steel. Pressure-cooked rice is far superior to boiled rice for everyday use, since many nutrients are lost after boiling over a period of time. In the case of wheat, whole-wheat berries are rather tough and somewhat difficult to chew so they are usually ground into flour, which is baked into bread. Bread should ideally be baked from freshly ground flour without the addition of yeast. Grains may also be eaten in the form of pasta or noodles, especially buckwheat (soba) and whole wheat (udon) noodles. In general, the majority of grain dishes should be eaten primarily in complete whole form rather than in cracked or processed form such as bulgur, corn grits, or rolled oats. Bread and flour products tend to be more difficult than whole grains to digest and tend to be mucus producing. Next to grain in whole-form, chapatis, tortillas, and other traditional flat breads are most highly recommended as well as sourdough wheat or rye. Grain products such as seitan (also known as wheat meat or gluten) may be consumed a few times a week as a source of protein.

SOUP

About 5 to 10 percent (one to two bowls) of daily intake may be in the form of soup. Soup broth can be made with miso or tamari soy sauce, which are prepared from naturally fermented soybeans, sea salt, and grains, to which several varieties of land and sea vegetables, especially wakame or kombu and green vegetables, may be added during cooking. The taste of miso or tamari broth soup should be mild, not too salty or too bland. Soups made with grains, beans, or vegetables can also be served from time to time. For instance, delicious seasonal varieties can be made such as corn soup in the summer or squash soup in the fall.

VEGETABLE DISHES

About 25 to 30 percent of our daily food should be fresh vegetable dishes, which can be prepared in a wide variety of cooking styles: sautéing, steaming, boiling, baking, and pressure-cooking. Among root and stem vegetables, carrots, onions, daikon (white radish), turnip, red radish, burdock, lotus root, rutabaga, parsnip, and salsify are excellent. When preparing root vegetables, cook both the root and leaf portions so as to achieve a proper balance of nutrients by using the whole food. Among vegetables from the ground, cabbage, cauliflower, broccoli, brussels sprouts, Chinese cabbage, acorn squash, butternut squash, buttercup squash, and pumpkin are quite nutritious and may be used daily. Among green and white leafy vegetables, watercress, kale, parsley, leeks, scallions, dandelion, collards, bok choy, carrot greens, daikon greens, turnip greens, and mustard greens are fine for regular use. Vegetables for occasional use include cucumber, lettuce, string beans, celery, sprouts, yellow squash, peas, Swiss chard, red cabbage, mushrooms (usual and shiitake), kohlrabi, endive, escarole, and Jerusalem artichoke. In general, up to one third of vegetable intake may be eaten raw in the form of salad or traditionally prepared pickles. However, it is better to avoid mayonnaise and commercial salad dressings. Vegetables that originated historically in tropical or semitropical environments such as eggplant, potatoes, tomatoes, asparagus, spinach, beets, sweet potatoes, yams, zucchini, avocado, artichoke, green and red peppers, and other varieties that tend to produce acid should be avoided or minimized unless you live in a hot and humid climate.

BEANS AND SEA VEGETABLES

From 5 to 10 percent of daily intake may be eaten in the form of cooked beans and sea vegetables. Beans for daily use are azuki (small red) beans, chickpeas, and lentils. Other beans may be used occasionally: soybeans, pinto, white, black turtle, navy, kidney, lima, split peas, and black-eyed peas. Soybean products such as tofu, tempeh, and natto may be used in moderation. Sea vegetables including kombu (kelp), wakame, hijiki, arame, nori, dulse, agar-agar, and Irish moss are rich in minerals and should be used in small volume on a daily basis in soups, cooked with vegetables or beans, or prepared as a side dish. These dishes may be seasoned with a moderate amount of tamari soy sauce, sea salt, or grain-based vinegar such as brown rice vinegar.

SUPPLEMENTARY FOODS

Persons in usually good health may wish to include some of the following additional supplementary foods in their diet:

Animal Food

A small volume of white-meat fish or seafood may be eaten a few times per week. White-meat fish generally contain less fat than red-meat or blue-skin varieties. Saltwater fish also usually have fewer chemical pollutants in their systems than freshwater varieties. Whole small dried fish (iriko), which can be consumed entirely including bones, may also be used occasionally as a dish with vegetables, in soup, or as a seasoning. Avoid or drastically limit all other animal products including beef, lamb, pork, veal, chicken, turkey, duck, goose, wild game, and eggs. Avoid or drastically limit all dairy foods including cheese, butter, milk, skim milk, buttermilk, yogurt, ice cream, cream, sour cream, whipped cream, margarine, and kefir.

Fruit

Fresh fruit may be eaten a few times a week—preferably cooked or naturally dried—as a supplement or dessert, provided the fruits grow in the local climatic zone. Fresh fruits can also be consumed in moderate volume occasionally during their growing season. In temperate areas these include apples, strawberries, cherries, peaches, pears, plums, grapes, apricots, prunes, blueberries, blackberries, raspberries, cantaloupe, honeydew melons, watermelon, and tangerines. In these climates, avoid or curtail tropical or semitropical fruits such as bananas, oranges, grapefruits, pineapples, mangoes, papayas, figs, dates, coconut, and kiwi, even though they are cooked or dried, unless for a short period for specific medicinal purposes. In tropical and semitropical regions, these fruits may be consumed infrequently in small volume. Fruit juice is generally too concentrated for regular use, although occasional consumption in very hot weather is allowable as is apple cider, preferably warmed, in the fall. Dried fruit may be eaten on occasion so long as it is from the same climatic region.

Desserts

Dessert may be eaten in moderate volume two or three times a week and may include cookies, pudding, cake, pie, and other sweet dishes prepared with natural ingredients. Often desserts can be prepared from apples, fall and winter squashes, pumpkins, azuki beans, or dried fruit and other naturally sweet foods without adding a sweetener. However, for dishes that need one, recommended sweeteners include rice syrup, barley malt, amasake (a fermented sweet rice beverage), chestnuts, apple juice and cider, and dried fruits such as raisins. Avoid white sugar, brown sugar, raw sugar, turbinado sugar, molasses, honey, corn syrup, maple syrup, chocolate, carob, fructose, saccharine, and other concentrated or artificial sweeteners. For custards, whipped toppings, and frosting, tofu, tahini (sesame butter), and other vegetable ingredients should be used instead of eggs, cream, milk, and similar animal products. A delicious sea vegetable gelatin made of agar-agar called kanten can be seasoned with fresh fruit, apple juice, and other natural sweeteners.

Snacks

Roasted seeds and nuts, lightly salted with sea salt or seasoned with tamari soy sauce, may be enjoyed occasionally as snacks. Suitable seeds and nuts include sesame seeds, sunflower seeds, pumpkin seeds, almonds, walnuts, pecans, filberts, and peanuts. It is preferable not to overconsume nuts and nut butters as they are difficult to digest and high in fats. Other snacks may include rice cakes, popcorn (without butter), and roasted beans and grains.

BEVERAGES

Recommended daily beverages include roasted bancha (kukicha) twig tea, roasted brown rice tea, roasted barley tea, dandelion tea, cereal grain coffee, and kelp and other sea vegetable teas. Any traditional tea that does not have an aromatic fragrance or a stimulant effect can also be used. However, coffee, black tea, and aromatic herb teas such as peppermint, rose hips, and chamomile should be avoided unless used medicinally as a stimulant. Daily beverages should preferably be prepared with spring or well water. For thirst, small amounts of this water may also be taken. Ice-cold water should be avoided. Beer or sake (rice wine) that has been made without additives or sugar and fermented by a traditional natural process may be taken in moderate volume, if desired, on occasion. However, alcoholic beverages generally should be limited or preferably avoided.

ADDITIONAL DIETARY SUGGESTIONS

Cooking Oil

For daily use, only unrefined sesame, corn, or mustard seed oil in moderate amounts is recommended. Other unrefined vegetable oils such as safflower, sunflower, soy, and olive may be used occasionally.

Avoid all chemically processed vegetable oils, butter, lard, shortening, and egg or soy margarines.

Salt

Naturally processed, mineral-rich sea salt and traditional, non-chemicalized miso and tamari soy sauce may be used as seasoning. Daily meals, however, should not have an overly salty flavor, and seasonings should generally be added during cooking and not at the table except for condiments and garnishes.

Pickles

A small volume of home-made pickles may be eaten each day to aid in digestion. In macrobiotic food preparation, this naturally fermented type of food is made with a variety of root and round vegetables, such as daikon or radish, turnips, carrots, cabbage, and cauliflower, and preserved in sea salt, rice or wheat bran, tamari soy sauce, umeboshi, or miso. Spices, sugar, and vinegar are avoided. Short-time, lighter pickles are recommended in warmer weather or for persons who need to reduce their salt intake. Long-time, saltier pickles can be eaten during colder weather or by those with a weakened condition. Different jars, crocks, and kegs can be used in their preparation, and aging varies from several hours to weeks, months, and even years. Principal types include *quick tamari pickles*, made by soaking thinly sliced root or round vegetables in a mixture of one-half tamari soy sauce and one-half water and serving after 2 to 3 hours; *tamari pickles*, made in the same way and aged for 3 to 5 days; *umeboshi pickles*, made by placing vegetables for 3 to 5 days in water in which umeboshi plums have soaked for several hours; *brine pickles*, made from soaking kombu and sliced vegetables in a jar with cool saltwater for 2 to 3 days; *rice bran* (nuka) *pickles*, made by layering roasted rice or wheat bran, sea salt, and vegetables in a crock and aging from 1 to 2 weeks or 3 to 5 months; *daikon and daikon leaf bran pickles* (takuwan), strongly salted white radish and tops that have aged from six months to several years.

Condiments

Condiments for daily use include *gomashio* (sesame salt), made usually from ten to fourteen parts roasted sesame seeds to one part roasted sea salt and half-grinding together in a small earthenware bowl called a suribachi; *roasted kombu* (kelp) or *wakame powder,* made from baking these sea vegetables in the oven until black and crushing in a suribachi and storing in a small container or jar; *umeboshi plums,* small salt plums that have been dried and pickled for many months with sea salt and flavored with shiso (beefsteak) leaves; *tekka,* a combination of carrot, burdock, and lotus root that has been finely chopped and sautéed in sesame oil and miso for many hours; *tamari soy sauce,* which is traditionally processed natural soy sauce; *shio nori,* squares of a paper-thin sea vegetable cooked with spring water and tamari soy sauce; and *shio kombu,* strips or squares of kelp cooked with water, tamari soy sauce, and grated ginger.

Garnishes

Seasonings for occasional use include grated ginger, pickled ginger, horseradish, grated daikon or radish, finely cut fresh scallions or onions, green mustard, and sauerkraut. They are used especially for detoxifying fish and seafood, as well as a supplement to buckwheat or other heavy tasting dishes. For daily use, stimulants should be avoided, especially strong spices (cayenne, cumin, black pepper, etc.), aromatic herbs, vinegar (except for grain vinegar), and ginseng.

WAY OF EATING

You may eat regularly two to three times per day, as much as is comfortable, provided the proportion of each category of food is generally correct and in daily consumption each mouthful is thoroughly chewed. Proper chewing is essential to digestion and it is recommended that each mouthful of food be chewed fifty tmes or more or until it becomes liquid in form. Eat when you are hungry, but it is best to leave the table feeling satisfied but not full. Similarly, drink only when thirsty. Avoid eating for three hours before sleeping as this causes stagnation in the intestines and throughout the body. Before and after each meal, express your gratitude verbally or silently to nature, the universe, or God who created the food and reflect on the health and happiness it is dedicated to achieving. This acknowledgment may take the form of grace, prayer, chanting, or a moment of silence. Express your thanks to parents, grandparents, and past generations who nourished us and whose dream we embody, to the vegetables or animals who gave their lives so we may live, and to the farmer, shopkeeper, and cook who contributed their energies to making the food available.

OBTAINING NATURAL FOODS

In selecting your foods it is important to obtain the freshest and highest quality natural foods. Of course, growing your own grains and vegetables is ideal, and you may want to make your own miso, tofu, or seitan at home. For many people, however, especially those living in the city, the local natural foods, health food, or grocery and produce store will be the primary source of their daily food. Applied to food, the word *natural* means whole and unprocessed or processed by natural methods. The term *organic*, when further applied to natural foods, is understood to mean food that is grown without the use of chemical fertilizers, herbicides, pesticides, or other artificial sprays. Since it is fairly difficult to distinguish organic foods from nonorganic except by taste, you may need to rely on the reputation of the local store or the distributor. Many suppliers have been certified by an organic growers' association, which makes on-site inspections, performs lab tests on soil and product samples, and offers educational guidance to farmers and consumers.

The harmful effects of chemical farming on human health as well as on the topsoil and the environment have been well documented. As long ago as the end of the nineteenth century, Dr. Julius Hensel, a German agricultural chemist, warned that the introduction of synthetic fertilizers, insecticides, the forced fattening of livestock, and other modern practices were resulting in the degeneration of the human blood and lymph and giving rise to a host of degenerative diseases. In 1893, he wrote in his book *Bread from Stones:*

> Agriculture has entered into the sign of cancer. . . . [We] cannot be indifferent [to] what kind of crops we raise for our nourishment and with what substances our fields are fertilized. It cannot be all sufficient that great quantities are harvested, but the great quantity must also be of *good quality*. It is indisputable that by merely fertilizing with marl, i.e., with carbonate of lime, such a large yield may be gained as to make a man inclined to always content himself with marl, but with such a one-sided fertilization slowly but surely evil effects of various kinds will develop; these have

given rise to the axiom of experience: "Manuring with lime makes rich fathers but poor sons." . . . As our present fine flour, freed from bran, is furnished almost entirely devoid of [nutrients], we need not wonder at the great number of modern maladies.

Organic foods are not always available nor can they always be afforded because of their higher price. In this case, the next best available produce should be obtained and thoroughly cleaned and properly cooked to eliminate potentially harmful chemicals. For better health, it is also wise to avoid all industrially mass-produced foods including instant food, canned foods, frozen foods, refined grains or flour, sprayed foods, dyed foods, irradiated foods, and all foods made with chemicals, additives, preservatives, stabilizers, emulsifiers, and artificial coloring.

NUTRITIONAL STUDIES

Over the last decade, modern society has gradually become aware of the limits of chemical agriculture and food technology. Recent medical studies show that most of the foods in the macrobiotic diet protect against cancer and other degenerative diseases. In Part II we summarize several hundred of these research reports and classify them under the forms of cancer to which they especially apply. However, as we have seen, cancer is not an isolated phenomenon, but a disease of the whole body. These foods will substantially help reduce the risk of cancer in general. Briefly, let us look at the major medical findings as they apply to the basic categories of food in the Cancer-Prevention Diet.

1. Whole Grains—A wide variety of epidemiological, laboratory, and case-control studies show that as part of a balanced diet whole grains, high in fiber and bran, protect against nearly all forms of cancer. The Senate Select Committee's report *Dietary Goals*, the Surgeon General's document *Healthy People*, the National Academy of Sciences' report *Diet, Nutrition, and Cancer*, and many others all call for substantial increases in the daily consumption of whole grains such as brown rice, millet, barley, oats, and whole wheat.

2. Soup—A ten-year study completed in 1981 by the National Cancer Center of Japan reported that people who ate miso soup daily were 33 percent less likely to contract stomach cancer than those who

never ate miso soup. The study also found that miso was effective in preventing against heart and liver diseases.

3. Vegetables—A wide range of international population studies shows that regular consumption of cooked vegetables, particularly dark green and dark yellow vegetables such as broccoli, carrots, and cabbage, helps protect against cancer. In Japan, a 1970 laboratory study reported that shiitake mushrooms had a strong antitumor effect and no toxic side effects. "The dietary changes now under way appear to be reducing our dependence on foods from animal sources," the National Academy of Sciences panel commented, looking into the future of the American diet. "It is likely that there will be continued reduction in fats from animal sources and an increasing dependence on vegetable and other plant products for protein supplies. Hence, diets may contain increasing amounts of vegetable products, some of which may be protective against cancer."

4. Beans and Sea Vegetables—Epidemiological studies indicate that regular consumption of pulses, such as lentils, reduces the risk of cancer. In addition, soybeans, a major source of protein in the macrobiotic diet, have been singled out as especially effective in reducing tumors. The active ingredient in soybeans is called a protease inhibitor. Laboratory tests show that soybeans and certain other beans and seeds containing this factor added to the diet prevent the development of breast, stomach, and skin tumors. Whole soybeans and soy products, including miso, tamari soy sauce, tofu, tempeh, and natto, are staples of the macrobiotic diet. In addition, several medical studies and case-history reports indicate that sea vegetables help discharge radioactive elements and other heavy particles from the body. For instance, studies beginning in 1964 at McGill University in Canada showed that a substance in kelp and other common sea vegetables could reduce by 50 to 80 percent the amount of radioactive strontium absorbed through the intestine. At St. Luke's Hospital in Nagasaki, a group of macrobiotic doctors and patients who had survived the atomic bombing on August 9, 1945 subsequently protected themselves against potentially lethal doses of radiation on a diet of brown rice, miso soup, sea vegetables, and sea salt. Nuclear energy and nuclear weapons testing pose a serious health hazard today to almost everyone. (For further information on the protective effects of these foods against nuclear radiation, see Chapter 16 on leukemia in Part II.)

The following chart summarizes the major types of food and environmental influences that can combine over a long period of time and cause or enhance cancer, as well as those factors that can protect against and relieve it. This list is based on the dietary research and macrobiotic case histories presented in Part II, as well as generally accepted environmental studies.

CANCER, DIET, AND OTHER FACTORS

CANCER	HIGH RISK		LOW RISK
	Primary Factors	*Contributing Factors*	*Protective Factors*
Bladder	meat, eggs, poultry, oil, fat, dairy, sugar	white flour, fruit, soft drinks, coffee, chlorinated water, artificial sweeteners, air pollution	whole grains, beans, green and yellow vegetables, sea vegetables, spring water
Bone	meat, eggs, hard fat, refined salt	sugar, dairy, stimulants, radiation	whole grains, beans, vegetables, sea vegetables, shiitake mushrooms, sea salt
Brain (inner region)	meat, dairy, poultry, eggs, oily fish	sugar, oil, fruit, juices, spices, stimulants, drugs, medications, pesticides	whole grains, beans, vegetables, sea vegetables
Brain (outer region)	oil, fat, sugar, dairy, spices, soft drinks, chemicals, medications, drugs	animal food, vinyl chloride and other plastics, synthetic clothing	whole grains, beans, vegetables, sea vegetables
Breast	oil, fat, sugar, dairy, white flour	meat, eggs, poultry, spices, soft drinks, drugs, medications, x-rays, hair dyes, synthetic clothing	whole grains, beans, soyfoods, leafy green and white vegetables, sea vegetables, breastfeeding
Cervix	meat, eggs, poultry, hard fat, dairy, oil, fruit, juices	white flour, sugar, stimulants, chemicals, medications, DES	whole grains, beans, vegetables, sea vegetables

Endome-trium	oil, fat, sugar, meat, dairy, white flour	fruit, chemicals, birth-control pills, estrogens	whole grains, beans, vegetables, sea vegetables
Esophagus	oil, fat, sugar, dairy, spices, chemicals, soft drinks	animal food, especially cured meats, ham, bacon; alcohol; tobacco; radiation	whole grains, lentils and beans, green and yellow vegetables, sea vegetables
Kidney	fats, oil, meat, dairy	fruit, juices, sugar, spices, soft drinks, stimulants, chemicals, drugs, medications	whole grains, beans, vegetables, sea vegetables
Large Intestine (colon and rectum)	meat, eggs, hard fats, poultry, white flour	sugar, dairy, oil, spices, soft drinks, beer, chemicals, drugs, medications	whole grains, fiber, beans and lentils, leafy green vegetables, sea vegetables, thorough chewing
Leukemia	oil, fat, sugar, soft drinks, stimulants, chemicals	animal food, fruit, spices, pesticides, radiation, x-rays, industrial pollutants	whole grains, miso soup, beans, vegetables, sea vegetables, sea salt
Liver	meat, eggs, hard fat, animal protein, oil, white flour	sugar, spices, dairy, alcohol, pesticides, birth-control pills, drugs, medications	whole grains, beans, vegetables, sea vegetables, shiitake mushrooms
Lung	meat, eggs, poultry, dairy, sugar, oil, white flour	spices, fruit, stimulants, drugs, tobacco, air pollution, asbestos	whole grains, leafy green and yellow vegetables, beans, sea vegetables, fresh air
Lymphoma & Hodg-kin's Disease	milk and other dairy, sugar, oil, fat, soft drinks, chemicals	animal food, spices, pesticides, benzene, radiation, x-rays, tonsillectomies	whole grains, pulses, beans, vegetables, seeds, nuts, sea vegetables
Melanoma	meat, sugar, poultry, eggs, dairy, oil, white flour	fruit, soft drinks, spices, stimulants, chemicals, medica-tions, PCB's	whole grains, beans, vegetables, sea vegetables

CANCER	HIGH RISK		LOW RISK
	Primary Factors	*Contributing Factors*	*Protective Factors*
Ovary	meat, hard fat, eggs, animal protein, dairy, oil	sugar, white flour, fruit, juices, stimulants, chemicals, birth-control pills	whole grains, beans, vegetables, sea vegetables, shiitake mushrooms
Pancreas	meat, eggs, poultry, cheese, fat, oil, sugar	milk and other dairy, white flour, spices, coffee, tobacco, radiation	whole grains, beans, vegetables, sea vegetables, shiitake mushrooms
Prostate & Testicular	hard fats, meat, eggs, cheese	oil, dairy, sugar, white flour, fruit, coffee, chemicals, drugs, medications	whole grains, beans, vegetables, sea vegetables, shiitake mushrooms
Skin	fat, oil, dairy, white flour, sugar, fruit, juices, spices, soft drinks, chemicals	animal food, sunlight, industrial pollutants	whole grains, beans, soyfoods, vegetables, sea vegetables, sunlight plus a low-fat diet
Stomach	white rice, white flour, oil, vinegar, stimulants, alcohol	animal food, dairy, industrial pollutants	whole grains, beans, miso soup, soyfoods, leafy green and white vegetables, sea vegetables

SWITCHING TO NATURAL FOODS

Over the last decade, hundreds of thousands of people in the United States, Canada, Europe, Latin America, the Middle East, Australia, and the Far East have adopted the Cancer-Prevention Diet and have found it nourishing, satisfying, and delicious. Most people find that soon after changing to whole unprocessed foods, their natural sense of taste returns. After years of eating refined foods and artificially flavored products, our taste buds begin to atrophy and we forget the rich flavors, subtle aromas, and variety of textures offered by grains and vegetables. Changing to natural foods ultimately results not only in improved health but also in recovery of our appetite for life itself.

In making the transition from a refined modern diet, it is important to proceed gradually and not try to make the change all at once. Meat and poultry are relatively easy to give up, and most people discover they have little or no desire to consume them after a few weeks. However, if cravings occur, seitan (wheat meat) or tempeh (soy meat) may be consumed more frequently in such forms as a grain- or soyburger. The wheat or soy meat tastes and looks like hamburger and many people cannot tell the difference.

Sugar and sweets are usually more difficult to give up than meat. A gradual transition to more natural sweeteners should be made to allow the body to adjust itself to a change in blood sugar levels. First, honey or maple syrup may be substituted for sugar. When balance begins to be restored, over a period of several weeks to several months, the change to the comparatively milder rice syrup, barley malt, or other grain-based sweetener can be easily made. When full health is restored, a single mouthful of food containing sugar, honey, or maple syrup will usually trigger an instant headache or discomfort as the body's natural defense system signals the ingestion of highly imbalanced food. Modern people, however, have consumed so much sugar and sweets over the years that their bodies have become dulled to these effects.

For psychological reasons, the third category of foods, dairy products, is the most difficult for people to give up. In many cases, dairy food was the original food of infants and children for several generations of mothers who avoided breastfeeding. We all have a strong emotional attachment to the food on which we were initially raised. In the case of cow's milk and other dairy products, it often takes a long time for modern people, including otherwise nutritionally aware individuals, to overcome this unconscious dependency. Soyfoods and other bean products, which have little saturated fat and no cholesterol, provide an excellent alternative to dairy products. In the natural foods kitchen, a wide variety of foods that have a taste and texture similar to dairy products can be prepared for those in transition, including soy milk, soy ice cream, soy yogurt, tofu cheese, and tofu cheesecake.

Depending upon their condition, cancer patients and other people with serious illnesses may not have time to make this gradual transition and need to adopt a stricter, more medicinal form of the diet immediately. Information on how to accomplish this is presented in subsequent chapters of Part I and in Part II. In order to make a successful change in your way of eating, proper cooking is essential. Everyone, well or sick, is strongly encouraged to learn how to cook from qualified macrobiotic instructors. Until you have actually tasted the full range of macrobiotically prepared foods and seen how they are prepared, you may not fully appreciate the depth and scope of the diet or have a standard against which to measure your own cooking. Cooking is the supreme art and cookbooks, including this one, can only provide general guidance. You will save yourself endless confusion and mistakes by receiving introductory cooking instruction from one of the authorized macrobiotic educational institutions listed in Part III. Once you have mastered the fundamentals, then you can improvise and experiment on your own and ultimately learn to cook with only your intuitive sense of balance as your guide.

6.

Yin and Yang in the Development of Cancer

Everything in the universe is eternally changing, and this change proceeds according to the infinite order of the universe. This order of the universe has been discovered, understood, and expressed at different times and at varying places throughout human history, forming the universal and common basis for all great spiritual, philosophical, scientific, medical, and social traditions. The way to practice this universal and eternal order in daily life was taught by Lao Tzu, Confucius, Buddha, Moses, Jesus, Muhammad, and other great teachers in ancient times, and has been rediscovered, reapplied, and taught repeatedly in many lands and cultures over the past twenty centuries.

From observation of our day-to-day thought and activity, we can see that everything is in motion. Everything changes: Electrons spin around a central nucleus in the atom; the Earth rotates on its axis while orbiting the sun; the solar system is revolving around the galaxy; and galaxies are moving away from each other with enormous velocity as the universe continues to expand. Within this unceasing movement, however, an order or pattern is discernable. Opposites attract each other to achieve harmony, the similar repel each other to avoid disharmony. One tendency changes into its opposite, which shall return to the previous state. Thus summer changes into winter; youth changes into old age; action changes into rest; the mountain changes into the valley; day changes into night; hate changes into love; the poor change into the rich; civilization rises and falls; life appears and disappears; land changes into ocean; matter changes into energy; space changes into time. These cycles occur everywhere throughout nature and the universe.

Several thousand years ago in China, the universal process of change was called the Tao. Understanding the dynamic nature of reality formed the basis for the *I Ching* or *Book of Changes*, which was studied by thousands of people including Confucius and Lao Tzu. These two philosophers based their teachings on the underlying principle of yin and yang—the universal laws of harmony and relativity. Thus in most complete translations of the *I Ching*, such as the Wilhelm/Baynes edition, we find the Book of Commentaries, which was added by Confucius, in which he recorded his interpretation of the order of change. Lao Tzu wrote his own interpretation in the Tao Te Ching, the central verses of which read:

> Tao gave birth to One,
> One gave birth to Two,
> Two gave birth to Three,
> Three gave birth to all the myriad things.
> All the myriad things carry the Yin on their backs
>   and the Yang in their embrace,
> Deriving their vital harmony from the proper blending
>   of the two vital Breaths.

We find the same underlying principles in other Eastern philosophies. For instance, in Hinduism we find Brahman, or the Absolute, differentiating into Shiva and Parvati, the god and goddess whose cosmic dance animates and gives rise to all phenomena in the universe. The same concept is expressed in Shinto in the Kojiki or Book of Ancient Matters. In this version of the creation story, Ame-no-minakanushi, or Infinity, gives birth to Takami-musabi and Kami-musubi, or the gods of centrifugality and centripetality, and from these two deities the entire phenomenal universe arose. In Buddhism, the world of change is called samsara and is viewed as a revolving wheel turned by the forces of sorrow and compassion. The traditions and legends of most ancient societies, especially myths about twin brothers or brother and sister, all point to the same idea.

In the West, the unifying principle has also been expressed under a multitude of names and forms. In ancient Greece, the philosopher Empedocles held that the universe is the eternal playground of two forces, which he called Love and Strife. Although only fragments of his work survive, we find one passage that reminds us very much of the Tao Te Ching, which was composed about the same era:

I shall speak a double truth; at times
one alone comes into being;
at other times, out of one several things grow.
Double is the birth of mortal things and double
    demise . . .
They [Love and Strife] are for ever themselves,
    but running
through each other they become at times different,
    yet are for ever
and ever the same.

In the Old Testament, the rhythmic alternation of complementary energies is often expressed in terms of light and darkness and symbolized in the six-pointed Star of David, showing the balanced intersection of ascending and descending triangles. In the New Testament, we find evidence of an underlying teaching about two interrelated opposites in the story of the Sermon on the Mount where Jesus feeds the multitude with loaves of barley bread and two small fishes. The fishes can be seen to symbolize the two fundamental energies of the universe whose understanding satisfies our spiritual hunger and confers eternal life. In the recently discovered Gospel According to Thomas, we find further elaboration upon this theme. In this text, Jesus says to his disciples, "If they ask you, 'What is the sign of your Father in you,' say to them: 'It is a movement and a rest.'"

In more recent times, the unifying principle has been studied and applied, directly and indirectly by many great philosophers and scientists. In 1790 the English essayist Walking John Stuart observed, "Discover that moral and physical motion have the same double force, centripetal and centrifugal, and that, as the celestial bodies are detained in tranquil orbits . . . so moral bodies . . . move . . . in the orbit of society." In Ralph Waldo Emerson's writings, we find further development of this idea. For example, in his essay "History" he wrote, "As the air I breathe is drawn from the great repositories of nature, as the light on my book is yielded by a star a hundred millions of miles distant, as the poise of my body depends on the equilibrium of centrifugal and centripetal forces, so the hours should be instructed by the ages and the ages explained by the hours. Of the universal mind each individual man is one more incarnation."

Meanwhile, in Europe the German philosopher Hegel postulated that human affairs develop from a phase of unity, which he termed thesis, through a period of disunity, or antithesis, and on to a higher plane of reintegration, or synthesis. Hegel's principle of dialectics was, of course, later studied by Karl Marx and formed the basis of his philosophical speculations in the sphere of politics and economics. Unfortunately, Marx's system remained largely abstract and he did not apply dialectics to health and many aspects of daily life. As a result of chronic illness, he was unable to complete *Das Kapital*, and his wife, daughter, and associate Frederick Engels died of cancer.

In the twentieth century, Albert Einstein, among many other scientific thinkers, sensed the complementary antagonism between the visible world of matter and the invisible world of vibration, or energy. Based on this insight, he formulated the universal theory of relativity in which he stated that energy is constantly changing into matter and matter is continuously becoming energy. The present generation of scientists has discovered the nondual nature of reality under the electron microscope in the double helical structure of DNA. The coiled spirals of chromosomes in the nucleus remind us of the ancient caduceus, the intertwined snake or snakes which have long served as the symbol of Hermes, the god of healing, and the medical profession.

In the social sciences, historian Arnold Toynbee based his study of civilization on the alternating movement of two forces which he called challenge and response. In one of the early chapters of his multivolume *Study of History,* we read, "Of the various symbols in which different observers in different societies have expressed the alternation between a static condition and a dynamic activity in the rhythm of the Universe, Yin and Yang are the most apt, because they convey the measure of the rhythm directly and not through some metaphor derived from psychology or mechanics or mathematics. We will therefore use these Sinic [Chinese] symbols in this study henceforward."

By whatever name we call them, yin and yang govern all phenomena and produce either an outward or inward movement or tendency. Yin, or outward centrifugal movement, results in expansion, while yang or inward centripetal movement produces contraction. We can see these universal tendencies in the human body as the alternating expansion and contraction of the heart and lungs, for example, or in the stomach and intestines during the natural process of digestion. In the areas of astronomy and geophysics, these two forces are manifested as a downward, centripetal, or yang force generated inward to the center of the Earth by the sun, the stars, and far distant galaxies; and an upward, centrifugal, or yin force generated outward due to the rotation of the Earth. All phenomena on the Earth are created and maintained in balance by these two forces, which ancient people universally referred to as the forces of Heaven and Earth.

The following classifications of the antagonistic and complemental tendencies, yin and yang, show practical examples of these relative forces.

EXAMPLES OF YIN AND YANG

	YIN ▽*	YANG △*
Attribute	*Centrifugal force*	*Centripetal force*
Tendency	Expansion	Contraction
Function	Diffusion	Fusion
	Dispersion	Assimilation
	Separation	Gathering
	Decomposition	Organization
Movement	More inactive, slower	More active, faster
Vibration	Shorter wave and higher frequency	Longer wave and lower frequency
Direction	Ascent and vertical	Descent and horizontal
Position	More outward and peripheral	More inward and central
Weight	Lighter	Heavier
Temperature	Colder	Hotter
Light	Darker	Brighter
Humidity	Wetter	Drier
Density	Thinner	Thicker
Size	Larger	Smaller
Shape	More expansive and fragile	More contractive and harder
Form	Longer	Shorter
Texture	Softer	Harder
Atomic particle	Electron	Proton
Elements	N, O, P, Ca, etc.	H, C, Na, As, Mg, etc.
Environment	Vibration . . . Air . . . Water . . . Earth	
Climatic effects	Tropical climate	Colder climate
Biological	More vegetable quality	More animal quality
Sex	Female	Male

*For convenience, the symbols ▽ for Yin, and △ for Yang are used.

	YIN ▽*	YANG △*
Attribute	Centrifugal force	Centripetal force
Organ structure	More hollow and expansive	More compacted and condensed
Nerves	More peripheral, orthosympathetic	More central, parasympathetic
Attitude, emotion	More gentle, negative, defensive	More active, positive, aggressive
Work	More psychological and mental	More physical and social
Consciousness	More universal	More specific
Mental function	Dealing more with the future	Dealing more with the past
Culture	More spiritually oriented	More materially oriented
Dimension	Space	Time

CLASSIFYING FOODS INTO YIN AND YANG

As we saw in an earlier chapter, food is the mode of evolution, the way one species transforms into another. To eat is to take in the whole environment: sunlight, soil, water, and air. The classification of foods into categories of yin and yang is essential for the development of a balanced diet. Different factors in the growth and structure of foods indicate whether the food is predominantly yin or yang:

YIN Energy Creates:

Growth in a hot climate
Foods containing more water
Fruits and leaves
Growth upward high above the ground
Sour, bitter, sharply sweet, hot, and aromatic foods

YANG Energy Creates:

Growth in a cold climate
Drier foods
Stems, roots, and seeds
Growth downward below ground
Salty, plainly sweet, and pungent foods

To classify foods we must see the predominant factors, since all foods have both yin and yang qualities. One of the most accurate methods of classification is to observe the cycle of growth in food plants. During the winter, the climate is colder (yin); at this time of year the vegetal energy descends into the root system. Leaves wither and die as the sap descends to the roots and the vitality of the plant becomes more condensed. Plants used for food and grown in the late autumn and winter are drier and more concentrated. They can be kept for a long time without spoiling. Examples of these plants are carrots, parsnips, turnips, and cabbages. During the spring and early summer, the vegetal energy ascends and new greens appear as the weather becomes hotter (yang). These plants are more yin in nature. Summer vegetables are more watery and perish quickly. They provide a cooling effect, which is needed in warm months. In late summer, the vegetal energy has reached its zenith and the fruits become ripe. They are very watery and sweet and develop higher above the ground.

This yearly cycle shows the alternation between predominating yin and yang energies as the seasons turn. This same cycle can be applied to the part of the world in which a food originates. Foods that find their origin in hot tropical climates where the vegetation is lush and abundant are more yin, while foods originating in northern or colder climates are more yang. We can also generally classify plants according to color, although there are often exceptions, from the more yin colors—violet, indigo, green, and white—through the more yang colors—yellow, brown, and red. In addition, we should also consider the ratio of various chemical components such as sodium, which is yang or contractive, to potassium, which is yin or expansive, in determining the yin/yang qualities of vegetables and other foods.

In the practice of daily diet, we need to exercise proper selection of the kinds, quality, and volume of both vegetable and animal food. With some minor exceptions, most vegetable food is more yin than animal food because of the following factors:

1. Vegetable species are fixed or stationary, growing in one place, while animal species are independently mobile, able to cover a large space by their activity.

2. Vegetable species universally manifest their structure in an expanding form, the major portion growing from the ground upward toward the sky or spreading over the ground laterally. On the other hand, animal species generally form compact and separate unities.

Vegetables have more expanded forms, such as branches and leaves, growing outward while animal bodies are formed in a more inward direction with compact organs and cells.

3. The body temperatures of plants are cooler than some species of animals and generally they inhale carbon dioxide and exhale oxygen. Animal species generally inhale oxygen and exhale carbon dioxide. Vegetables are mainly represented by the color green, chlorophyll, while animals are manifested in the color red, hemoglobin. Their chemical structures resemble each other, yet their nuclei are, respectively, magnesium in the case of chlorophyll and iron in the case of hemoglobin.

Although vegetable species are more yin than animal species, there are different degrees even among the same species, and we can distinguish which vegetables are relatively more yin and which are yang. As a general principle, when we use plant foods in the warmer season of the year or in a warmer environment, it is safer to balance these yang factors with vegetables from the yin category. Conversely, when selecting plants in the colder season of the year or in colder regions, we can offset these yin environmental factors with a diet high in vegetable food from the yang category. Food can also be made more yang by increasing the length of cooking as well as increasing other factors such as heat, pressure, and salt.

Thus we are able to classify, from yin to yang or yang to yin, the entire scope of food as well as classify within each category. Generally speaking, animal food is extremely yang; fruits, dairy food, sugar, and spices are extremely yin; and grains, beans, and vegetables are more centered and fall in the middle of the spectrum. Within the category of extreme yang foods, we can further classify from most yang to less yang the following: salt, eggs, meat, poultry, salty cheeses, and fish. In the category of extreme yin foods, from less yin to most yin, we find milk and other dairy products; tropical vegetables and fruits; coffee and tea; alcohol; spices; honey, sugar, soft drinks, and other sweetened foods; all food prepared with chemicals or artificial additives; marijuana, cocaine, and other drugs; and most medications. In the center of the spectrum, relative to each other, cereal grains are more yang, followed by beans, seeds, root vegetables, leafy round vegetables, leafy expanded vegetables, nuts, and fruits grown in a temperate climate.

Since we need to maintain a continually dynamic balance and harmony between yin and yang in order to adapt to our immediate environment, when we eat foods from one extreme, we are naturally attracted to the other. For example, a diet consisting of large quantities of meats, eggs, and other animal foods, which are very yang, requires a correspondingly large intake of foods in the extreme yin category such as tropical fruits, sugar, alcohol, spices, and, in some cases, drugs. However, a diet based on such extremes is very difficult to balance, and often results in sickness, which is nothing but imbalance caused by excess of one of the two factors, or both.

Among our foods, the cereal grains are unique. As both seed and fruit, they combine the beginning and end of the vegetal cycle and provide the most balanced food for human consumption. It is for this evolutionary reason, as well as their well balanced nutritional contents and the great ability of cereals to combine well with other vegetables, that whole grains formed the principal food in all previous civilizations and cancer-free societies.

CLASSIFYING DISEASES INTO YIN AND YANG

The principle of yin and yang can also be used to understand the structure of the body and the origin and development of disease. In the human body, for example, the two branches of the autonomic nervous system—the orthosympathetic and parasympathetic—work in an antagonistic, yet complementary, manner to control the body's automatic functions. The endocrine system functions in a similar way. The pancreas, for example, secretes insulin, which controls the blood sugar level, and also secretes anti-insulin, which causes the level to rise.

Among sicknesses, some are caused by an overly expanding tendency; others result from an overly contracting tendency, while others result from an excessive combination of both. An example of a more yang sickness is a headache caused when the tissues and cells of the brain contract and press against each other, resulting in pain, while a more yin headache arises when the tissues and cells press against each other as the result of swelling or expansion. Therefore, similar symptoms can arise from opposite causes.

Cancer is characterized by a rapid increase in the number of cells and in this respect is a more expansive or yin phenomenon. However, the cause of cancer is more complex. As everyone knows, cancer can appear almost anywhere in the body. Skin, brain, liver, uterine, colon, lung, and bone cancer are just a few of the more common types. Each type has a slightly different cause.

To better understand this, let us consider the difference between prostate and breast cancer, both of which are increasing in incidence. Recently, female hormones have been used to control prostate cancer temporarily. At the same time, a male hormone has been found to have a similar controlling effect with breast cancer. Suppose, however, that female hormones were given to women with breast cancer. This would cause their cancers to develop more rapidly, while male hormones would accelerate the growth of prostate cancer. Therefore, women who have taken birth-control pills containing estrogen have a higher risk of developing breast cancer.

As we can see in the above example, breast and prostate cancer have opposite causes. Since more yin female hormones help neutralize prostate cancer, we can assume that this condition is caused by an excess of yang factors. Since breast cancer can be temporarily neutralized by more yang male hormones, this disorder has an opposite, or more yin, cause. In general, there are two types of cancer, which we can classify according to cause. The first results from excess consumption of foods in the extreme yang category including eggs, meat, fish, poultry, condensed types of dairy food such as cheese, other salty foods, and baked flour products. The second type of cancer is caused by excessive intake of foods in the extreme yin category including soft drinks, sugar, milk and ice cream, citrus fruit, stimulants, chemicals, refined flour, spices, and foods containing chemicals and artificial additives.

In general, if the cancer appears in the deeper or lower parts of the body or involves the more compact organs, it is caused by the overconsumption of yang foods. Yin cancers usually develop at the peripheral or upper parts of the body or in the more hollow, expanded organs. However, this classification is not absolute. Although cancer arises as the result of a predominance of one factor or another, the opposite factor is also involved, though to a lesser degree. For example, cancers resulting from the overconsumption of yang foods also require an intake of extreme yin, since this provides the stimulus for tumor growth.

Thus, among the Eskimos, whose diet largely consists of meat and fish, cancer was unknown until sugar and other refined products of modern civilization were introduced. The inclusion of these extremely yin items provided the necessary stimulus for their normally very yang diet to lead to the formation of a variety of malignant tumors.

Also, regions within each organ of the body have a more yin or more yang nature. For example, the stomach as a whole is classified as a yin organ because it is relatively hollow and expanded in comparison, say, to the pancreas, which is tight and compact. However, the stomach can be divided into the more expanded upper region, which secretes a strong acid (more yin), and the more compact lower region, which secretes a much weaker acid (less yin). The upper portion of the stomach known as the body is more yin, while the lower pylorus is more yang in structure. Cancers that appear in the upper stomach region result from the intake of foods such as sugar, monosodium glutamate (MSG), white rice, white flour, and other extremely yin products; while those tumors that develop in the pylorus result from the overconsumption of meat, eggs, fish, and other extremely yang products combined together with yin substances. Since these more yin foods are consumed widely in Japan, the people in that nation have a very high incidence of stomach cancer. Cancers of the large intestine, rectum, prostate, and ovaries, resulting from the intake of more yang foods including saturated fat, are predominant in America where more red meat and other animal foods are consumed. Other cancers, such as those of the lung, kidney, bladder, and more centrally located organs are usually caused by a combination of extreme yin and extreme yang foods, though more yang foods are the primary cause. A chart listing common varieties of cancer and their general classification according to yin and yang is presented on page 68. It should be kept in mind that different parts of each organ—e.g., the upper or lower part, the expanded or condensed part, the peripheral or central part, the ascending or descending part—differ respectively in their degree of yin and yang owing to various combinations of yin foods and yang foods.

To help offset the development of cancer, it is important to center the diet and avoid foods from both the extreme yin and yang categories. A more centrally balanced diet based on foods such as whole cereal grains, beans, and cooked vegetables can help protect against and relieve cancers caused by either more yin or yang factors. This does not mean, however, that the same dietary program should be adopted in every case. For a person in good health, the Cancer-Prevention Diet allows a wide variety of foods and cooking styles to be

GENERAL YIN AND YANG CLASSIFICATION
OF CANCER SITES

More Yin Cause	More Yang Cause	Yin and Yang Combined
Breast	Colon	Lung
Stomach (upper region)	Prostate	Bladder/Kidney
Skin	Rectum	Uterus
Mouth (except tongue)	Ovary	Liver
Esophagus	Bone	Spleen
Leukemia	Pancreas	Melanoma
Hodgkin's Disease	Brain (inner regions)	Tongue
Brain (outer regions)		Stomach (lower region)

selected according to a variety of factors including personal needs and enjoyment. For persons with cancer or a serious precancerous condition, a stricter diet needs to be followed at first until vitality is restored and gradually more and more foods can be added for variety.

7.

Relieving Cancer Naturally

In treating illness with dietary methods, it is important that the sickness be properly classified as predominantly yin or yang, or sometimes as a combination of both extremes. This is especially true with a life-threatening disease such as cancer. Once the determination is made, dietary recommendations can be more specifically aimed at alleviating the particular condition of excess.

Location of the tumor in the body generally determines whether a cancer is more yin or yang. However, in some cases, as we have seen, cancer in a specific organ can take either a yin or a yang form. In the case of a predominantly yang cancer, the general Cancer-Prevention Diet should be followed, slightly modified so as to accentuate more yin factors. The reverse is true in the case of more yin cancers. The standard diet should be followed and partially adjusted to emphasize more yang factors. For cancers caused by both extremes, a central way of eating is recommended. In all cases, however, all overly expansive and contractive food should be strictly avoided, as these items initially caused the cancer to appear.

By centering the diet and, if necessary, making nutritional adjustments emphasizing the complementary opposite quality, healthy balance can be restored. This common sense method underlies traditional healing and medicine in both East and West. For example, in Hippocrates' *The Nature of Man*, we read:

Diseases caused by overeating are cured by fasting, those caused by starvation are cured by feeding up. Diseases caused by exertion

69

are cured by rest; those caused by indolence are cured by exertion. To put it briefly: the physician should treat disease by the principle of opposition to the cause of the disease according to its form, its seasonal and age incidence, countering tenseness by relaxation, and vice versa. This will bring the patient most relief and seems to me to be the principle of healing.

In treating illness, the Hippocratic writings employ a variety of polarities and relativities to describe the organs of the body, the different foods that relieve illnesses, and varying human constitutions and conditions. These include strong/weak, fierce/tame, and elongated/hollow.

Over the last 2,500 years, the unifying principle has gradually disappeared from the Western scientific and medical vocabulary as ever smaller fragments of reality have been discovered under the magnifying glass and the microscope. Diseases are no longer looked at as wholes or parts of larger systems, but are broken down into cellular components. Instead of seeing sickness as a form of healthy adjustment, modern medicine sees health and disease as deadly enemies to one another. Instead of seeing that disease develops in one of two fundamentally different directions, modern medicine categorizes sickness into thousands of unrelated subgroupings and symptoms.

A failure to understand the distinction between the general tendencies of yin and yang illnesses explains why some people experience serious side effects from certain medications and others do not. It also explains why so many nutritional therapies and popular health diets produce mixed results or fail entirely. Vitamin C, for instance, is a yin substance that can benefit people with a cold caused by overconsumption of contractive yang foods. However, vitamin C taken in supplement form rather than in daily whole foods can further weaken persons with a cold caused by intake of excessive yin because it contributes further expansive energy to their system.

Across-the-board recommendations to take vitamin X, drug Y, or food Z to prevent or relieve cancer do not take into account the two opposite forms that illness may take. Nor do they always make room for differing human constitutions and conditions and varying geographical, social, and personal factors. Modern science is justified in rejecting alternative cancer remedies that ignore these variables. On the other hand, holistic medicine is correct in questioning modern science for focusing on quantity rather than quality. Eating whole foods containing vitamin C, such as broccoli, produces a different effect on the body than taking vitamin C pills, even though the actual amount of the nutrient may be the same.

DIETARY CONSIDERATIONS

On the whole, dietary suggestions should be directed primarily toward restoring the individual's excessively yin or yang condition to one that is less extreme. Once a more natural, balanced condition has been established and stabilized, the person's body will no longer need to accumulate toxic excess in the form of cancer. If we keep this holistic view in mind, we can avoid being caught up in an endless maze of symptoms.

If there is any uncertainty about whether the cause of a cancer is more yin or yang, we can safely recommend the central Cancer-Prevention Diet, which minimizes both tendencies.

Since cancer is a disease of excess, someone with cancer should be careful not to overeat. To prevent this, two important practices are advised. The first is to chew very well, at least 50 and preferably 100 times per mouthful until the food becomes liquefied. A person may eat as much food as he or she wants, provided it is well chewed and thoroughly mixed with saliva. Proper chewing releases an important enzyme in the mouth, which is essential for digestion. The second point of caution is not to eat for at least three hours before going to bed. Food eaten during that time often becomes surplus and will serve to accelerate indigestion, gas, mucus and fat formation, and enhance the development of cancer. Regarding liquid intake, the individual should drink moderately and only when thirsty.

For both yin and yang cancers, all intake of fatty animal foods, including meat, eggs, poultry, and dairy food, and other oily, greasy foods (including those of vegetable quality) should be strictly avoided. A person with more yin cancer, however, may have a very small quantity of fish once or twice a week if he or she craves it. In such instances, cooking a small portion of small dried fish in a soup may be appropriate. A person with yang cancer should stay away from all animal food, including fish, at least for the initial period of a few months. Nuts, on the other hand, should be completely avoided by someone with yin cancer, whereas a person with yang cancer may have a small quantity if desired. In both cases, nut butters should be avoided or limited because they are very oily and contain excess protein. It is also advisable for an individual with a more yin cancer to avoid or limit fruit and dessert completely. A person with a more yang cancer may occasionally have small amounts of cooked, dried, and, in some instances, fresh fruit, but only when craved.

The cooking of vegetables should be different for yin and yang cancers. In the case of yang cancer, one advisable method is to chop the vegetables while bringing water to a boil; add the vegetables to the boiling water for a few minutes or even one minute, then remove; a small amount of tamari soy sauce may be added for taste. Another method is to sauté the vegetables quickly for about two to three minutes on a high flame, adding a pinch of sea salt. These styles of cooking will preserve the crispness, freshness, and slightly more yin qualities of the vegetables. For yin cancer, vegetables should be cooked in a slower, longer, and more thorough manner, and tamari soy sauce or miso seasoning may be a little stronger. An emphasis on green leafy vegetables such as watercress or kale produces a slightly more yin effect; an emphasis on root vegetables such as carrot or turnip will produce a slightly more yang effect; an emphasis on round vegetables such as onion or acorn squash will result in a slightly more centered effect.

As for daily beverages, there are now several varieties of bancha tea available in natural foods and health food stores, including green tea, usual bancha tea, and bancha stem tea. Bancha stem tea is also commonly known as kukicha tea. All are produced from the same tea bush. Green tea is harvested in the summer and consists of the green leaves taken from the upper parts of the bush. However, some leaves are left on the plant until fall, at which time they become harder, drier, and darker in color. These leaves are used to produce the usual bancha tea. Bancha stem tea is made from the branches and stems of the plant, which are then dry roasted. More yin green tea contains plenty of vitamin C and can be used to help offset the toxic effects resulting from the overconsumption of animal foods, while more yang bancha stem tea contains less vitamin C, but plenty of calcium and minerals. It is advisable for all cancer patients to use bancha stem tea (kukicha) as their usual beverage. However, persons with more yang cancers may occasionally use the green tea from time to time for a short duration only. Green tea is not recommended for persons with other types of cancer. Of course, dyed black tea and aromatic herbal teas, especially those that have been cultivated and processed chemically, are not recommended for use even by healthy persons.

Among some daily condiments such as gomashio (sesame salt) or umeboshi salt plums, slight adjustments in use may also need to be made depending upon the form of cancer. The specific dietary recommendations for each major form of cancer are listed in detail in Part II and recipes and sample menus are provided in Part III.

ENVIRONMENT AND LIFESTYLE

In addition to dietary change, several other measures are important in cancer recovery. To promote better circulation of the body's natural flow of energy, direct contact with the elements of nature is advisable. Walking outdoors on the grass, soil, or beach, preferably barefoot, is an excellent therapeutic measure. Regular exercise, including Do-in (Oriental self-massage), yoga, or the martial arts, can also be beneficial. A person should be as active as his or her health allows without becoming tired or overworked.

The discoveries and inventions of modern science and industry have contributed substantial convenience and efficiency to our daily life. However, at the same time, many technological applications are hazardous to our health and spiritual well-being. Artificial electromagnetic energy in our environment changes the atmospheric charge surrounding us, producing various effects on our physical and mental condition. Often we may notice a general fatigue, mental irritability, and unnatural metabolism as the result of high voltage lines, electrical appliances, and other communications equipment in our vicinity. Cooking on an electric range or in a microwave oven especially contributes to undesirable effects on our digestion and nourishment and should preferably be avoided. Synthetic home furnishings and artificial building materials may prevent healthy relaxation. When we start to change our blood to a healthy quality by eating a more centrally balanced diet, we naturally begin to reduce our reliance upon technological comforts in our environment. Our natural defense mechanism is restored and our bodies adjust more easily to extremes of hot and cold, necessitating less dependence on central heating in winter and air conditioning in summer. We appreciate, value, and continue to use some of the technological advances that modern civilization offers. However, we should reduce our reliance on the use of excessive mechanical or electronic conveniences that may hinder the smooth exchange of energy between ourselves and the natural environment. We especially try to avoid those features of modern life that may contribute to the development of sickness or make the recovery from sickness more difficult.

Synthetic clothing, such as that made of nylon, polyester, and acrylic, especially impedes the regular flow of energy through the body. It is therefore advisable not to wear these types of fabrics directly next to the skin. Undergarments of cotton are the ideal alternative, and as we gradually replace our wardrobe we begin to feel more comfortable in all natural clothing such as 100 percent cotton, linen, or silk. Synthetic sheets, blankets, and other furnishings should be avoided if possible. Excessive metallic accessories, such as rings, pendants, and other jewelry, should be kept to a minimum as well.

Free circulation of air and open sunshine should be encouraged in the patient's room; the addition of several green plants will also help to stimulate deeper breathing and stronger metabolism. Television, particularly color television, exerts a draining influence on the organism, and should be viewed moderately to minimize radiation. Long hot baths or showers, which deplete the supply of minerals in the body, should also be reduced. In general, the patient's environment should be open, happy, and free of any dark or heavy features. This should also extend to such influences as reading material or conversation.

OUTLOOK AND SPIRITUAL PRACTICE

Mental attitude is, of course, very important. A person with cancer must understand that he or she was directly responsible for the development of the disease, through his or her daily diet, manner of thinking, and way of life. The patient should be encouraged to reflect deeply, to examine those aspects of modern mentality that have produced the problem of cancer and a host of other unhappy situations. These reflections should include a review of the rich heritage of traditional wisdom developed by many cultures over thousands of years, an appreciation of the endless wonders of the natural world, including the body's marvelous self-protective and recuperative mechanisms, and a respect for the order of the universe that produces these phenomena.

Prayer, meditation, and visualization (in which the mind focuses on images of healing) will also contribute to improving the person's course of recovery. Several recent medical tests have shown that mental relaxation, emotional support, and awareness of being part of a larger community can help reduce tumor development. However, it is important that these methods serve as an adjunct and not a replacement for fundamental dietary change. The following chart summarizes the interrelationship among these factors:

A HOLISTIC APPROACH TO CANCER

Way of Life	Healthy	Degenerative
Daily Food (primary factor)	Whole	Processed
	Natural	Artificial
	Organic	Chemical
	Unrefined	Refined
	Balanced	Extreme
	Seasonal	Unseasonal
	Locally Grown	Transcontinental
	Home-Cooked	Pre-cooked
Environment & Lifestyle (contributing factor)	Clean	Polluted
	Orderly	Disorderly
	Active	Sedentary
	Real	Synthetic
Outlook (contributing factor)	Peaceful	Complaining
	Grateful	Arrogant
	Flexible	Rigid
	Cooperative	Competitive

All of us must realize that without food there is no life; without food we cannot create healthy blood; and without healthy blood, there is no cell formation, including the formation of healthy brain cells. The strength of our minds, emotions, and spirits is conditioned by the daily food we take, and these, in turn, reciprocally influence the health and vitality of our physical being. However, this relationship has often been misunderstood, and disease has been equated with sin and health with saintliness. To the eye of the universe, however, moral sanctity does not necessarily protect from sickness or disability.

For example, my wife and I recently returned from giving seminars on cancer and diet in Spain and Portugal. While in Spain, I saw many sick people who were seeking macrobiotic advice. One Catholic nun, about thirty-five years old, was among them. She attended my seminars, and when I saw her privately, she confessed that she was suffering from breast cancer. I asked her how many nuns were in her convent, and she replied that about three hundred were living there. I then asked how many had developed cancer, and she told me that sixty nuns had developed the disease, and of these thirty had already died. Thirteen women had entered the convent when she did, and, of this original group, twelve had died from cancer and she was the only one left. In some instances, prayer may have prolonged the lives of these unfortunate women. However, only by changing the convent's daily way of eating would their lives be completely saved. (For inspiring accounts of how spiritual practices have been combined with the Cancer-Prevention Diet, see the story of John Jodziewicz in the chapter on male cancers and the story of Neil Scott in the large intestine section in Part II.)

GETTING STARTED

Once the decision has been made to reverse the cancerous condition by embracing a more balanced way of life, combining diet, physical activity, and self-reflection, the person should forget about the sickness and live as happily, actively, and normally as possible. Cancer patients are often depressed; once the person begins to eat a healthier diet, he or she should be strongly encouraged not to worry and to maintain an optimistic attitude.

A more complex situation occurs when a person with cancer has received chemotherapy, cobalt radiation, or undergone surgery. In such cases, recovery may be somewhat more difficult, but is still possible so long as the patient has normal appetite, good vitality, and the will to live. In such a situation, it is particularly vital for both the patient and the members of his or her family to understand the importance of properly implementing the dietary recommendations. Ideally, they should spend several days, or preferably weeks, learning how to cook macrobiotically and should seek qualified individual advice on the correct manner of cooking and eating for their particular situation. (For the macrobiotic education center nearest you offering cooking classes and health and dietary counselling, contact the national headquarters of the East West Foundation, 17 Station St., Brookline, MA 02146, (617) 731-0564.)

Among the different types of cancer, breast, cervical, colon, pancreas, liver, bone, and skin cancer tend to respond more readily to this dietary method, whereas cancer of the lung is more difficult to change. Cancers caused by eating eggs are among the most difficult, particularly when they appear deep within the body such as in the ovaries or testicles.

Cases that are even more serious—so-called terminal cases—require additional attention. In these situations, the cancer may be rapidly spreading and the patient may be in great pain, with an accompanying loss of appetite. Such cases require the use of external applications along with the proper way of eating. Food should be cooked to the normal texture and consistency, provided the patient is able to chew and swallow. If the patient has difficulty eating in this manner, it is advisable to mash the foods after they have been cooked. It may also be necessary to cook the food with more water than usual, to arrive at a softer, more creamy consistency. Grains, vegetables, beans, and other foods can be cooked in this way and then mashed by hand in a traditional Japanese mortar called a suribachi. An electric blender should not be used.

The most important home-care techniques are the ginger compress, the taro potato plaster, and the buckwheat plaster. The methods for preparing these and their proper uses are given in Part III. Most cancers can be dealt with successfully without the use of such external treatments. It is only the 20 to 30 percent that are considered terminal or that have been complicated by previous treatment that require these special methods. These external applications are also effective for the relief of a variety of precancerous conditions, benign tumors, and cysts including fibroid tumors, ovarian cysts, and breast cysts.

Simple, safe, and effective solutions to the problem of cancer and other degenerative diseases already exist. These methods extend back to the common roots of traditional medicine in East and West, including home remedies and folk medicine, and are now being successfully practiced by hundreds of thousands of people around the world to improve their health. Whether we are able practically to implement these approaches as a society will determine whether modern civilization continues to degenerate biologically or whether we create a sound and healthy future for ourselves, our children, and all humanity.

8.

Diagnosing Cancer Safely

Early detection of cancer and accurate classification into categories of yin and yang make adjusting the diet and lifestyle easier and contribute to a smoother recovery. One of the universal features of modern life is that we have lost the natural ability to diagnose and treat disease without recourse to complex, expensive, and often dangerous technology.

However, over the last several years, the limits of this approach to sickness, and to cancer in particular, have become more widely recognized. Mammograms have been implicated in causing as much cancer as they protect against, and other diagnostic x-rays may also be hazardous. Cervical Pap smears sometimes show the presence of cancer where none exists or vice versa. Tissue samples taken in biopsies are subject to contamination and distortion in the operating room and can be misjudged under the microscope. Surgical procedures to remove tumors have actually helped some cancers spread. Radiation therapy can damage healthy tissue and lead to acute or chronic secondary disorders. Chemotherapy can poison normal as well as toxic cells and cause a host of blood-deficiency diseases leading to massive infection.

Hormone treatments have resulted in impotence or sterility. Anesthetics and painkillers frequently weaken the body's immune system and make healing more difficult. Today's miracle cure for cancer, such as Interferon, turns out to be tomorrow's tumor promoter. Even the chemical solution in which surgical instruments are routinely cleaned and the plastic tubing for intravenous feeding have been implicated in medical tests as cancer causing.

Despite the most optimistic predictions and interpretation of the statistics, the casualties in the war on cancer continue to mount. As a result of this dilemma, the concept of a cure for cancer has undergone a significant change during this century. In cancer treatment, cure no longer carries the usual dictionary definition of restoration to a healthy and sound condition, but signifies only that the patient is still alive five years from the time the tumor was originally treated. *Control* is a more appropriate word than *cure,* and over the last few decades the slight increase in the control rate has reflected advances in surgery, blood transfusions, and antibiotics more than break-throughs in actual cancer treatment.

The challenge to modern cancer therapy was underscored in an address to a panel of the American Cancer Society in 1969 by Dr. Hardin Jones, a professor of medical physics at the University of California in Berkeley and an expert on statistics and the effects of surgery, drugs, and radiation:

My studies have proven conclusively that untested cancer victims actually live up to four times longer than treated individuals. For a typical type of cancer, people who refused treatment lived for an average 12½ years. Those who accepted surgery and other kinds of treatment lived an average of only three years. . . . I attribute this to the traumatic effect of surgery on the body's natural defense mechanism. The body has a natural defense against every type of cancer.

Dr. Hardin's conclusions echo Hippocrates' warning that cancer patients who are treated with incision die, but those who are not treated with the knife live a relatively long time. Three hundred years ago, on the eve of the scientific revolution, the French author Molière observed laconically, "If we leave Nature alone, she recovers gently from the disorder into which she has fallen. It is our anxiety, our impatience, which spoils all; and nearly all men die of their remedies, not of their diseases."

From reports such as Dr. Hardin's, some people have concluded that modern medicine is iatrogenic (disease-causing) and will no longer see a doctor or go to a hospital under any circumstances. However, this is to overlook the many positive advances in emergency treatment and in the control and relief of pain that have developed over the decades. In general, we recommend avoiding those features of modern medicine that treat symptoms rather than underlying causes and that are potentially harmful. However, under a few special circumstances, it may be necessary to take advantage of the lifesaving apparatus and techniques afforded by hospitals. For example, if a cancer patient can no longer eat and is rapidly losing weight, it may be necessary to supply intravenous glucose injections until body metabolism is stabilized. Meanwhile, soft grains and mashed vegetables can be prepared and given the patient in the hospital room as her or his appetite returns. Similarly, there may be emergency situations when surgery or radiation treatment are advisable, such as obstructions in the digestive system that totally block ingestion of food of any kind.

Except in these types of lifesaving situations, we do not encourage patients to combine the Cancer-Prevention Diet with surgery, radiation, or chemotherapy. However, occasionally when some cancer patients first hear about macrobiotics, they initially lack confidence in the dietary approach because it seems new. If they decide to pursue the diet along with conventional therapy, their recovery might be slower. This approach can work temporarily, but once a patient improves, it is better to begin reducing the frequency of outside treatment. This transitional period might last from one to four months.

COOPERATING WITH THE MEDICAL PROFESSION

Closely related is the question of medication and whether a patient who decides to change his or her way of eating and thinking should stop taking drugs and other prescription or nonprescription preparations. The general rule is to reduce reliance on medicines slowly rather than all at once. Most of these substances fall into one of three general categories. First are those medications that keep vital body functions going and that, if stopped, would result in immediate death or severe disability. These include certain hormone replacements. As the way of eating changes and improvements in health and vitality are noticed, the medications may slowly be tapered off, preferably under medical supervision, over a period usually ranging from three to six months. Sometimes, as in the case of insulin, this may take longer, up to one or two years depending on the case. In the event that an essential organ has been removed, the supply of medications or hormones may need to be continued for a lifetime.

Secondly come those medicines that affect or control bodily conditions such as blood pressure: anticonvulsives, antibiotics, asthma medication, cortisone, and others. As health improves on the new diet, these items can gradually be withdrawn over a period of about one to four months.

The third category includes sedatives, tranquilizers, stimulants, and nutritional supplements. Examples are thorazine, sleeping pills, vitamin capsules, and mineral tablets. These kind of aids may be stopped much sooner, within ten days to two months.

These time periods are only an average guideline. Each individual case is different and must be judged on its own merits. Until the blood quality begins to change through proper eating, the patient needs to proceed slowly in making the transition. Normally it takes the blood plasma ten days to change in quality. Within this period on the Cancer-Prevention Diet, the patient should experience relief in digestive and respiratory functions as well as disappearance of bodily pain. After about two weeks on the diet, circulatory and excretory changes are felt, the emotions begin to change, and the patient will generally feel less depressed and less angry. Nervous functions improve after about a month and thinking tends to become clearer and more focused. After three to four months, the body's red blood cells have completely changed in quality, and the skin, bones, organs, and tissues begin to heal. At this time the person's relations with family and friends often become gentler, more respectful, and loving. Nervous cells take three seasons or approximately nine months to alter, and after this time the person's view of life may become broader, more flexible, and more understanding. Total harmony can take three to seven years or more to achieve, at which time universal consciousness begins to develop. Once again, these are very general averages, and the actual time it will take to restore full health will vary with each individual.

In general, we advise cancer patients to consult with and keep their regular doctors informed of their progress on the Cancer-Prevention Diet and have periodic medical checks. Full medical records documenting the progressive reduction of the tumor and restoration of normal bodily functions can prove helpful to future medical and nutritional researchers. Ideally, the macrobiotic consultant and the medical doctor—who may sometimes be the same person—will work together to monitor the patient's condition. In this way, the best possible dietary treatment and emergency medical relief are available. The patient, the family, the hospital, and the macrobiotic adviser can learn from each other as they cooperate to ensure a smooth recovery.

The crisis of faith in modern medicine's ability to cure cancer reflects a deeper loss of awareness and judgment we all share regarding our health and well-being. Every day we hear about someone who is active and seemingly fit discovering in a routine medical examination that his body is riddled with tumors. How often we hear of someone who dies of a heart attack shortly after being given a clean bill of health by his or her doctor, or read in the newspapers about a tragic crime that has been committed by someone with a serious mental or emotional disorder that has escaped the attention of his or her family, neighbors, and co-workers. Our most sophisticated technology can reveal the chemical structure of our blood and brain tissue, but it cannot tell us very long in advance whether we are developing a serious physical, mental, or emotional ailment. It is increasingly acknowledged that cancer takes many years, perhaps decades, to develop. However, approximately 50 percent of tumors are not discovered until after they have spread from the primary site to other regions or organs of the body.

Clearly we need to supplement our health care with a medicine that is preventive in direction and humane and economical in application. The traditional medicine of China, Japan, and other countries of the Far East, as well as folk medicine and home cares, can contribute greatly to filling this need.

The Yellow Emperor's Classic of Internal Medicine, the Caraka Samhita, and other standard Oriental medical texts on the causes of disease stressed the relationship between an individual's health and his or her diet, activity, spiritual development, and total environment. No single aspect of human life was considered separate from another aspect. The biological, psychological, and spiritual were seen as interrelated aspects of the totality. The medical practitioner was an adviser and teacher who could point out the source of a potential sickness and give practical suggestions for changes in diet and lifestyle that could eliminate the problem before visible symptoms occurred.

Modern medicine diagnoses a disease principally by observing physical symptoms. The experienced macrobiotic counselor, however, can foresee the development of sickness before pain, fever, rash, or other symptoms surface. In former times, Oriental physicians were ordinarily paid by a family so long as the family members remained in good health. In cases of sickness, the doctor received no stipend because he or she should have foreseen the ailment and prevented it through proper dietary adjustments. This was the traditional test of a good healer.

DIAGNOSIS BY PHYSIOGNOMY

The principal tool of macrobiotic diagnosis is physiognomy, which the *Oxford English Dictionary* defines as "the art of judging character and disposition from the features of the face or the form and lineaments of the body generally." The basic premise of physiognomy is that each of us represents a living encyclopedia of our entire physical, mental, emotional, and spiritual development. The strengths and weaknesses of our parents, the environment we grew up in, and the food we have eaten are all expressed in our present condition. Our posture, the color of our skin, the tone of our voice, and other traits are external manifestations of our blood quality, inner organs, nervous system, and skeletal structure. These, in turn, are the result of our heredity, diet, environment, daily activity, thoughts, and feelings.

The secret of diagnostic skill is to recognize the signs of a particular set of changes before they become serious—to see visual clues on the face or in the eyes that stones are developing in the kidneys, that the heart is expanding, or that a cancer is developing—even before these symptoms bring pain or discomfort. This type of diagnosis depends completely on the practitioner developing his or her own sensitivity and understanding fully the principles that underlie the techniques, together with his or her life experience.

The study of physiognomy originally developed in the West as well as in the East and served as an integral part of everyday life and medicine in the ancient Hellenistic world and in Europe through the Renaissance. In the Zohar, a book of Jewish teachings from the Middle Ages, we read, "The character of a man is revealed in the hair, the forehead, the eyes, the lips, the features of the face, the lines of the hands, and even the ears. By these seven the different types of men can be recognized." Leonardo da Vinci's notebooks contain numerous material on physiognomy. For example, he compiled a reference dictionary for his own use of heads, eyes, mouths, chins, necks, throats, shoulders, and noses upon which he drew for his famous anatomical sketches and character studies. Western literature abounds with references to physiognomy, and until the nineteenth century many great authors drew upon their knowledge of this art for development of their characters. In *Ivanhoe*, for instance, we find this description of Prince John:

> Those who remarked in the physiognomy of the Prince a dissolute audacity, mingled with extreme indifference to the feelings of others, could not yet deny to his countenance that sort of comeliness which belongs to an open set of features, well formed by nature, modelled by art to the usual rules of courtesy, yet so far frank and honest, that they seemed as if they disclaimed to conceal the natural workings of the soul.

The general principles of physiognomy can be found in a macrobiotic text—or a novel like Scott's. However, development of the art requires that the practitioner's own health and judgment be refined and involves much study and patience. My own practical study of physiognomy began in the early 1950's shortly after I arrived in the United States and settled in New York. I used to stand on Forty-second Street and Broadway and along Fifth Avenue observing thousands of people: their body structure, their way of walking, their way of expression, their faces, their behavior, and their thinking. In cafeterias and restaurants, theaters and amusement parks, trains and subways, shops and schools, every day I observed the countless variety of human faces and forms.

Week by week, month by month, year by year, it became apparent that all physical, psychological, social, and cultural manifestations of human activity depend upon our environment and dietary habits. It became clear that hereditary factors are nothing but the result of the past environment in which our ancestors lived and the food they observed in their daily diet. The constitution we inherit at birth is largely influenced by the food our mothers ate during pregnancy. Leonardo succinctly summed up this relationship in his writings on the embryo: "The mother desires a certain food and the child bears the mark of it."

During the embryonic period, all major systems of the body gather and form the entire facial structure. These include the digestive and respiratory systems, the nervous system, and the circulatory and excretory systems. As the fetus grows, the upper and lower parts of the body develop in parallel. Following birth, each area of the face correlates with an inner organ and its functions. These major correlations are discussed below.

Correlation of Inner Organs and Facial Features

The condition of the cheeks shows the condition of the chest cavity, including the lungs and breasts and their functions. The tip of the nose represents the heart and its functions, while the nostrils represent the bronchi connecting the lungs. The middle part of the nose represents the stomach, and the middle to upper part of the nose the pancreas. The eyes represent the kidneys as well as the condition of the ovaries in the case of a woman and the testicles in the case of a man. Also, the left eye represents the condition of the spleen and pancreas, and the right eye the liver and gallbladder. The irises and whites of the eyes reflect the condition of the entire body. The area on the lower forehead between the eyebrows shows the condition of the liver, and the temples on both sides the condition of the spleen. The forehead as a whole represents the small intestines, and the peripheral region of the forehead represents the large intestines. The upper part of the forehead shows the condition of the bladder. The ears represent the kidneys: the left ear the left kidney, and the right ear the right kidney. The mouth as a whole shows the condition of the entire digestive tract. More specifically, the upper lip shows the stomach; the lower lip shows the small intestines at the inner part of the lip and the large intestine at the more peripheral part of the lip. The corners of the lips show the condition of the duodenum. The area around the mouth represents the sexual organs and their functions.

Lines, spots, moles, swellings, discolorations, and other abnormalities in any of these locations indicate specific malfunctions in the corresponding inner organs as a result of improper food consumption. The markings of the hands, feet, chest, back, and all other parts of the body also offer clues to the internal physiological condition of the individual as well as mental and psychological tendencies. On the basis of these observations and other simple, safe techniques, the person's overall health can be ascertained and season-to-season, week-to-week, or day-to-day fluctuations can be monitored.

Identification of Diseased Conditions

In this way chronic ailments or precancerous conditions can be identified long before they develop and appropriate dietary adjustments taken. For example, developing obstructions, cysts, and tumors can be diagnosed through careful observation of the eye-whites, which represent the condition of the whole body. Precancerous conditions often correlate with the following markings:

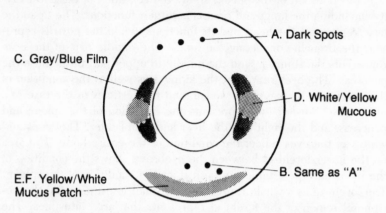

A. Calcified deposits in the sinuses are frequently indicated by dark spots in the upper portion of the eye-white.

B. Kidney stones and ovarian cysts are often indicated by dark spots in the lower eye-white.

C. and D. The accumulation of mucus and fat in the centrally located organs (liver, gallbladder, spleen, and pancreas) frequently appears in the form of a blue, green, or brownish shade, or white patches, in the eye-white on either side of the iris, often indicating reduced functioning in these organs.

E. Accumulation of fat and mucus in and around the prostate are often indicated by a yellow or white coating on the lower part of the eyeball.

F. Fat and mucus accumulating in the female sex organs are frequently indicated by a yellow coating in the same area of the eye as E above. Vaginal discharges, ovarian cysts, fibroid tumors, and similar disorders are also possibly shown as white/gray mucus.

Another clue to approaching cancer is a change in skin color. When cancer develops, a greenish shade will often appear in certain areas on the skin. The appearance of this color represents a process of biological degeneration. To better understand this, let us consider the order of colors in the natural world. Among the seven primary colors, red has the longest wavelength and is the warmest, brightest, and most active. Therefore we classify red as yang. The opposite colors—purple, blue, and green—have shorter wavelengths and are cooler, darker, and more still or passive. We therefore classify them as yin. Red is the color of the more yang animal kingdom and is readily apparent in the color of the blood and the general pigmentation of the skin. On the other hand, green is the color of the more yin vegetable realm and is the color of chlorophyll. Eating represents the process whereby we transform green vegetable-quality life into red animal-quality blood. It is based on the ability to change magnesium, which lies at the center of the chlorophyll molecule, into iron, the element that forms the basis of the hemoglobin in our blood.

▽ Purple — Blue — **Green** — Yellow — Brown — Orange — **Red** △

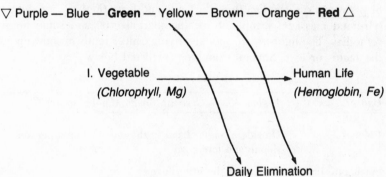

I. Vegetable _____ Human Life
(Chlorophyll, Mg)   (Hemoglobin, Fe)

Daily Elimination

II. Cancer ◄———————————————— Body Cell

The above diagram depicts the classification of basic colors from yang (△) to yin (▽). The process of humanization (I) represents the transformation of green vegetable life into human blood and body cells. Cancer represents a reverse process (II) in which body cells decompose, often producing a greenish shade on the skin.

The more yin colors—purple, blue, or gray—appear in the sky and atmosphere, both of which are more expanded or yin components of the environment, as well as often near the time of death. The more yang colors—yellow, brown, and orange—appear in the more compact world of minerals. During the transformation of vegetable life into human blood and cells, waste products are eliminated through functions such as urination and bowel movements. These represent in-between stages in the transformation of vegetable into human life and therefore are yellow and brown, the colors that lie in between green and red in the color spectrum.

Cancer represents a reverse evolutionary process in which body cells decompose and change back toward more primordial vegetable life. Multiplication of these degenerating cells gives rise to tumors and manifests in a greenish shade appearing on the skin. This shading does not appear on the entire body or near the tumor itself, but in certain areas along the respective meridians of electromagnetic energy corresponding with the location of the cancer. These meridians or pathways run the length of the body and form the basis for shiatsu (Oriental massage), acupuncture, the martial arts, and some home remedies. The light-green color signifying cancer tends to show up on the hands or feet. Several examples are listed below:

Cancer Type	Region Where Greenish Shade Might Appear
Colon	Outside of either hand in the indented area between thumb and forefinger
Small Intestine	Outside of the little finger
Lung/Breast	Either or both cheeks and on the inside of the wrists
Stomach	Along the outside front of either leg, especially below the knee or in the extended area of the second and third toes
Bladder/Uterus Ovaries/Prostate	Around either ankle on the outside of the leg
Liver/Gallbladder	Around the top of the foot in the outside central area, with its area extending to the fourth toe
Spleen/Lymph	Inside of the foot from the outer root of the big toe toward the area below the anklebone

SEASONAL APPEARANCE OF SYMPTOMS

The season of the year in which symptoms first appear or the time of day in which discomfort is greatest can also help us determine the nature and location of the sickness. Heart and small-intestine ailments arise more frequently in summer and in the late morning or noontime of the day. Spleen, stomach, pancreas, and lymph related disorders arise more during the late summer or in the afternoon. Lung and large intestine troubles often surface in autumn and during the middle to late afternoon. Kidney, bladder, and reproductive difficulties are particularly prevalent in wintertime and during the evening or night. Gallbladder and liver disorders commonly arise in spring and are especially noticeable in early morning. In general, the incidence of cancer increases with cold weather in autumn to early winter as excess accumulation from the summer is manifested in the formation of tumors. At this time of year, breast, skin, and other more yin type cancers appear because of the high volume of sugar, soft drinks, and dairy food that are consumed in the summertime. Conversely, in winter people tend to eat more meat, poultry, eggs, and other strong yang foods, giving rise to proportionately more yang cancers in the spring including those of the colon, liver, ovaries, and prostate. Of course, these are not absolute, but general tendencies. Cancer may appear in any specific form at any time of the year.

There are many other factors to consider and other traditional diagnostic procedures we may use to help detect cancer before it develops or if it has already appeared before it spreads further. These supplementary methods include taking pulses on both wrists and touching the pressure points on the skin along the meridians of electromagnetic energy.

In contrast to modern medicine, traditional diagnosis does not require an elaborate or expensive technology and the methods employed are simple, safe, and accurate. Our own senses are the only tools employed. As our understanding of physiognomy develops, we realize that we are our own machines, and our own intuition and judgment is superior to the most advanced computer. What we see, hear, smell, taste, and touch can tell us the story of an individual's past, present, and probable future. The outer echoes the inner; the inner mirrors the outer. Learning to perceive the development of just one person can lead us to begin to understand the destiny of humanity. The person to begin with is oneself.

9.

Medically Terminal or Macrobiotically Hopeful?

I have met thousands of people with cancer over the last fifteen years. Of these 90 percent or more had already received chemotherapy, radiation, surgery, or some other treatment. Many were considered terminally ill. In some cases there was nothing that modern medicine could do for them; in others, all possible treatments had already been tried and met with no success.

Patients who have received treatment often take longer to recover than those who have not, and their recovery is often more complicated and difficult. With macrobiotics we try to change the quality of the blood and cells through living a natural daily life. However, when violent or artificial treatments have first been applied, a person must recover not only from the cancer, but also from the toxic and unnatural effects of the treatment.

This brings us to the difference between cases considered to be *medically terminal* and those considered to be *macrobiotically terminal*. A medically terminal case is one for which present treatments offer no hope of recovery. In some cases, an exploratory operation is performed and the patient is told that no treatment will be applied. Persons in this situation often have a better possibility of recovery on the Cancer-Prevention Diet than those who were considered hopeful by modern medicine and who received conventional treatment.

In determining the likelihood of relieving cancer by dietary means, there are several factors that may interfere with the natural process of recovery.

LACK OF GRATITUDE

A spirit of thankfulness is essential to the healing process. The person needs to see that his or her past way of eating and living created the cancer and that he is fortunate to have the opportunity to change his diet and lifestyle. However, many cancer patients—as well as many relatively healthy people—constantly complain when the new diet is introduced. They frequently say or think: "These vegetables are tasteless." "Only Chinese eat rice every day." "This looks like bird feed." "Why can't I have a glass of milk?" "How long do I have to stay on this diet?" Such persons think that cancer happened to them accidentally and that they have done nothing to deserve it. They blame their disease on a virus, a gene they inherited from their parents, a carcinogen in their workplace or environment, stress produced by their spouse or landlord, malpractice by their doctor, nuclear fallout from Russia, or a hostile universe. This type of person has no understanding of himself, nature, or God, and is incapable of self-reflection. Even if he or she temporarily improves on the diet, he will return to meat and sugar, cheese and wine, and milk and cookies as soon as the slightest improvement is experienced. For such people, macrobiotics is just another pill to be taken and then discarded when their symptoms disappear. They may survive for a while, but will never fundamentally heal themselves or be happy. The death certificate will say cancer, heart attack, or the flu, but the real cause is arrogance.

INACCURATE DIETARY PRACTICE

In some cases, the macrobiotic dietary recommendations are not well understood or carefully practiced. For example, when we advise, "Eat 50 to 60 percent whole grains every day, prepare rice in a pressure-cooker or with a heavy cover, and add a pinch of sea salt," most people indicate that they understand. However, upon returning home, some might cook with plenty of salt and others with no salt. They may use too much water or not enough. Rather than buying a pressure-cooker for the price of about one hospital x-ray, they steam or bake their rice. Still others apply the conventional wisdom that if a little is good, a lot is better and eat 100 percent grain instead of 50 percent. As a result, their condition becomes excessively contracted and soon they are consuming desserts, salad, fruit juice, and other excessively expansive foods to restore balance. Naturally, these practices hinder recovery.

Another mistake is to confuse the macrobiotic approach with other dietary or nutritional approaches to cancer and "to be on the safe side" try to combine them all. Moreover, some people new to natural foods assume that everything that is sold in the health food store is safe to eat. These misconceptions must be overcome or the way of eating will become chaotic and disorderly.

The need to learn proper cooking cannot be overemphasized. When we advise people to take classes in macrobiotic cooking, they sometimes reply that they already know how to cook. The person thinks, "I went to a cooking school," "I've been cooking for my family for twenty years and my husband loves my cooking," "I'm already vegetarian and know how to prepare natural foods." No matter how tasty, appealing, or meatless, the previous style of cooking was one of the major factors that caused the cancer to develop. Persons who feel they already know how to cook often have more difficulty with the Cancer-Prevention Diet than people who have never cooked before or cooked very little.

Macrobiotic cooking is actually very simple once the basic techniques have been mastered. However, before learning the basics, it is easy to make mistakes, even while consulting various books and publications. It is very important to attend cooking classes in order to actually see and taste the foods that you wish to prepare. It isn't necessary to spend a great deal of time attending classes. If you are able to learn at least ten or twenty basic dishes, you can go on to develop your own cooking style. When beginning the diet, seek the advice of friends with experience who live near you. Don't hesitate to show them dishes you have prepared and ask for their advice and suggestions.

One mistake common among cancer patients is the overconsumption of flour products. As much as possible, it is better to eat grains in their whole form rather than in the form of flour. Especially in the case of cancer flour products easily create mucus and intestinal stagnation, and for this reason it is better to avoid items like muffins, pancakes, and biscuits. Even high-quality whole-grain bread should be eaten only several times per week, and not on a daily basis. It is also advisable for cancer patients to avoid heavily baked or grilled foods.

LACK OF WILL

In some cases persons who have no desire to live are introduced to the Cancer-Prevention Diet, often by some well-intentioned family member or friend. Such persons, who frequently ignore the advice they are given, have a very slight chance of recovery. We can continue to extend to them our love, sympathy, and prayers, but ultimately we must respect a person's decision to die.

LACK OF FAMILY SUPPORT

Among the many patients whom I have counselled were a number of middle-aged men who, although they were married, visited us by themselves. When asked why their wives had not come, they often replied that their wives did not agree with their desire to begin macrobiotics. When asked who would cook, more often than not they replied that they would try to do it. When asked what would the wife and children eat, they usually replied that the rest of the family would continue to cook for themselves and eat steak, french fries, and ice cream. I have also met many women who did not have the support of their husbands or children whose parents were not sympathetic.

I sympathize very much with these people because in a real sense they are alone. Their families lack the understanding, love, and care that are essential for their recovery. In many cases, they have never cooked for themselves at all prior to this time. Despite their courage, the chances of succeeding are low. Among all the cancer patients I have met, those who recovered were primarily single and cooked for themselves or had the full support of their families, even to the extent that the other family members also started the diet and learned to cook macrobiotically. A kitchen divided against itself cannot long stand. Therefore, the cancer patient in this situation should investigate the possibility of temporarily living separately from his or her spouse. This may take the form of living alone in an apartment for a few months, moving in with friends or relatives who are sympathetic, or entering some health-care facility that provides macrobiotic food.

To help meet the growing need for this kind of service, the East West Foundation and Kushi Institute have established a Cook Referral Service (Box 1100, Brookline Village, Mass. 02147, (617) 731-0564) to recommend trained and certified macrobiotic cooks. These individ-

uals are available to visit the home for a few days and orient the
patient and family to the new diet, give elementary cooking lessons,
and show how to prepare the ginger compress, taro potato plaster,
and other home-care equipment that may be necessary. In some
cases, full-time live-in cooks can be arranged.

LOSS OF NATURAL HEALING ABILITY

Extensive chemotherapy or radiation tends to diminish the body's
self-healing abilities and interferes with the natural process of recovery. Sometimes, for example, the kidneys are seriously damaged or a
major section of the digestive tract has been removed. If a person has
completely lost her self-healing abilities through such treatments, it is
doubtful that the Cancer-Prevention Diet can help her recover.

A case can be considered macrobiotically terminal when any of
the five factors just discussed is present, regardless of the actual stage
of the tumor. However, it is still worthwhile for these persons to
begin the diet, since it can help reduce much unnecessary pain and
suffering. There have been several instances where people near death
have started eating nourishing food and after several weeks have become very peaceful and experienced the disappearance of pain. Then,
when the end came, they were able to die in a calm and dignified
manner. Family or friends can contribute to the serenity of the person's last days by their loving presence, peaceful thoughts, and
prayers.

Conversely, there are several factors that contribute to ready acceptance of the diet and make recovery more likely.

SPIRITUAL AWARENESS

There are some people who are genuinely grateful for their illness
and what it has to teach them. They do not complain and blame
others, but look within themselves for the source of their troubles.
They realize their past way of eating and living was ignorant or foolish
and they are happy to make a fresh start and change. Such people
often have a deep faith in something larger than themselves, such as
God, nature, or the universe, and they experience the coming of
macrobiotics into their lives as an expression of that faith. As their
health improves, they grow closer to their original religious heritage,

whether it is Catholicism, Judaism, Protestantism, or Buddhism, and their appreciation of other spiritual traditions deepens. After healing themselves, such people go on to help many others. Looking back on their illness, they often say that cancer was one of the best things that ever happened to them because of the changes it brought in their understanding of life.

DEEP SUFFERING

People who have experienced the full range of pain and fear and who truly want to be free from suffering readily embrace the diet. They have tried many different symptomatic approaches and been disappointed. They are now ready to give up their defensive way of life, their stubbornness, and their rigidity to find freedom and regain their health. They have developed the ability to self-reflect and embarked on a personal search for truth. When they discover the unifying principle of yin and yang, they learn how to transmute sickness into health and sorrow into joy.

WILL AND DETERMINATION

People who have cancer but still retain their cheerfulness, humor, and will to live also have a high likelihood of success. These people usually have very strong native constitutions inherited from their mothers, grandparents, and ancestors who ate grains and vegetables as a major portion of their diet. This shows up in such features as a large head, firm bone structure (especially in men), steady well-focused eyes, proportionately large hands, and large ears that lie flat against the side of the head and have long, detached lobes. Even though such persons spoiled their health in later life, they have reservoirs of strength from their embryological development and early childhood. They also have a foundation of common sense and appreciation, which they have lately forgotten. They only need to be reminded.

LOVE AND CARE OF FAMILY
AND FRIENDS

With the close cooperation and support of the patient's immediate family, a successful outcome is greatly enhanced. The patient's family should clearly understand the situation and begin to eat in a similar manner, while extending their love and support to the patient in every possible way.

When caring for others, we should always keep in mind that the object of healing is to improve our own health and judgment as well as the patient's. Dealing with serious illness can be draining. However, at some level we are receiving as much energy as we give out. Helping someone with cancer is a supreme challenge to our own understanding of the universe as well as our physical stamina, mental clarity, and emotional strength.

The approach offered in this book provides a clear and hopeful direction. However, it is usually up to the immediate family members to help the patient implement that direction, make day-to-day decisions about what to cook, when to give a compress, and how to handle the disagreements and crises that inevitably crop up. Family members or friends taking care of the person with cancer must also constantly self-reflect and consider whether their advice is sound. As we develop as healers and teachers, we will face many difficulties and frustrations. However, as our own way of eating improves and our intuition develops, we are able to help more and more people.

CANCER AND SOCIETY

Finally, we should all realize that cancer is not solely the concern of cancer patients, their families, or the medical profession. Cancer is merely one dramatic symptom, out of many, of the deep misconceptions and ultimately self-destructive tendencies upon which we have built modern civilization. In a very real sense, we all have cancer and will continue to be affected by the disease until a new, peaceful way of life is established in place of the old.

Cancer, as we have seen, is not a disease of certain cells or certain organs but the means of self-protection for an entire diseased organism. If the cancer is artificially removed without changing the underlying way of eating and life that gives rise to the disease, this balance is disrupted and the whole may collapse. In modern society there are many parallels between the way we approach cancer and the way we approach relations between men and women, the break-up of the family, crime and social disorder, and international conflict.

In the Book of Isaiah and the Psalms, we find the earliest reference to the term "staff of life." In this deeply divided world, there is a growing recognition that we must turn our weapons into plowshares if we are to survive. As we do so let us also recognize that those plowshares were primarily used to grow whole grains and vegetables and on this foundation the whole of Western and Eastern civilization rests. The disappearance of the staff of life in today's world poses as lethal a threat to the future of humanity as atomic or hydrogen bombs. If we can learn to recover from cancer naturally, we may consider that a lasting solution to the multiple ills of society itself will be on the horizon.

10.

The Myth of Carcinogens

The history of nutritional experiments goes back at least as far as the Bible. In the Book of Daniel we read that during the Babylonian Captivity, King Nebuchadnezzar commanded several of the most gifted children of Israel be brought to court to enter the royal service. The king instructed the master of his household to feed the young Israelites the best meat and wine from the royal table. The rich food was set out before Daniel and his three companions, but to the surprise of the steward they refused to eat and instead asked for the simple food they were accustomed to. The steward replied that he would lose his head if the king saw Daniel and his friends undernourished in comparison to the other young Babylonians their age also in training for royal service. Daniel replied:

"Submit us to this test for ten days. Give us only vegetables* to eat and water to drink; then compare our looks with those of the young men who have lived on the food assigned by the king, and be guided in your treatment of us by what you see." The guard listened to what they said and tested them for ten days. At the end of ten days they looked healthier and were better nourished than all the young men who had lived on the food assigned them by the king. So the guard took away the assignment of food and the wine they were to drink, and gave them only the vegetables.

*This text is from the New English Bible. The King James Version translates the food Daniel requested as "pulses." The original Hebrew word means "things sown" and signifies grains, seeds, and small beans. The food that Daniel ate probably consisted primarily of barley, wheat, lentils, and chickpeas.

Daniel and his companions went on to become trusted advisers to the king, and we read that "whenever the king consulted them on any matter calling for insight and judgment, he found them ten times better than all the magicians and exorcists in his whole kingdom."

The story in the Book of Daniel, the first recorded nutritional experiment in history, has many of the features of modern-day medical testing. There is the statistically significant number of subjects, the four Israelites; a control group, the young men on the royal Babylonian diet; a measurable period of time, ten days; observed behavioral effects, healthier and better nourished; and quantified results, ten times higher insight and judgment than the court soothsayers.

Since Babylonian times our daily way of eating has become even richer, and today's diet contains thousands of foodstuffs, chemicals, and artificial ingredients never dreamed of by Daniel or the well-fed king.

THE CARCINOGEN QUESTION

As cancer rates began to climb in the early part of this century, some scientists speculated that pollutants in the food supply or environment might be associated with the spread of the disease. In 1915 two Japanese researchers induced skin tumors in rabbits by applying a sample of coal tar on their ears over a period of six months. This experiment inaugurated the era of modern animal experimentation and gave rise to the concept of carcinogenicity. A carcinogen is defined as any agent that increases tumor promotion in humans or animals.

In recent decades, the list of carcinogens has grown to include thousands of chemicals, metals, and foodstuffs, as well as tobacco, certain styles of cooking such as grilling at high temperatures, and even the rays of the sun. Suspected cancer-causing chemicals—benzene, chlorine, DES, nitrosamines, PCB's, and vinyl chloride—have become household words, and many of the consumer and industrial products of the modern way of life are linked to the disease. These include kitchenwares, home furnishings, building materials, cosmetics, synthetic clothing and fabric, farm and garden sprays, smoke detectors and other radioactive devices. Millions of people are fearful of getting cancer from prolonged exposure to these materials and some of them go to great lengths to avoid the disease. For example, some cancer specialists are presently encouraging women who are healthy but who fear cancer because they are in high-risk categories to have their breasts surgically removed as a preventive measure. In a recent column, Ann Landers concurred with one doctor who recommended that some women fearful of cancer replace healthy breast tissue with silicone implants: "On balance, the peace of mind is worth the time, trouble, and discomfort."

If this kind of tragedy is to be avoided on a national scale, the myth of carcinogens must be dispelled. The unifying principle of yin and yang can guide us through this maze of fear and help us understand the relationship of individual chemicals, elements, and compounds to the origin and development of cancer.

Let's start with the classical coal-tar experiment. When rubbed on rabbits' ears over a six-month period, a tumor started to develop, and the scientists concluded that the tar must be responsible. However, tar is not in and of itself a cancer-causing factor. In structure, tar is a more condensed or yang compound. It constricts or inhibits rapid growth—the dominant feature of cancer—rather than enhancing it. However, by continuously applying a more yang factor such as tar to the rabbit's ear, the cells on the skin became inflamed and drew opposite, expansive yin factors from the bloodstream, which started to spread and form the tumor. This process is simply an illustration of a dynamic natural law that yin attracts yang; yang attracts yin—opposite factors attract each other—and at the extreme, yang produces yin; yin produces yang.

Over a half century ago, some researchers began to question the validity of carcinogen experiments. For example, in the January 1931 *American Journal of Cancer*, K. Wolkoff asserted: "The writer thinks that the results show that food influences the development of tar cancer in mice, and that, therefore, cancer is not wholly a local disease, but has something to do with the conditions of nutrition. . . . The appearance of carcinomata of the skin at a distance from the tarred area implies that a carcinomatous condition must first develop before the tumors appear. In order to produce tumors in mice, an excess of lipoids [fat and cholesterol] should be administered."

Similar doubts have periodically surfaced in the scientific literature. In "Relevance of Animal Studies to Human Disease" in the November 1975 *Cancer Research*, journal of the American Association for Cancer Researchers, D. Mark Hegsted, professor of nutrition at Harvard School of Public Health and a principal influence on the Senate Select Committee's report *Dietary Goals*, stated: "Sufficient examples are available to demonstrate that the outcome of some experiments may be determined by the nature of the diet fed as well as the nature of the toxic material under test. . . . It is rather frightening to contemplate the possibility that some of the results of the extensive testing program may be erroneous because of unexplored dietary effects."

Similarly to coal tar, the sun has often been accused of causing skin cancer, and many modern people are afraid to go out in the heat of the day. The sun is warm, bright, and intense—all yang characteristics. For millennia people living in the sunnier and warmer tropical climates of the world have never appreciably suffered from skin cancer. However, in the less sunny northern regions, skin cancer has sharply risen in recent decades, especially among people who work outdoors like pilots and farmers. We have to consider whether this is the result of some solar phenomenon (including certain rays or radiation) that affects only industrialized latitudes, whether there is something unique to industrial civilization itself that is giving rise to this effect, or whether as many scientists believe there is something in the pigmentation of the skin or other genetic factors responsible. The solution lies in observing the difference in diet and lifestyle between traditional and modern cultures. People in industrial society eat large amounts of fat, sugar, dairy products, and other greasy and oily foods, as well as soft drinks, drugs, and medications, which create an acidic or extremely yin condition in their blood. Repeated exposure to a strong yang factor such as the sun brings these extreme yin items to the surface and a skin tumor or rupture results. These refined foods provide the underlying basis for skin cancer, a more yin disorder. The sunlight serves only as a catalyst to localize this toxic excess on the skin. People in tropical society eating a balanced diet of grains, tubers, seeds, vegetables, locally grown fruit, and a small volume of animal food will not get skin cancer no matter how long they are out in the sun because their blood and tissues do not carry the toxic excess.

To take another example, several years ago it was discovered that the fat and protein molecules contained in grilled meat or fish often appear to produce cancerous cells in a process known as pyrolosis. However, people have been eating foods such as grilled sardines, fish, and meat for thousands of years, yet rarely developed cancer. What is the difference? Traditionally these foods were eaten in much smaller quantities and balanced with plenty of fresh green vegetables.

This created a complementary balance that prevented cancer from developing.

BALANCING YIN AND YANG

In themselves, none of these factors is cancer causing. In judging whether something is safe or dangerous for human consumption, we need to look at two things. First, we need to examine its relative balance of yin expanding and yang contracting qualities. Secondly, we need to examine its relation to other factors in our diet and lifestyle and the overall balance of yin and yang. For example, salt is made up chiefly of sodium and chlorine. Sodium is a very yang element and chlorine is a very yin element. Taken individually, each of these elements is poisonous to the human body. However, combined in salt, the toxic effects of sodium and chlorine are neutralized. Overall, salt is classified as yang among the food categories because it has a relatively high proportion of sodium to chlorine relative to other foods. We experience a contractive yang effect when we put a few grains of salt on our tongue. However, if we take too much salt, we get thirsty and naturally rebalance by taking water, beer, or something else yin. This is a good example of something in excess producing its opposite. We must also consider the quality of the salt. Modern table salt has been chemically refined so that many of the trace minerals found in natural sea salt are missing. Artificial salt has a different balance of yin and yang than real salt, and we usually require more of it in order to make up for the minerals that have been left out. The entire secret of selecting and preparing foods is to understand that by changing the quantity of what we eat we change the quality. Conversely, by taking only the highest quality foods to begin with, we don't need to eat so much volume to obtain proper nourishment.

The ideal proportion of yang to yin in foods for human consumption fluctuates according to climate. In polar and cooler regions of the world, we naturally adapt ourselves to the environment by making our food more yang in quality, applying heavier cooking, and even using animal foods to some degree. The ratio of yang to yin is about one to five or one to seven, analyzing foodstuffs according to their proportion of sodium and other yang elements to potassium and other yin elements. On the other hand, people who live in the tropical or semitropical areas of the world naturally eat little if any animal food, consume more raw vegetables and fruits, and apply lighter cooking.

The ratio of yang to yin varies from about one to eight to one to twelve or more. In the temperate zones, where it fluctuates from warm to hot to cool to cold, people naturally tend to eat in between the extremes, consume more cooked grains and vegetables, and take only a small volume of animal food. The proportion of yang to yin falls between one to six and one to eight and averages one to seven.

Most of the foods in the modern diet, however, do not fall within the central part of the spectrum. They consist of a combination of foods that are more appropriate for a semipolar and a semitropical climate. Of course, the body cannot adjust to these two extremes at the same time, nor are they appropriate for a temperate region. In addition, many chemicals, artificial ingredients, and other compounds have been added to the food directly or have found their way into the food system indirectly through pesticide use or environmental pollution. The yang to yin ratio of these substances is much higher than one to twelve. It is often one to eighteen or more. On this scale, chemicals, drugs, and medications are imbalanced in themselves and imbalanced in combination with other items in the diet. Such substances can be considered toxic and unsafe for human consumption in any form and quantity.

As cancer research shifts toward nutrition, tests will increasingly show some factors in our diet that at times appear to protect against cancer and other times seem to enhance it. These factors include vitamin A, selenium, protein, and cholesterol. The researchers say they are unable to explain the divergent results except that they appear to be related to dosage. The theorem that yin or yang, at its extreme, turns into its opposite once again accounts for this behavior.

In traditional Oriental medicine, foods on the yin end of the food spectrum, in order of increasing potency, are fruit, dairy food, alcohol, and drugs. The results of modern carcinogen testing tend to follow the same pattern. For instance, lactose produces tumors at 50 PPM (parts per million per kilogram of the animal's body weight), while fructose takes 5,000 PPM. This finding suggests that dairy sugar (lactose) is much more concentrated than fruit sugar (fructose) and conforms to the traditional yin/yang classification noted above. Recent international studies, moreover, show that about 75 percent of the world's population are lactose-intolerant and cannot digest milk or dairy products. There is no comparable trouble digesting fruit. In laboratory testing, both fructose and lactose are considered very weak in relative toxicity compared to most drugs and chemicals. On the basis of such comparisons, we can begin to make sense of carcinogen tests, not to blacklist any substance, but to classify foods in an orderly way and discover the quantitative thresholds at which they begin to change quality.

IMMUNITY TO CANCER

Related to dosage is the subject of natural immunity. Some individuals remain immune to cancer and other serious illness even though they consume large amounts of extreme foods and are exposed to toxic chemicals in their environment. Why is this so? Usually, the individuals' inherited constitutions are very strong and well-built, rich in various minerals. Their mothers and forebears ate plenty of grains and vegetables and passed along sound digestive, circulatory, and nervous systems that can withstand heavy abuse. Other people who do not necessarily have strong constitutions but who appear immune to illness frequently have unusually strong day-to-day energy and vitality from activities and exercises, which they have cultivated over many years of balanced living. These people too can absorb and neutralize almost any extreme factor up to a certain point. For example, in Nagasaki following the atomic bombing in August 1945, a group of surviving macrobiotic doctors and patients avoided radiation sickness by eating brown rice, sea salt, miso soup, sea vegetables, and other very yang traditional foods. Meanwhile, many other survivors in Nagasaki eating the modern Japanese diet of white rice, heavy animal food, and sugar died of atomic sickness within a few days or of leukemia in subsequent years.

CANCER AT THE CELLULAR LEVEL

The unifying principle can also be used to understand the mechanism of cancer at the cellular level. As we have seen, nature is organized according to a system of complementary and antagonistic qualities such as inner and outer, front and back, and centripetal and centrifugal energy. At the molecular level, this manifests in the cell as the more dense, central nucleus, which we can classify as yang, and the more expanded peripheral cytoplasm, which is more yin. In turn, these structures can be further subdivided into twin interrelated components. In the nucleus we find the more condensed (yang) DNA, which functions as the template for replication, and the more diffuse (yin) RNA, which transmits information to the outside. The cytoplasm too can be arranged into the more compact (yang) organelles and the surrounding, less dense (yin) plasm.

The movement of materials across the cell membrane is divided into active (yang) and passive (yin) processes. Active processes such as active transport, endocytosis, and exocytosis require energy to be supplied by the cell, thereby contracting it. Passive processes such as diffusion, osmosis, and dialysis involve energy coming into a cell and expanding it. In this way, the structures and functions of cellular metabolism can be continuously divided and subdivided into ever smaller pairs of complementary opposites until we come to the atomic level. The world of elements follows a similar pattern. On the basis of their structure, atomic weight, color, spin, and other properties, we find that the elements hydrogen, carbon, sodium, and magnesium fall into the centripetal or yang category, while nitrogen, oxygen, calcium, and potassium can be grouped together as more centrifugal or yin.

Nearly all modern medical research is involved in investigating disease at the cellular and subcellular levels. The assumption is that since cancer is a disease characterized by abnormal cell multiplication, there must be some substance or process within the cell that causes or "triggers" uncontrolled cell growth. The theory assumes that if this specific factor can be isolated, a biochemical means can be found to prevent its harmful effects. Conventional treatments for cancer such as surgery, radiation, and chemotherapy attempt to eliminate the disease by excision, irradiation, poisoning, or other form of "blocking." Since there are thousands of components in the cell, cancer researchers around the world are looking at many different stimuli and processes. For instance, chemotherapy drugs commonly include alkylating agents, which inhibit cell growth by cross-linking molecules of DNA; antimetabolites, which inhibit essential enzymes and block DNA formation; alkaloids, which hinder cell division or mitosis; and hormones, which can either suppress or accelerate cell growth to prevent the tumor from spreading.

However, as we have seen, cancer is not caused by any single factor that spontaneously mutates, but by a combination of many factors that create an imbalance in the whole organism over a long period of time. The place to start searching for the origin of cancer is not inside the cell but outside, in the blood, in the lymph, in the interrelated organs and systems of the body, in the refrigerator, in the topsoil, in the quality of the air and water, in our way of looking at the world.

Over a century ago in 1845, a British physician wrote a book on cancer and explained that one of the commonsense places to look for the origin of the disease was in the daily food that the patient ate. In *The General Nature and Treatment of Tumours,* George Macilwain proposed that doctors ". . . examine the food, the various organs which represent the various stages, which I have included in the word assimilation; and to test the properties of both one and the other by any knowledge we may have of their natural effects, habits, and propensities. . . ." Using an analogy from the emerging Industrial Revolution, he went on:

This is just what we should do with a manufacture; if a raw material—wool, for example—were put into an elaborate machinery, which carried it through various processes, which were to result in the production of a beautiful cloth; and we were to find that the cloth, instead of exhibiting its usual texture, was disfigured by various irregularities; the manufacturer would at once conclude either that the fault was in the raw material, the machinery to which it had been submitted, or both. But we know that, in examining this, he would not examine *solely* either one or the other, much less would he confine his examination to one point in the machinery; least of all would he seek to correct the error either in the wool or the machinery, by throwing in oil, or dye, or iodine, or any other substance, until he had instituted the examination in question. He would, on the contrary, institute a thorough examination until he had discovered and tested the cause of this defect.

Modern medical research is well meaning and carried out by compassionate and devoted individuals. However, it is engaged primarily in investigating isolated parts of the body's machinery and throwing in the modern pharmaceutical equivalent to oil, dye, and iodine. With some notable exceptions, modern medicine is involved in examining effects, not causes. And at the cellular level, it is examining the effects of effects. So long as modern cancer specialists continue to look in the wrong place, there can be no hope of curing the disease. The advances that have been made in treating leukemia, certain reproductive cancers that are responsive to hormones, and other tumors with chemotherapy can be explained in terms of yin and yang by looking at complementary and antagonistic reactions between the drugs and factors in the blood and endocrine system. For instance, the alkylating agents have a contractive (yang) or blocking effect on cell growth, which is an expansive (yin) process. However, at the cellular level, these are controlling mechanisms, not curative ones. The cancerous effects and subeffects may be suppressed or altered by drugs, hormone injections, monoclonal antibodies, and other substances but the underlying cause will remain. The symptoms will only be driven to deeper and deeper levels of the body and eventually surface somewhere else, requiring another round of artificial intervention and biochemical blocking.

ALTERNATIVE TREATMENTS TO CANCER

The failure of the modern medical approach to cancer has generated a variety of alternative treatments. These usually include a nutritional program emphasizing a specific substance such as laetrile, vitamin C, selenium, hydrazine sulfate, and various enzymatic and mineral preparations. The results of these therapies have been mixed. In some cases they seem to retard tumor development, in others they produce little apparent effect, and in still others they enhance the disease. The unifying principle of yin and yang—the natural laws of relativity and harmony between the antagonistic and complemental factors— once again helps us to understand these divergent results. Because of the difference in cause, no single dietary approach is beneficial for all cancers. The alternative cancer clinics in Mexico, southern California, and Texas, which offer some of these substances such as laetrile along with a diet of tropical juices, raw salads, and other uncooked foods, can help relieve the symptoms of yang types of cancer. However, if a person with a more yin form of cancer such as leukemia were to follow such a diet, the results could be tragic. In common with modern medicine, many of these therapies assume that there is some specific cellular mechanism responsible for all types of cancer. However, instead of trying to root out the cancer with toxic methods, these therapies have adopted a more holistic approach, in which balance is restored to the diseased body by supplying the deficient vitamin, mineral, or other nutrient in combination with a more natural way of life. This is an improvement over the conventional approach. However, alternative cancer therapies need to begin focusing on the whole rather than parts and to recognize that not all cancers are the same in their origin or development.

CONSIDERATIONS IN ANIMAL TESTING

The rise of the holistic health movement, the Senate Select Committee's report, *Dietary Goals,* and increasing public awareness of diet have occasioned more medical researchers to study the effects of different foods and chemical additives on laboratory animals. These tests are aimed in the right direction. However, they suffer many theoretical limitations, which often affect their results. The usual procedure is to administer increasingly high doses of a suspected cancer-causing agent to an animal until tumors are produced and then go back and determine statistically what percentage of subjects would contract cancer from smaller doses. Several problems arise here. For example, scientists are unable to agree among themselves whether dosage should be measured according to the animal's body weight, body surface area, or accumulated intake of the substance over the animal's lifetime. Moreover, data can be interpolated from high doses to low doses on a variety of scales. A difference in linear or logarithmic measurement can result in findings that differ by 3, 40, and, in one common test, 70,000 times.

In research circles, this has prompted a search for scientific models of acceptable levels of risk for toxic compounds. The controversy is similar to the debate about whether there are any safe thresholds for exposure to low-level ionizing radiation and, if so, what they are and how they are to be measured. In its 1982 report, *Diet, Nutrition, and Cancer,* the National Academy of Sciences reviewed this problem and agreed with an earlier government study that concluded, "The ultimate choice of a model for high- to low-dose interpolation is, therefore, arbitrary. Not only is there great uncertainty in the mathematical modeling procedures, but also there is no sound biological basis for any of them."

The second major consideration in animal testing involves extrapolating the data from the test species to human beings. For example, tests indicate that humans are 60 times more sensitive to the drug thalidomide than mice and 100 times more than rats. Furthermore, some substances cause tumors in some animals, but not in others. A nitrogenous coloring agent can induce cancer of the liver in rats, but not in rabbits or guinea pigs. Modern science has no unified theory to explain this.

Once again we can turn to the unifying principle of yin and yang to try and make order out of these conflicting results. In the case of thalidomide, mice are gentler, more timid, and less carnivorous than rats. Compared to rats, mice can be classified as more yin. Their genetic structure is more susceptible than that of the rats to a powerful expansive drug such as thalidomide. This is an example of the principle that yin plus yin produces excessive yin conditions, resulting in the expansive growth of cells. However, in comparison to humans, mice are much more compact, active, and carnivorous and can be considered yang. Therefore, they are less sensitive to the drug than we are. In the case of the artificial food coloring, the carnivorous rat is also more yang than the vegetarian rabbit and shy guinea pig. The rat's liver, a compact yang organ situated deep in the body, would naturally attract a moderately strong yin toxin such as the food additive. In this case, the livers of the rabbit and guinea pig would not be as affected as the liver of the rat since the food coloring is proportionately less toxic than a powerful yin substance such as the mutagen thalidomide. This is an example of the general law that yin repels yin—that similar factors repel each other. The attraction and repulsion among phenomena are proportional to the difference of the complementary and antagonistic energies. This law holds true for star systems and galaxies as well as the realm of subatomic particles, for the structure among plants and animals as well as the order and development of human affairs.

In general, cancer tests based on observing the reactions of mice, rats, guinea pigs, rabbits, and even bacteria (the common Ames Test) are not very accurate barometers of human health. In addition to overlooking evolutionary order, there are other variables affecting laboratory experiments that are seldom taken into consideration. These include the quality of the animal's diet. Is the food organically grown or chemically grown? Are the grains refined or unrefined? Is the salt chemically processed or natural sea salt? Are the oil and fat from unrefined lipids or refined lipids? Is the food cooked by gas heat or on an electric range or by microwave? All of these factors can produce conflicting results.

We must also consider the psychological health of the animal. Is it unhappy being in a cage all day? Has it been taken away from its family? Does it have a family or is it artificially bred? How does it interact with other animals? Does it interact with other animals or is it kept in isolation? Modern science assumes that animals have no appreciable thoughts or feelings. However, common sense tells us otherwise, and current studies with dolphins, whales, and chimpanzees are beginning to change this attitude. Several years ago, for example, researchers at Ohio State University were studying the incidence of heart disease in different batches of rabbits. They noticed that one test group consistently showed 60 percent less atherosclerotic changes than the other groups. They were very puzzled. As it turned out, the person who fed the healthier group of rabbits regularly took them out of their cages and petted, stroked, and talked to them. In this way, the scientists discovered an unforeseem variable, the handler and rabbits' affections.

Then there are vibrational considerations. Is there high-voltage equipment in the laboratory? Is there radiation from other medical apparatus nearby? Are there fumes from stored chemicals or a lack of natural lighting? Recently, doctors at the Medical School of the University of Minnesota tried to duplicate a cancer experiment, but could not after several attempts. They concluded that there must have been an error in the protocols or test procedures. However, it was later discovered that the original experiment was conducted with full-spectrum lighting, while the subsequent test used light admitting only a narrow part of the spectrum. When the lighting was changed, similar findings resulted.

LIMITATIONS OF SCIENTIFIC METHOD

The problem with modern scientific testing is not primarily that it overlooks crucial variables. The major drawback to laboratory experiments is that they are conducted in an artificial environment to begin with. A laboratory does not recreate conditions in the natural world. It can only simulate them. Living animals and persons do not eat test tubes of protein, fat, carbohydrates, and vitamins. For the most part, they eat real food. It has taken cosmological evolution at least six- to eight-billion years or more to create the natural environment in which we live. The most advanced computers will never be able to duplicate a living ecosystem and all of its measurable and immeasurable energies.

Moreover, living things have real thoughts and feelings that affect and shape their health and well-being. Since the seventeenth century, modern scientific method has progressively eliminated the mental, emotional, and spiritual aspects of our lives from investigation because they cannot be quantified by existing technology. No two persons, for example, have exactly the same thoughts or emotions—

unless perhaps in the event that they are in love. How do we measure insight, understanding, and compassion with our senses? The
scientific inventions and discoveries of this era are only extensions of
our sight, our hearing, and our sense of touch. Yet it is our dream
that gives meaning to our existence. Our intuition and judgment tell
us that life itself is unrepeatable and can never be artificially controlled. The riddle of cancer has challenged this materialist trend of
the last 400 years and put the assumptions of modern science under
the microscope.

The animal kingdom has a lot to teach us about our health and
environment. The proper place to observe mice, hamsters, and
monkeys is in their natural habitat. One of the most valuable cancer
experiments with animals was conducted in the early part of the
twentieth century by a doctor in Holland named Cornelius Moerman.
After finishing medical school, Dr. Moerman decided to dedicate his
life to cancer research and wrote one of the big scientific supply com-
panies in Germany for equipment and supplies and mentioned that
he had decided to experiment with carrier pigeons. The scientific
supply house wrote back that in their experience it was a waste of
time to undertake this kind of experiment because they had as yet
been unable to infect healthy homing pigeons with cancer. Instead,
they recommended that he experiment with birds especially bred by
the laboratory for test purposes. Dr. Moerman reflected on this advice and decided that it contained an important clue to the enigma of
cancer. If healthy carrier pigeons in the wild could not be infected
with cancer, perhaps there was some factor that distinguished them
from the caged pigeons that could be infected with the disease.

Over a period of time he began observing the carrier pigeons in
their natural environment. He recorded everything they ate and noticed that they especially liked to nibble the grains in the Dutch
fields before they were harvested for milling. He also noticed that
they would go to the seashore and dip their beaks in the sand for
little bits of trace minerals that evidently washed up from seaweeds
and other life forms in the ocean. In this way, Dr. Moerman figured
out the natural diet of the carrier pigeons and found that it consisted
of whole grains and little bits of garden vegetables and orchard fruits,
while the birds in captivity were fed the refined grains, seeds, and
other foods preferred by modern Hollanders.

After several years of this experiment, Dr. Moerman was ap-
proached by a man who had been diagnosed as terminally ill with

cancer. A famous surgeon had operated on him and sent him home to die. The man agreed to be Dr. Moerman's subject and see whether the kind of diet that kept the carrier pigeons healthy could also help humans. The man began eating unrefined barley, millet, and whole-wheat bread, as well as the fresh vegetables and fruits that grew in the countryside. Within six months, the man's cancer had disappeared.

There are many other examples like this from the natural world. We need only clear our minds and take the time to observe and listen rather than intervene and manipulate.

MEASURING THE HUMAN DIET

The safest and most useful medical studies measure human dietary consumption. These include epidemiological surveys that compare nutritional intake among different populations and case-control studies in which two groups are directly compared. The test in the Book of Daniel was a case-control study.

Analysis of dietary data, however, is still in its infancy, and scientists employ a variety of different methods to determine and measure what people are actually eating. For instance, data may be classified in terms of foods or nutrients—is the variable vitamin C or citrus fruits, carotene or grams of dark green and deep yellow vegetables? Do we measure total calories from fat or the characteristics of specific kinds of fat? As with animal tests, most human nutritional tests currently fail to take into account such important variables as whether the food is organically grown or chemically grown, artificially processed or naturally prepared, cooked with gas heat or electricity. For example, in some food studies brown rice and cane sugar are grouped together under the same classification as carbohydrate. In its cancer and diet report, in the chapter on methodology, the National Academy of Sciences pointed out the biases unintentionally concealed in many dietary studies: "The nature of the hypothesis determines the nature of the classification used for data collection. This explains much of the discrepant data from different investigations of the same cancer site, although the source of the discrepancy may not be immediately apparent from even the most careful perusal of the published reports." In other words, researchers find what they are looking for.

Still, human food studies offer the most promising direction in cancer research. In the years ahead, we can expect the focus of epidemiological and case-control studies to shift to monitoring and comparing people eating the usual modern diet, the macrobiotic diet, and other more vegetarian diets. At the theoretical level, statisticians will continue to develop concepts of cocarcinogenecity, synergy, and initiation/promotion, which are now in the formative stages, to explain conflicting results and describe complementary and antagonistic relationships. During the next several decades, science will move toward adopting a modern form of the traditional yin/yang principle, and a new prevention-oriented medicine, centered on nutrition, will develop. "Just as it was once difficult for investigators to recognize that a symptom complex could be caused by a lack of a nutrient," the National Academy of Sciences' report commented on the shift in scientific thinking under way, "so until recently has it been difficult for scientists to recognize that certain pathological conditions might result from an abundant and apparently normal diet."

BACK TO BABYLON

In the span of 2,500 years, the pendulum of dietary testing has returned to where it began in ancient Babylon. Like Daniel, who in later life found himself undergoing another test in the lion's den, we are confronted with a powerful and lethal force—the modern spread of cancer—against which it is impossible to put up a violent fight. However, by maintaining our faith in God or the infinite universe and eating a diet in harmony with our environment, we too can emerge unscathed from our trial, and our understanding of life and the laws of nature will be strengthened.

In ancient literature we occasionally read about women who mutilated themselves in fits of frenzy and about men who worshipped the darkness. We shake our heads in amazement. Today millions of modern women are considering having their uteruses, ovaries, and breasts removed as preventive measures against cancer. Millions of men are reluctant to work outside in the heat of the day unexposed for fear of skin cancer.

There is not much time to regain our health, insight, and judgment. Over the last few decades countless researchers, doctors, nurses, nutritionists, and environmentalists, as well as many ordinary people, have devoted their lives to understanding cancer. There have been notable successes, sorrowful failures, and many experiences in between. Some investigators have come close to the mark, many have missed it. A few patients have cured themselves, far too many have suffered a tragic death. However, everyone has a little piece of the puzzle and contributed in some way to the change in collective thinking about the disease that is beginning to take place.

We may think that we are experimenting with nature. However, the truth is that evolution is testing us. The present biological degeneration of humanity is challenging us to join together and tame the lion of cancer before it devours us all. Let us go forward into the light as one humanity and together raise a new generation of Daniels.

PART II

A Guide to Different Cancers

Introduction

This section of the book is intended to serve as a guide to relieving the more common types of cancer. The fifteen chapters may be read together as a complementary unit to the first part of the book, which emphasizes cancer prevention. Chapters may also be read individually for information on how to approach cancer in a particular organ or body system. Since many similar foods and home cares are recommended, the actual recipes and instructions have all been gathered together in Part III.

It should be pointed out that the guidelines suggested here are general in nature and will differ slightly for each person. After reading this book, it is best for cancer patients and their families who wish to pursue this approach to see a qualified macrobiotic teacher and counselor or a medical doctor who has been trained in this way of life. He or she will be able to provide an accurate evaluation of the person's condition and help formulate dietary guidelines suited to the individual's unique situation, condition, and needs. These advisers may be contacted through the authorized macrobiotic educational centers listed on pages 361-362.

In this section, each type of cancer will be described under the following headings:

Frequency notes the extent of the disease, standard forms of medical treatment, and the current five-year survival rate for patients treated with surgery, radiation, and chemotherapy. Mortality figures, remission rates, and other statistics are from the latest reports of the National Cancer Institute, the American Cancer Society, and U.S. Vital Statistics.

Structure examines in brief the physiology of the organ or body system. A fuller treatment of anatomy and illness in general can be found in my book, *The Macrobiotic Way of Natural Healing* (New York: Japan Publications, 1979).

Cause of Cancer discusses the progressive development of disease and the types of food, beverages, and other substances that commonly give rise to a specific form of cancer. Usually no one food can be said to cause cancer; rather, it is the overall way of eating that has persisted over a long period of time that needs to be changed. Yin and yang are used as analytical tools to help explain this process. A full explanation of these terms is presented in Chapter 6 of Part I.

The major categories of food are summarized as follows:

Strong Yang Foods

Refined Salt	Poultry
Eggs	Fish
Meat	Seafood
Cheese	

Balanced Foods

Whole-Cereal Grains	Root, Round, and Leafy
Seeds	Vegetables
Beans and Bean Products	Spring or Well Water
Nuts	Nonaromatic, Nonstimulant Teas
Sea Vegetables	Natural Sea Salt

Strong Yin Foods

Temperate-Climate Fruit	Honey, Sugar, and Refined
White Rice, White Flour	Sweeteners
Tropical Fruits and Vegetables	Alcohol
Milk, Cream, Yogurt	Foods containing Chemicals,
Oils	Preservatives, Dyes,
Spices (pepper, curry, nutmeg, etc.)	Pesticides
	Drugs (marijuana, cocaine, etc.)
Aromatic and Stimulant	Medications (tranquilizers, anti-
Beverages (coffee, black tea, mint tea, etc.)	depressants, etc.)

Medical Evidence presents data from epidemiological (population) studies, laboratory tests on animals, and clinical studies on human patients pertaining to cancer and diet. In most instances, the items relate to the specific cancer under consideration. However, a few of the older historical materials do not distinguish among different forms of cancer and are included because they are relevant to cancer in general (or its absence in a traditional society) or because they introduce a factor (e.g., protein or fat) that subsequent investigation has associated with the type of tumor under review. It should further be noted that current medical research has concentrated on the more common cancers, such as those of the breast, large intestine, lung, prostate, ovary, esophagus, and bladder. Based on the preponderance of evidence, not just a single study, the dietary link is considered strong for most of these forms of cancer. On the other hand, nutritional studies are comparatively rare for bone, brain, and liver cancer and for leukemia, lymphomas and Hodgkin's disease, and for skin cancer and malignant melanoma. In most of these cases, scientists consider the dietary association not yet firmly established. Sources after each item give the author or principal researcher's name (et al. means "and others"), the book or professional medical journal in which the material appeared, volume and page numbers, and the date of publication if not included in the general discussion. The strengths and weaknesses of scientific testing are discussed in Chapter 10 of Part I and should be kept in mind.

Diagnosis contrasts modern hospital techniques with simple visual methods of detection. The diagnostic methods described here are part of my observations based on the living tradition of the Far East and are explained more fully in Chapter 7 of Part I and in my book, *How to See Your Health: Book of Oriental Diagnosis* (New York: Japan Publications, 1980).

Dietary Recommendations explains how to relieve a particular form of cancer by changing the daily way of eating. These guidelines are offered for people living in temperate climates. Those living in other areas may need to make climatic and seasonal adjustments and should consult a qualified macrobiotic teacher and counselor in their region for advice. There are also a variety of less common cancers not discussed in this book. If it cannot be clearly determined whether the tumor is more yin or yang in origin, a centrally balanced Cancer-Prevention Diet may safely be followed, such as that described in the chapter on lung cancer. Macrobiotic cooking instruction is essential for orientation to the new diet.

In the event a cancer patient has received or is currently undergoing surgery, chemotherapy, radiation therapy, or hormone therapy, as well as certain nutritional therapies, the dietary guidelines may need to be further modified to balance the effects of the medical treatment as well as the effects of cancer. Therefore, it is advisable for such a patient to consult his or her medical doctor, nutritional consultant, or other appropriate professional on how to adjust the Cancer-Prevention Diet to his or her unique medical situation and nutritional needs. Together with proper food preparation and cooking, it may be necessary to continue periodic medical checkups to monitor the patient's changing condition as these adjustments are implemented. These dietary modifications may include proportionately increasing the volume of food consumed, especially protein, complex carbohydrate, minerals, vitamins, or saturated fat of vegetable or animal quality. For example, some patients with low energy or weight loss may initially need to increase the amount of fish consumed or use more unrefined vegetable oil in cooking. In this way, the Cancer-Prevention Diet can be adjusted to compensate for diminished blood quality and other possible results of prior or ongoing medical attention.

Home Cares lists various compresses and other applications that can be prepared in the home to reduce pain and help discharge toxic materials through the skin or urine. These remedies are inexpensive, easy to prepare, and, if used properly, totally safe. However, if unnecessarily applied, overused, or incorrectly administered, they may be slightly counterproductive. Their application will differ a little with the individual, and it is recommended to consult an experienced macrobiotic counselor or medical professional. Instructions on how to prepare home cares are given in Part III.

Other Considerations offers some way-of-life suggestions and other types of activity that may be used in conjunction with the dietary approach. For further information on supplementary breathing, fitness, or meditative exercises, see my book *The Book of Do-In: Exercise for Physical and Spiritual Development* (New York: Japan Publications, 1979).

Personal Experience looks at actual accounts of men, women, and young adults who have relieved or are currently relieving cancer and cancer-related disorders using the diet and methods presented in this book. Many of these people have sought guidance from me in recent years and after restoring their health gone on to become teachers or counselors. Their stories are drawn largely from case histories published by the East West Foundation and *East West Journal*. While these accounts are largely anecdotal, with varying degrees of medical documentation, we hope that they provide an impetus for cancer researchers to conduct fully supervised studies to measure the effectiveness of the Cancer-Prevention Diet and propose modifications in light of evolving clinical experience. We would like to cooperate in these investigations and evaluations as we have done over the last decade on research on diet and heart disease at Harvard Medical School. As we go to press, the School of Public Health and Tropical Medicine of Tulane University has expressed interest in conducting a "Longitudinal Study of Macrobiotics and Cancer Survival." This case-control study would involve 500 patients in the New Orleans area with cancer of the colon, breast, stomach, prostate, uterus, or ovaries.

11.

Bone Cancer

FREQUENCY

In 1983 an estimated 10,300 Americans will die of bone cancer and connective tissue tumors and 16,300 new cases will surface. Bone cancer appears in a variety of forms. The most lethal is *multiple myeloma,* accounting for about two thirds of bone-cancer deaths. Multiple myeloma affects both bone tissue and the plasma cells of the blood and usually develops in adults over fifty. This condition is characterized by the spontaneous fracture of the bones, including the vertebrae, ribs, pelvis, and skull as cancer cells replace normal cells. Other bone cancers include *osteogenic sarcoma,* a tumor affecting children and young adults, which begins in the bone and cartilage and often spreads to the bone marrow, muscles, liver, and lungs; *Ewing's sarcoma,* another cancer of childhood, which appears in the marrow of the longer bones and spreads to other bones and organs; *chondrosarcoma,* a slow-growing tumor, which originates in the cartilage of the large bones and affects primarily middle-aged persons; *chordoma,* a rare tumor found at the base of the skull or end of the spine; and *rhabdomyosarcoma,* a soft-tissue tumor in the fat and muscles, which spreads rapidly and usually affects children mostly between the ages of two and six. Primary bone cancer is comparatively rare. However, the bones are frequently the site of cancer spreading from other sites.

Amputation is prescribed for many bone cancers, though most myelomas are too advanced for surgery. Radiation therapy and chemotherapy are often used as supplemental treatments. The five-year survival rate for multiple myeloma is 16 to 17 percent. For other bone cancer, it varies with the type and reaches up to 50 percent.

STRUCTURE

The skeletal and muscular system supports the body framework and governs mobility and physical interaction with the environment. The bones also serve to protect vital inner organs and store calcium, phosphorous, and other minerals that are needed for metabolism. Bone is considered both a tissue and an organ and is composed of specialized cells called osteocytes, which are imbedded in a matrix. The matrix includes small fibers and an adhering substance made up of mineral salts. The skeletal structure is also composed of cartilage, which is more flexible than bone; joints, which are junctions between two or more bones; muscles, which control tension and body movement and make up half the body weight; and tendons, which connect muscles and bones.

Bone tissue is made up of thin layers called lamellae. In fully developed bone, these lamellae are classified as either spongy or compact. The skull and ribs, for instance, are more porous or spongelike in structure, while the long bones of the legs and arms consist of a central canal surrounded by concentrically arranged plates of bone tissue. Blood vessels and nerves run through the canals, transporting nutrients and wastes to and from the osteocytes. The bone marrow consists of the soft tissues in the medullary canals of the compact bones and in the interstices of spongy bones.

Bone tissue is constantly changing in order to adapt to stress and varying environmental factors. The bones of infants and children are softer than adults and more subject to malformation or fracture. In the course of aging, the proportion of inorganic mineral salts in the bones increases, slowing their growth. In elderly people, this can cause bones to become brittle and break more easily.

CAUSE OF CANCER

The dense, compact bones are classified as yang in structure, and tumors in this part of the body arise primarily from excess accumulation of refined salt and minerals in combination with excessive animal-quality protein and saturated fat. Foods that can produce this overly contracted condition include meat, eggs, poultry, fish and sea-food, and hard, salty cheese.

In addition to these yang influences, strong yin factors are also sometimes involved in bone-cancer formation, especially in the case of multiple myeloma. In this disease, the cells of the bone marrow revert to red blood cells, enhancing the susceptibility of the skeletal system to fracture. This condition reflects stagnated intestinal activity caused by excessive consumption of extreme foods in both the yang and yin categories. The latter includes dairy food, refined flour products, sugar and other sweets, coffee and stimulants, soft drinks, tropical fruits and vegetables, drugs and medications, and all kinds of chemicalized or artificially processed foods. The bones and deep inner organs are particularly susceptible to radioactive substances, such as strontium 90, which displace calcium and other minerals in the tissue. Radioactive elements accumulate in the food chain and are consumed principally in animal foods, such as milk and beef. (For a complete description of the relationship between cancer and radiation, see the chapter on leukemia.)

MEDICAL EVIDENCE

• In 1968 Canadian researchers reported that sea vegetables contained a polysaccharide substance that selectively bound radioactive strontium and helped eliminate it from the body. In laboratory experiments, sodium alginate prepared from kelp, kombu, and other brown seaweeds off the Atlantic and Pacific coasts was introduced along with strontium and calcium into rats. The reduction of radioactive particles in bone uptake, measured in the femur, reached as high as 80 percent, with little interference with calcium absorption. "The evaluation of biological activity of different marine algae is important because of their practical significance in preventing absorption of radioactive products of atomic fission as well as in their use as possible natural decontaminators." Source: Y. Tanaka et al., "Studies on Inhibition of Intestinal Absorption of Radio-Active Strontium," *Canadian Medical Association Journal* 99:169–75.

• In 1970 Japanese scientists at the National Cancer Center Research Institute reported that shiitake mushrooms had a strong antitumor effect. In experiments with mice, polysaccharide preparations from various natural sources, including the shiitake mushroom commonly available in Tokyo markets, markedly inhibited the growth of induced sarcomas resulting in "almost complete regression of tumors . . . with no sign of toxicity." Source: G. Chihara et al., "Fractionation and Purification of the Polysaccharides with Marked Antitumor Activity, Especially Lentinan, from *Lentinus edodes* (Berk.) Sing. (An Edible Mushroom)," *Cancer Research* 30:2776–81.

• In 1974 Japanese scientists reported that several varieties of kombu and mojaban, common sea vegetables eaten in Asia and traditionally used as a decoction for cancer in Chinese herbal medicine, were effective in the treatment of tumors in laboratory experiments. In three of four samples tested, inhibition rates in mice with implanted sarcomas ranged from 89 to 95 percent. The researchers reported that "the tumor underwent complete regression in more than half of the mice of each treated group." Similar experiments on mice with leukemia showed promising results. Source: I. Yamamoto et al., "Antitumor Effect of Seaweeds," *Japanese Journal of Experimental Medicine* 44:543–46.

• In 1979, 64 veterans or widows of U.S. soldiers stationed in Hiroshima and Nagasaki in 1945 to help clean up the A-bombed cities filed claims asserting that their exposure to radiation had contributed to serious or fatal illness, including bone cancer, leukemia, and blood-related diseases. Source: Harvey Wasserman and Norman Soloman, *Killing Our Own* (New York: Delta, 1982, pp. 14–15).

DIAGNOSIS

Modern medicine commonly tests for bone cancer by a variety of methods including chest and skeletal surveys, acid and alkaline phosphatase tests, serum calcium tests, and a bone biopsy. For multiple myeloma, detection usually includes a myelogram. In this procedure, a dye is injected into the spinal fluid and x-rayed for possible malignancies.

Traditional Oriental diagnosis avoids technological methods of detection that can be harmful to health in favor of simple visual observations, acupressure techniques involving touching certain spots on the body, and other safe but accurate procedures. In this way, development of serious illness, including cancer, can be diagnosed long before it reaches a critical stage and corrective dietary adjustments taken.

In general, the quality of a person's native constitution can be seen in the bone structure, while the quality of the individual's year-to-year, month-to-month, or day-to-day condition appears more in the muscles, skin, and other peripheral areas of the body. The constitution can be judged by feeling the bones, especially in the area of the shoulders, arms, and legs. Stronger and bolder bones indicate a stronger, more yang constitution, while thinner and weaker bones indicate a more yin, weak and fragile condition. The former type of person has a tendency to be more active in physical and social life, while the latter tends to be more active in mental and artistic life.

Softer muscles show a more yin constitution, nourished by fluid, vegetables, and fruits, while tighter muscles show a more yang constitution, nourished by grains, beans, and animal food, with more minerals. The condition of the skin is also an indication. However, in comparison with the bones, the condition of the muscles and skin are more changeable through diet and exercise, since they are composed of more protein and fat, while the bones are composed of more minerals. Accordingly, while the muscles and skin show the constitution developed during the periods of pregnancy and growth, they also show the present physical and mental conditions. Softer muscles and fine skin indicate a more adaptable and mentally oriented nature, while tighter and harder muscles and skin show a nature that is more physically oriented and active.

These are general tendencies and differ depending upon the individual. In visual diagnosis, both constitution and condition are taken into account in determining relative health or sickness and are examined in assessing the digestive, circulatory, nervous, and excretory systems as well as the skeletal and musculature system.

Bone cancer is a yang disorder and especially affects those who are sturdy in build or lean with very strong constitutions. The development of this form of malignancy can be determined by a variety of observations. Facial color is either red-brown or milky-white, and in both cases, facial and body skin appears oily.

In bone cancer cases, a green coloration often appears along the spleen meridian, especially from the inside of the big toe up the outside of the leg. Also, in some cases, fatty spots with a green shade appear on the outside of the foot below the ankle. The inside of the wrist may also show a dark green or dark blue color. The outer edge of the palm may become red-white, while the edge on the back of the hand may be green.

In many cases of bone cancer, the toenails may become white or cracked, and often callouses appear on the tips of or between the toes. Hard mucus accumulation and calcification also arise on the forehead and are a possible indication of this condition. A yellow-white color, also showing mucus buildup, often appears on the lower eye-whites. The finger tips, especially the second section, often become white, and the second and third set of knuckles tend to be hard. From these and other signs, developing bone cancer can be detected and protected against naturally.

DIETARY RECOMMENDATIONS

Bone cancer is caused primarily by longtime overconsumption of animal food, especially beef, pork, poultry, eggs, cheese, other dairy food, and fish and seafood—especially those processed with large amounts of salt. These and other animal foods high in fat, protein, and salt should be discontinued. At the same time, contributing to bone cancer is the overconsumption of all fatty and oily foods, both of animal and vegetable quality, including sugar, honey, chocolate, carob, and other sweeteners, spices, stimulants, and aromatic foods and drinks, as well as foods that form fat and mucus such as flour products. These should be limited or avoided completely. Soft drinks, chemical additives, alcohol, and all artificially processed food and beverages are to be avoided as they are considered possible contributing factors.

The following are general dietary guidelines for the relief and prevention of bone cancer:

• Fifty to sixty percent, by volume, whole-cereal grains. Pressure-cooked brown rice is recommended as the principal daily food, barley the next most frequently used food. All other grains may also be used occasionally with the exception of buckwheat, which is better avoided for an initial period of several months. Bread and other flour products are to be limited, though unleavened whole-wheat or whole-rye bread can be consumed occasionally when desired. Whole-wheat pasta may be consumed but only occasionally and in limited amounts. Buckwheat noodles are to be avoided for the initial period. Once or twice a week, fried rice or noodles may be consumed.

• Five to ten percent soup, consisting of one or two bowls of miso (especially barley miso) or tamari soy sauce soup, may be consumed daily. Soups can be made with wakame or kombu sea vegetables and green and white leafy vegetables. To help relieve this condition, pieces of fresh daikon, turnip, or radish can be added almost daily. Often or frequently, small pieces of shiitake mushroom may also be cooked with the soup. In addition to these regular soups, grain or bean soups may be eaten occasionally. The taste of the soup should be milder than usual.

• Twenty to thirty percent vegetable dishes. All regular round, leafy, and root vegetables can be used to produce various dishes, and cooking methods may include boiling, steaming, and sautéing. Of course, avoid all vegetables initially of tropical origin such as potatoes, eggplant, and tomatoes. While oil is not usually recommended for most cancer patients, for bone cancer one dish of sautéed vegetables cooked with unrefined sesame oil should be eaten daily or every other day. Sweet vegetables such as cabbages, onions, pumpkins, and winter squashes can be used most often, though root and leafy vegetables are also to be used regularly. Vegetables may be seasoned during cooking with sea salt, miso, or tamari soy sauce, and the taste should be milder than usual.

• Five to ten percent beans and bean products. All regular beans are recommended, though smaller ones such as azuki beans, lentils, and chickpeas are preferred for frequent use. Black soy beans are also highly recommended for regular use for this form of cancer. Beans can be cooked with 10 to 20 percent kombu or other sea vegetable, 30 to 50 percent fall-season squash, or 10 to 30 percent onions and carrots. Season lightly with sea salt, miso, or tamari soy sauce. Bean products such as tempeh, tofu (cooked), and natto may be used a few times per week in moderate volume.

• Five percent or less sea vegetables to be eaten daily. These may be prepared as a small side dish in addition to the sea vegetables cooked in soups, vegetable dishes, and beans. Hiziki, arame, and kombu should be used most often, though all others should be consumed as well. Sea vegetables may occasionally be cooked with 1 to 2 drops of sesame oil. A moderate volume of tamari soy sauce may be used for seasoning.

As for supplemental dishes and foods, fish and seafood are to be limited or preferably avoided completely for the initial few months. If craved, a small portion of nonfat white-meat fish may be served together with a small dish of grated daikon, radish, or ginger, with a taste of tamari soy sauce, in order to detoxify the effects of the fish on the body.

Fruits are also to be avoided if possible for the initial few months. If craved, however, dried or cooked fruit, in season, may be consumed in moderate volume.

Nuts are also to be avoided, though roasted unsalted seeds, such as pumpkin, sunflower, or sesame, may be used occasionally in moderate volume as a snack.

A sweet taste may be acquired from naturally sweet vegetables including carrots, cabbages, onions, fall-season squash, and chestnuts. However, if craved, a stronger taste can be obtained from grain-based sweeteners such as rice syrup or barley malt.

A sour taste can be provided by umeboshi plums or their juice, sauerkraut, and brown rice or sweet brown rice vinegar.

Seasonings and condiments may follow the general guidelines for cancer prevention, though volume should be moderate and slightly milder in taste.

There are a variety of special dishes and condiments for bone cancer. These include shiso (beefsteak) powder, made from roasting and grinding the dried leaves that umeboshi plums usually come prepared with. One-half to 1 teaspoon of shiso powder can be sprinkled daily on grain and vegetable dishes.

A cup of kuzu drink is also beneficial for this condition and may be consumed frequently. Prepare by dissolving 1 teaspoon of kuzu powder in a cup of hot water and cook briefly with 2 teaspoons of grated daikon or radish and a little tamari soy sauce for taste.

Ume-sho-bancha tea with half a sheet of crushed, toasted nori sea vegetable can be consumed up to 1 cup a day, a few times a week.

For strength, bone cancer patients may prepare occasionally carp soup (koi koku). Mochi or tempeh may also be added to miso soup frequently to restore vitality and generate energy.

Beverages and all other dietary practices may follow the general guidelines. Thorough chewing of each mouthful of food until liquefied is essential, and overconsumption and eating within three hours before sleep should be avoided.

As explained in the introduction to Part II, cancer patients who have received or who are currently undergoing medical treatment may need to make further dietary modifications.

HOME CARES

• A ginger compress for 5 to 10 minutes, followed by a taro potato plaster (mixed 50/50 with grated fresh lotus root) for 3 to 4 hours, may be applied on the affected region to help reduce the tumor. Use daily for up to 2 to 4 weeks.

• Scrubbing the entire body each day with a hot towel soaked in hot grated gingerroot water is beneficial to promoting circulation.

• In case of pains and aches, the ginger compress and taro plaster are helpful. Also, a plaster can be made with cabbages and white potato crushed in a 50/50 mixture. Apply on the affected area until it becomes warm, generally 2 to 3 hours, and then repeat.

OTHER CONSIDERATIONS

• Bone cancer patients should particularly avoid damp and humid environments.

• Fresh green plants in the house will stimulate air and energy flow.

• Avoid artificial electromagnetic radiation, such as from color television, cooking appliances, and other devices. Avoid nuclear installations as well.

• Wear cotton clothing, especially next to the skin, and use natural fabrics for sheets, blankets, and other furnishings insofar as possible.

PERSONAL EXPERIENCE

Metatastic Bone Cancer

In the course of a checkup for a pain in his lower body, Joseph Koenig, a sixty-six-year-old machinist from Port Jervis, New York, was diagnosed with terminal cancer on September 21, 1979. "I'm sorry, the prostate is filled with cancer, and it has already spread to all the bones," the doctor told his wife. "Your husband has only three months to live."

Except for intermittent arthritis for many years, Koenig felt that he was in relatively good health and never dreamed that he had cancer. That summer he had been looking forward to his retirement and while cutting wood on his farm began to experience a pain in his groin that grew sharper each day. The doctors gave him pain killers and recommended various medical treatments to relieve his suffering, including the drug Stilbestrol, a female hormone. However, he developed a blood clot as a result of taking this drug and had to be hospitalized.

Meanwhile, one of his daughters-in-law had attended a natural foods convention and noticed a booth dispensing information on alternative therapies. Following the unpleasant stay in the hospital, Koenig decided to start Laetrile treatments. These consisted of intravenous injections of Laetrile and vitamin C administered in a doctor's office filled with patients going there for the same treatment. The procedure took four to five hours, three times a week. Over the next 13 months, Koenig continued to take Laetrile along with a raw foods diet, which included four to six glasses of fresh squeezed carrot and vegetable juices a day, 60 vitamin and enzyme pills, and a coffee enema each morning. These were supplemented with visualization exercises, in which he saw himself getting well, and with prayers with the rest of the family.

The treatment and supplementary exercises seemed to control the cancer from spreading. However, he had no energy and spent most of the time in bed when he wasn't commuting to the doctor's office. The Laetrile treatments had cost almost $15,000 and were exhausting the Koenigs' retirement funds. Meanwhile, a new urologist advised him to have his testicles surgically removed and to start chemotherapy. From another direction, one of his daughter's high school teachers sent home a copy of a recent article in the *Saturday Evening Post* describing how a medical doctor with terminal cancer healed himself with the help of the macrobiotic diet. Mrs. Koenig read the article to her husband but he did not want to try something new.

While at this crossroads, destiny seemed to intervene. One day, after returning from a Laetrile treatment, the Koenigs' car skidded on a patch of snow and Koenig suffered a compression fracture in his back. "My faith began to waver at this point," his wife later wrote, "but, praise the Lord, He had a plan for us and good was going to come out of all this. After another two weeks in the hospital, Joe was put in a back brace and couldn't sit very long, so we discontinued going back to Nyack for [Laetrile] treatment. He then became weaker and weaker and began passing out. Many times I had to pick him up from the floor and put him in bed."

One night, at home, Koenig passed out and began throwing up and moving his bowels in bed. When he awoke, both he and his wife recognized that he was dying. Mrs. Koenig again brought out the article in the *Saturday Evening Post* and suggested going to Boston to attend an East West Foundation seminar on cancer and diet. The next seminar was only six days away and they weren't sure he could make the trip. Calling the Kushi Institute, they were advised to start eating brown rice and miso soup immediately. "We both ate the soup and loved it," Mrs. Koenig noted. "We were told to chew the rice 50 to 100 times each mouthful. Joe did start to feel more energy returning to his pain-wracked body and we were able to go to the seminar. We learned all about the reasons for sickness and how we are all responsible for our own health. Cooking classes were given and I must say my head was spinning from hearing all these strange names of foods. But we learned so much that weekend. It truly was the turning point of our lives."

As Koenig ate the new food, he began to gain strength. After 16 months on the Cancer-Prevention Diet, he is now able to do all the things he had planned to do in retirement. He drives the car and tractor, plows, plants, and harvests. "Sometimes when I can't find him," his wife says, "he's up on the barn repairing leaks or in his beloved shop making tools or parts. We work together now and our life has taken on a whole new quality."

In July 1982, Koenig went to see his urologist, who examined him and took blood tests. Coming back into his office with an amazed look on his face, the doctor asked Koenig if he was taking any medication or vitamins. "No, sir," Koenig replied. "Then you really believe your healing is from the food you eat?" the doctor asked. "Yes, sir," Koenig answered. The doctor then told him that the prostate was absolutely normal and the blood test (Acid Phosphatase) was only one point above normal.

"The other day Joe's doctor called up," his wife wrote in conclusion, "and I saw a smile come over Joe's face. When he got off the phone, he said to me, 'Guess what, my doctor would like a copy of my diet.' Praise God." Source: *East West Journal*, "Mending Shattered Dreams," March 1983.

12.

Brain Cancer

FREQUENCY

Brain tumors and cancer of the central nervous system will kill an estimated 10,800 Americans in 1983, and 12,600 new cases will develop. Men, between fifty and sixty, are most at risk, but brain tumors are on the rise in children and now account for about 35 percent of all cancer deaths in both males and females under fifteen.

A majority of brain tumors affect the brain tissue itself and are called gliomas. These are subdivided into four main types: 1) *glioblastoma multiforme,* a malignant tumor affecting both children and adults and one that may spread quickly through the cerebrum, cerebellum, brain stem, and spinal cord; 2) *astrocytoma,* a tumor found mostly in children, affecting the cerebellum and brain stem; 3) *ependymoma,* another childhood tumor, which grows in the ventricles of the brain; 4) *oligodendroglioma,* a slow-growing tumor that affects the white matter in the frontal lobe and is found in both children and adults.

Other brain tumors include *medulloblastoma,* a childhood cancer that spreads from the cerebellum to other regions of the brain and central nervous system; *meningioma,* a tumor affecting the membrane covering the brain and spinal cord; *pituitary adenoma,* a tumor that affects the hypothalamus and optic nerve; *gaulioneuroblastoma,* a malignancy that spreads quickly through the nerve cells; *neurofibrosarcoma,* a cancer affecting the peripheral nervous system; and *neuroblastoma,* a tumor that affects children three years old or younger and spreads through the nervous network in various regions including the chest, neck, abdomen, lower back, eye, and adrenal glands. About 15 percent of brain tumors have metastasized from other organs, especially the lungs, kidney, breast, or the lymph nodes in the case of Hodgkin's disease.

Because of their location within one of the most sensitive parts of the body, many brain tumors are considered untreatable by modern science. However, depending on the type and staging, surgery and radiation therapy are often employed. The operation is called a craniotomy and involves removing part of the skull, removing the malignant tissue, and putting back the excised bone. The risk of damaging the brain during such a procedure is high.

When surgery is ruled out, radiation is commonly used, especially for medulloblastomas and ependymomas. However, x-ray treatments may cause permanent damage to the spinal cord, especially in children. Hormone therapy is sometimes used in conjunction with surgery to decrease the swelling or control metastases. Steroids are given and followed up by drugs such as prednisone, which may be administered intravenously or intramuscularly for the rest of the patient's life. Other methods of treating brain tumors include hypothermia (lowering the temperature of the brain or body), cryosurgery (freezing), and implanting radiosensitizers to enhance radiation therapy. The present survival rate for all forms of brain tumors is 25 percent for males and 33 percent for females.

STRUCTURE

The human nervous system has two anatomical divisions: the central nervous system, which includes the brain and spinal cord, and the peripheral nervous system, which includes all of the nervous structures outside of the skull and vertebral canal, such as the craniospinal nerves and the orthosympathetic branch of the autonomic nervous system. The central nervous system acts as a switchboard for incoming impulses from receptors and outgoing impulses to effectors; it regulates all body activities except for chemically controlled ones and is the seat for the higher consciousness processes.

The autonomic nervous system is not considered to be an anatomical division, but a functional unit, which handles the involuntary, unconscious body activities, such as the beating of the heart, breathing, digestive peristalsis, and so on. The autonomic system is, in turn, composed of two antagonistic branches: the parasympathetic (yang) and the orthosympathetic (yin). The parasympathetic nerves have a more central position of origin in the body, beginning in the brain stem and sacral region of the spinal cord, and passing outward through four pairs of cranial nerves and three pairs of sacral nerves. The orthosympathetic nerves have a more peripheral position, beginning in the central section of the spine and passing outward through the corresponding spinal nerves. In almost all organs, tissues, and smooth muscles, there are pairs of autonomic nerves, one ortho- and one parasympathetic, which act in opposite ways. When the parasympathetic nerves act on expanded (yin) organs, such as the bronchi of the lungs or the wall of the digestive tract, there is naturally a resultant contraction. Their action on compact organs (yang), such as the iris of the eye or cardiac muscles, brings about expansion or dilation. The orthosympathetic nerves have a complementary, opposite effect. They inhibit hollow organs, such as the bladder, and stimulate compact ones, such as the uterus, during pregnancy.

The two major divisions of the brain are the large forebrain, including the cerebrum, and the more compact hindbrain, including the cerebellum. Since the forebrain is more open and expanded, it is classified as yin, while the smaller, more compact hindbrain is yang. The brain can also be divided into its more central region, known as the midbrain, and more peripheral region, called the cortex. In order for communication to proceed smoothly, incoming and outgoing impulses need to be balanced. Within the brain, the more compact or central regions tend to be areas where images and impulses are received, while outgoing communication originates in the more peripheral or expanded areas. Thus, nervous impulses from the eyes, ears, nose, skin, and other sense organs gather in the midbrain, while images, dreams, and thoughts are dispatched outward from the more peripheral cortex region. Also in terms of receiving and dispatching, the hindbrain receives incoming vibrations and stores them as memory, while outgoing vibrations, including our images of the future, arise in the forebrain.

CAUSE OF CANCER

In the last several years there has been considerable research concerning the relationship between the right and left hemispheres of the brain. Studies show that the right hemisphere in most people is the origin of more simple or mechanical action and consciousness, while the left hemisphere produces more complex and creative thinking. In terms of language, more simple or basic expressions originate in the right hemisphere, while the left hemisphere creates more refined and original expression. Imagination, which is based mostly on futuristic thinking, develops more in the left hemisphere, while analytical thinking, based more on actual past experiences, arises in the right hemisphere.

Our modern technological civilization has arisen due to the active development of right-hemisphere thinking. This more focused, yang type of thinking and activity has resulted from a way of eating centered around meat, dairy food, and other animal products. Imbalance in one direction produces a corresponding pull in the other. To balance the increasing amounts of animal food, modern society has witnessed a proliferation of extreme substances in the yin category including alcohol, spices, coffee and other stimulants, refined sugar, imported tropical fruits and vegetables, chemical additives, and a variety of drugs including tranquilizers, birth-control pills, and hallucinogens.

Within many modern countries, especially during the last fifteen or twenty years, young people have been exposed to these types of food from birth, and many have experimented and become regular users of marijuana, hashish, cocaine, or LSD. These extremely yin substances have produced a rapid shift in thinking from the right side of the brain, which is predominant in modern society, toward the left side, and also from the back of the brain more toward the front. As a result, many young people started looking more toward the future, while neglecting or forgetting previous traditions, including the relationship with their parents, elders, and ancestors. Similarly, they lost interest in school, business or professional careers, and the political and economic condition of society. Instead they turned to music, the arts, spiritual teachers from the East, and other nonlinear pursuits.

In many cases, the continuous intake of yin type foods and drugs has led to very unbalanced conditions and expression. By moving to the other extreme, vegetarians who eat primarily fruits, juices, and raw foods and members of the psychedelic counterculture risk a variety of illnesses. These include mental disease, herpes, multiple sclerosis, leukemia, and brain cancer.

Tumors that affect the outer regions of the brain or the nerve cells of the peripheral nervous system are caused primarily by foods, drinks, and medications or drugs in the yin category. These forms of brain malfunction or nervous disorders are more commonly found in children or young adults who have grown up on sugar-coated breakfast cereals, honey, chocolate, and other sweeteners, orange juice, soda pop, ice cream, oily and greasy foods as well as many chemical additives in conjunction with constant intake of milk, butter, and other dairy foods.

Tumors in the inner region of the brain or spinal cord are more yang in structure and location. They arise primarily from consumption of excess animal food including meat, poultry, eggs, and cheese and refined salt and thus tend to affect older persons. As a whole, the brain and central nervous system are extremely compact (yang) and therefore a magnet to attract drugs, medications, synthetic vitamins, food and mineral supplements, and other extremely expansive (yin) substances. By avoiding these things and centering the diet, the brain and nervous system can maintain their normal functions.

MEDICAL EVIDENCE

• In 1845 British physician George Macilwain wrote a book on cancer in which diet played a prominent role in preventing and relieving the disease. "[If] I see a man with a huge bump on his face, knowing that it is not a natural appendage to him, . . . I am at least certain of this, that either the food contains something unusual, or that some of the assimilating organs are acting on it in some unusual manner, or both. This seems indisputable. It does not indeed unveil to us the causes of tumours; but it immediately points to at least one mode of looking for them. That is to examine the food, the various organs which represent the various stages, which I have included in the word assimilation; and to test the properties of both one and the other by any knowledge we may have of their natural effects, habits, and propensities, respectively." Macilwain presents case histories of several of his patients whose tumors of various kinds were eliminated or reduced by a simple diet high in vegetables and cereal grains, low in meat and animal products, and who maintained "the rigid exclusion of sugar, and grease of all kinds." Source: George Macilwain, *The General Nature and Treatment of Tumours* (London, 1845, pp. 30-31).

• A 1974 study reported an increase in brain tumors and other cancers in men who had been occupationally exposed to vinyl chloride for at least one year. Vinyl chloride is widely used in plastic wrapping for packaging and storing foods. The FDA classifies it as an indirect food additive and its residues are found in many foods. Source: I.R. Tabershaw and W.R. Gaffey, "Mortality Study of Workers in the Manufacture of Vinyl Chloride and Its Polymers," *Journal of Occupational Medicine* 16:509–18.

• In 1978 researchers reported fourteen cases of neuroblastoma, a brain tumor, over a sixteen-month period in people exposed to chemical pesticides. Five cases were children who were unintentionally exposed before or after birth to chlordane formulations. These pesticide residues tend to accumulate in high-fat foods such as meat, poultry, dairy products, and fish. Source: P.F. Infante et al., "Blood Dyscrasias and Childhood Tumors and Exposure to Chlordane and Heptachlor," *Scandinavian Journal of Work and Environmental Health* 4:137–50.

• In 1981 medical doctors reported a unique approach to brain tumor therapy regulating plasma levels of an essential amino acid and putting the terminal brain cancer patients on a natural foods diet. Developed at the University of Tennessee Center for Health Sciences, the experiment was conducted on three patients with glioblastomas beginning in 1975. Two of the three showed marked improvement. The first lived 15 months and the tumor initially disappeared before reappearing. The second lived 23 months. The third survived 8 months. In contrast, the mean survival for patients with this disease is 4 to 6 months. Source: C.R. Greer et al., "Surgery, Irradiation, and Metabolic Control of Brain Tumors" (letter), *American Journal of Clinical Nutrition* 34:600–01.

• In a follow-up to the above study, researchers at the University of Tennessee reported on the safety and feasibility of dietary management for brain cancer. Six patients with glioblastomas who had been treated with surgery and irradiation were put on a natural foods diet high in foods such as oatmeal, corn, carrots, and zucchini and a dietary supplement that restricted an essential amino acid. The regime was low in meat, dairy products, and other high-protein foods. "Amino acid restriction resulted in no additional patient morbidity," the researchers concluded. "There were no alterations in laboratory values to indicate the need for [medical] intervention. Quality of life for the patients did not diminish." Source: J.B. Burgess et al., *Nutrition and Cancer* 1(4):16–21.

• In laboratory tests beginning in 1973, rats fed aspartame in their diet at various levels for up to two years had greater incidences of brain tumors than controls. However, aspartame, a chemical 180 times stronger than sugar, was approved by the USFDA in 1981 for use as a sweetener and flavoring agent in certain foods after other tests showed no significant increase in tumors. Source: *Diet, Nutrition, and Cancer* (Washington, D.C.: National Academy of Sciences, 1982, pp. 14:7–8).

DIAGNOSIS

Brain tumors are commonly detected by x-rays or CAT scans to the skull, spinal cord, and chest. Other medical techniques may include an electroencephalogram, cerebral angiogram, brian scan, spinal puncture, and myelogram.

Oriental medicine uses a variety of simple observations to ascertain the condition of the nervous system. A purplish-red color around the eyes shows an overworked nervous system caused mainly by consumption of drugs, chemicals, medications, refined simple sugars, and other extreme foods and drinks from the yin category. The parasympathetic system is especially affected by these substances. However, the orthosympathetic system will also be weakened, making all body reflexes and functions less sharp. The immediate effect can often be seen in the eyes, where the pupils contract, and in the vascular system, where the blood vessels dilate. After continued drug use, however, the parasympathetic nerves become worn out, expanding more and more. The pupils then dilate and the vessels contract.

The middle region of the forehead also shows the condition of the nervous system. A red color here shows nervousness, oversensitivity, excitability, and instability due to the overconsumption of yin type foods, drinks, stimulants, and drugs. A white color is caused by excess intake of dairy products, especially milk, cream, and yogurt, together with excessive liquid. Nervous functions are generally slow and dull, and mental activities are cloudy and unclear. A yellow color indicates alertness but a tendency toward narrow-mindedness and inflexibility. The major cause is excessive intake of eggs, poultry, and dairy food. Dark spots or patches on the forehead indicate elimination of excessive sugars, fruits, honey, milk sugar, and other sweets as well as chemicals and drugs. Red pimples or spots on the middle forehead show the elimination of sugar and fruits combined with refined white flour products or dairy products.

The middle layer or ridge of the ear reflects the condition of the entire nervous system. A red color here indicates nervous disorders.

The earlobe corresponds to the brain, and pimples, discolorations, or other abnormalities in this region may show developing cysts or tumors.

A loose mouth shows a variety of disorders, including nervous-system malfunctions. This condition usually also reflects trouble in the small intestine, the brain's complementary opposite organ.

The coloring on the back of the hand may also indicate nervous problems. If marijuana, hashish, or other hallucinogenic substances, as well as medications, are used repeatedly for some time, the body will begin to discharge these toxins and the color of the hands and fingers will change to red or purple.

Rough skin also shows nervous disorders caused by extreme yin type foods or drugs. This condition may be accompanied by an irregular pulse, excessive sweating, frequent urination, diarrhea, vertigo, excessive sensitivity, and emotional instability.

The sensitively trained hand can also locate the approximate region of brain tumors and cancer by detecting vibrations produced and discharged from each part of the brain. In some cases, brain tumors may cause paralysis, seizure, loss of sight, and loss of physical and mental coordination. By examining the paralyzed parts and functions of the body, indirect detection of the area of the brain affected can be done.

Generally, brain tumors are comparatively easier than other cancers to relieve through proper eating. This is because they tend to grow slowly in this very compact region, and the abundance of blood supply to the brain means that a change in blood quality from an altered diet will quickly affect the condition of the brain and nervous system.

DIETARY RECOMMENDATIONS

The formation of brain tumors usually results from the overconsumption of protein and fat, especially of animal quality. Animal products, including eggs, meat, poultry, dairy food, and oily, fatty fish, should be strictly avoided. The formation of brain tumors also results from ingestion of chemicals in artificially processed food as well as exposure to industrial pollutants. It is therefore advisable to avoid the continued use of all synthetic food products and for patients with this condition to restore their health in a relatively fresh and clean atmospheric environment. Furthermore, sugar and other sweeteners such as honey, chocolate, carob, and foods and beverages containing these items are not to be consumed. Although they are not direct causes of brain tumors, fruits, fruit juices, spices, stimulants, alcohol, and aromatic beverages and substances are to be avoided because they tend to accelerate tumor growth. Because of their potential for contributing to cancer creation and growth, flour products, especially refined flour treated with oil, fat, and sweets, as well as overconsumption of liquid, are also to be avoided.

Nutritional advice for infants and young children, including those with brain tumors, is given in "Baby Food Suggestions" in Part III. Following are general dietary guidelines for older children and adults:

• Fifty to sixty percent whole-cereal grains consisting primarily of pressure-cooked whole grains. Brown rice, millet, and barley can be used as staples and other grains may be substituted occasionally. Flour products should be minimized. However, whole unrefined flour products such as unyeasted whole-wheat or rye bread and whole-wheat and buckwheat noodles may be used occasionally in limited volume a few times a week.

• Five to ten percent soup prepared with miso or tamari soy sauce in which sea vegetables and hard land vegetables are cooked. One or two bowls may be eaten daily. Whole-cereal grain soup may be substituted occasionally. The miso or tamari soy sauce should be fermented naturally for a period of at least one-and-a-half years.

• Twenty to thirty percent vegetables. All vegetables should be cooked, though they may be prepared in various styles. However, the use of oil for sautéing vegetables is to be limited to occasional use of very small volumes of sesame or corn oil. The kinds of vegetables can be varied—including root, round, and leafy ones—with an emphasis on those that are harder and rich in fiber. Fresh raw salads are to be avoided, though a boiled salad may frequently be prepared by cooking the vegetables in boiling water for one to two minutes. A small volume of long-time pickles, even though raw, may be frequently consumed.

• Five percent beans and bean products. Smaller beans such as azuki beans, lentils, and chickpeas are preferred to larger beans. They can be cooked with 10 to 20 percent (by volume) sea vegetables, chopped carrots and onions, or fall-season squash (such as acorn or buttercup squash). Bean products such as tempeh, natto, and dried or cooked tofu may occasionally be substituted for beans. A moderate volume of sea salt or tamari soy sauce may be used for seasoning.

• Five percent or less sea vegetables. Any type is recommended

for daily consumption, though arame and nori are especially beneficial and may be used more frequently than others.

In addition, persons with brain tumors can help improve their
condition by consuming frequently—several times a week—a small
side dish of burdock and carrot roots sautéed with a small amount of
sesame oil and seasoned lightly with tamari soy sauce. This dish is
called kimpira. Dried, shredded daikon cooked with kombu may also
be taken frequently as one of the regular side dishes.

Condiments to be taken with the meals include one to two teaspoons a day of sliced lotus root cooked together with kombu and a bit
of grated ginger, seasoned with tamari soy sauce. Several small pieces
of kombu cooked with tamari soy sauce can also be helpful if consumed
daily with any meal. This is called shio kombu or salty kombu.

In general, saltiness from such seasonings as sea salt, tamari soy
sauce, and salty condiments should be moderate in order to avoid the
unnecessary desire for excessive liquids, fruits, fruit juices, and
sweeteners.

The overconsumption of liquids in any form, even good-quality
beverages, should be avoided. Intake of fruit, fruit juices, nuts, nut
butters, and any other food rich in fat and sugar is to be minimized
and kept to a limited volume.

Fish and seafood are to be generally avoided, though small portions of nonfatty white-meat fish may be consumed with 1 or 2 tablespoons of grated daikon or radish, if craved.

Chewing very well until food substances become liquefied in the
mouth is highly recommended. Consuming food and beverages in the
evening, especially before sleeping, should be avoided. As a whole, it
is better to consume a lesser volume of food than an excess volume.
This amount, of course, should be reasonable to maintain normal
physical activities. All other dietary practice may follow the general
recommendations for cancer prevention listed in the guidelines and
recipes in Part III.

As explained in the introduction to Part II, cancer patients who
have received or who are currently undergoing medical treatment
may need to make further dietary modifications.

HOME CARES

• Daily scrubbing of the whole body, including neck, face, head
regions, as well as feet and toes, with a towel inserted in very hot

ginger water is very helpful to activate circulation of blood, lymph, and other bodily fluids and energies.

• Heavy pressures and pains in the head or brain can be relieved by reducing the consumption of fruit, juices, beverages, or temporary avoidance of salty food. A lotus-root plaster, consisting of a 50/50 mixture of grated fresh lotus root and mashed cabbage leaves or other greens, with 10 to 20 percent white flour and 5 percent grated ginger, is also helpful if applied directly on the region and kept there about three hours.

• Brain tumors and cancer can be accelerated if the intestinal functions are stagnated as in the case of constipation or menstrual difficulties in the case of women. Accordingly, keeping the bowels smooth and the menstrual function regular is very helpful and can also help relieve pressure and pain in the head regions. An enema for inducing elimination may be needed as well as a massage or ginger compress applied on the abdomen. Douching to eliminate stagnated fat and mucus in the uterine region may also be necessary.

OTHER CONSIDERATIONS

• Avoid wearing shoes or socks while indoors. Walk barefoot or on the grass or soil outside, when possible, to stimulate the flow of electromagnetic energy from the earth to the nervous system.

• Avoid synthetic clothing, especially underwear, stockings, socks, hats, and scarves. Wigs or hair pieces should also be avoided. Synthetic rugs, curtains, furniture, blankets, and other home furnishings should gradually be replaced with more natural materials.

• Avoid medical x-rays, video terminals, color television, and other artificial sources of electromagnetic radiation that might affect the nervous system and brain.

• Long, hot baths or showers should be avoided in order to prevent depletion of minerals from the body. Limit bathing to a few times a week.

• Good physical exercise is always helpful.

• Brain and nervous disorders are often accompanied by excitability, hypersensitivity, despondency, or lowered will to live. Short but regular periods of meditation—including visualization, prayer, chanting, yoga, or other exercises—can help to calm the mind and center the thoughts.

• Mental nourishment is as important to self-development as physical sustenance. Avoid loud and frenzied music, chaotic art, brutal and violent films, and depressing magazines and literature. Within moderation, select strong, meaningful mental outlets. Reading, music, and arts that help to create a positive attitude should be selected.

PERSONAL EXPERIENCE

Brain Tumor

In May 1977, Jack Lackner, a thirty-three-year-old man living in Boston, entered the hospital for partial removal of a malignant astrocytoma. Over the next four months, he received thirty radiation treatments and five doses of chemotherapy. In January 1978, he adopted macrobiotics and discontinued all other forms of treatment.

During conventional treatment, doctors observed a slight increase in the size of the tumor. After implementing the Cancer-Prevention Diet, Lackner's tumor progressively diminished to about one half its size in July 1978. By January 1979, a CAT scan showed that the tumor had completely disappeared. Doctors recommended a review in six months. A subsequent CAT scan in July 1979 confirmed that the tumor was gone. Source: "Brain Cancer," *Cancer and Diet* (Brookline, Mass.: East West Foundation, 1980, p. 74).

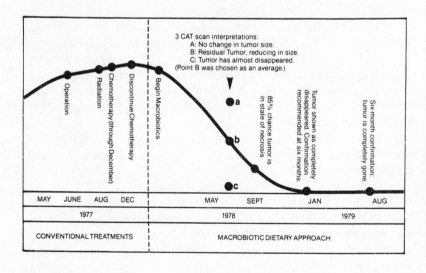

Reduction of Malignant Brain Tumor: Jack Lackner's CAT Scans

13.

Breast Cancer

FREQUENCY

Breast cancer is the most common form of cancer in American women and is on the rise. According to a recent article in the *Journal of the American Medical Association,* the incidence of diagnosed breast cancer showed an 18 percent increase between 1935 and 1965 and a 50 percent increase between 1965 and 1975. Breast cancer currently accounts for about 20 percent of female cancer deaths in the United States and is the leading cause of death for American women aged forty to forty-five. In 1983 an estimated 114,900 new cases will develop, and 37,500 people will die from the disease. In other parts of the world, breast-cancer incidence is much lower. For example, in Japan women are only one fifth as likely to die from mammary tumors as American women. A majority or more of patients with breast cancer develop metastases. Malignant tumors may spread to the lungs, bone, brain, or lymph nodes. Breast cancer may also occur in men, but it is rare.

Surgery is the most common method of treating breast cancer. The operation is called a mastectomy and includes several types of incisions depending on the development of the tumor and the age and condition of the patient. A *lumpectomy* excises the cancerous lump and a small amount of surrounding tissue. A *subcutaneous mastectomy* removes internal breast tissue, leaving the skin intact. A *simple mastectomy* removes the breast. A *modified mastectomy* removes the breast and lymph nodes in the armpit. A *Halsted radical mastectomy* removes the entire breast plus the lymph nodes and the pectoral muscles of the chest wall. In addition to these operations, the adrenal glands, pituitary gland, or ovaries are sometimes removed in order to regulate secretions and try to reduce tumor growth.

Radiation may be employed as an alternative or supplement to surgery. Chemotherapy is sometimes used to control metastases and to stop recurrence of the original tumor. Hormone therapy may be employed as an adjunct or alternative to chemotherapy: Estrogens, antiestrogens, progestins, androgens, or adrenocortical steroids are given to control tumor growth and metastases.

About 65 percent of women with breast cancer survive five years or more. In 1973 researchers at Italy's National Cancer Institute in Milan reported that studies showed no difference in survival or recurrence rates between women who had complete mastectomies and those who had partial ones. In 1977 Dr. Jan Stgersward, a Swiss cancer researcher, reported that breast-cancer patients who received no radiation therapy survived 10 percent longer than those who received radiation treatment. On March 15, 1980, *The Lancet*, a British medical journal, noted: "The overall survival of patients with primary breast cancer has not improved in the past ten years, despite increasing use of multiple-drug chemotherapy for treatment of metastases. Furthermore, there has been no improvement in survival from first metastasis, and survival may even have been shortened in some patients given chemotherapy."

STRUCTURE

The female breasts or mammary glands consist chiefly of a round, compressed mass of glandular tissue known as the corpus mammae. This tissue is made up of fifteen to twenty separate lobes connected by fat. Each lobe contains a milk duct, which leads to the nipple and is further subdivided into lobules and alveoli. The breast is encased in a layer of fat tissue called the adipose capsule and is attached to the chest wall by connective tissue.

CAUSE OF CANCER

If we continue to eat poorly over a long period of time, we eventually exhaust the body's ability to discharge excess wastes and toxins. This can be serious if an underlying layer of fat has developed under the skin, which prevents discharge toward the surface of the body. Repeated overconsumption of milk, cheese, and other dairy products, eggs, meat, poultry, and other fatty, oily, or greasy foods brings about this stage. When it has been reached, internal deposits of mucus or fat begin to form, initially in areas with some direct access to the outside such as the sinuses, the inner ear, the lungs, the kidneys, the reproductive organs, and the breasts.

The accumulation of excess in the breast often results in a hardening of the breasts and the formation of cysts. Excess usually accumulates here in the form of mucus and deposits of fatty acid, both of which take the form of a sticky or heavy liquid. These deposits develop into cysts in the same way that water solidifies into ice, and the process is accelerated by the intake of ice cream, milk, soft drinks, fruit juice, and other foods that produce a cooling or freezing effect.

Women who have breastfed are less likely to develop breast cysts or tumors. Women who do not nurse their children miss this opportunity to discharge through the breasts and therefore face a greater possibility of accumulating excess in this region of their bodies.

Many nutritionists and doctors are now aware of the relationship between the intake of saturated fats, cholesterol, and degenerative disease but often overlook the effects of sugar and dairy products, both of which contribute greatly to heart disease, cancer, and other illnesses. (See the section on pancreatic cancer for a discussion of sugar metabolism and the role of refined sugars in tumor formation, including breast cancer.)

The consumption of milk and other dairy foods in our society usually begins in infancy or early childhood. One of the major biological changes in modern times has been the progressive decline of breastfeeding. In traditional cultures, mothers usually nurse their babies for one year or more. At the beginning of the twentieth century, about 60 percent of the babies in the United States were breastfed. By the 1970's that number had fallen sharply. A 1968 survey showed that only 11 percent of American mothers attempted to nurse their infants, and two-thirds of these mothers gave up in thirty to forty days.

In composition, cow's milk and human milk are very different. Cow's milk contains about four times as much calcium, three times as much protein, and two-thirds as much carbohydrate as human milk. The different structure and growth rate of calves and human babies account for the varying proportion of these ingredients. For example, at birth the brain and nervous system of the calf is fully developed, and the large amount of calcium and protein is needed to increase its bone structure and muscular development. A baby calf often puts on

75 pounds in the first six weeks. In contrast, the body of the human infant is designed to grow slowly, gaining only two to three pounds in the first six weeks. The infant's brain, however, is only 23 percent mature at birth, and the nutrients in mother's milk are needed to complete its central nervous system.

In addition, mother's milk contains antibodies that resist the growth of undesirable bacteria and viruses, provide immunity against disease and infection (especially against rickettsia, salmonella, polio, influenza, strep, and staph), promote strong white blood cells, which destroy harmful bacteria, and produce *B. bifidum*, a unique type of healthy bacteria found in the intestines of babies that creates resistance to a large variety of microorganisms. One study of 20,000 infants in the 1930's showed that in the first nine months of life, 1.5 of every 1,000 breastfed babies died of infant diseases, while 85 of every 1,000 fed cow's milk perished during that time.

Another ingredient in milk is lactose, a simple sugar that is digested by lactase, an enzyme produced in the intestine. In most traditional societies, lactase is no longer produced after the baby is weaned from its mother's milk between ages two and four. As a result, ingestion of dairy products after that age produces indigestion, diarrhea, cramps, allergy, or other illnesses. This condition is called lactose intolerance.

In the West, however, dairy products have become a dietary staple over the course of many generations. Biologically, lactase continues to be produced in the intestine after early childhood, allowing dairy foods to be consumed into adulthood and later life. Among Caucasians, lactose intolerance is low. Only 2 percent of Danes cannot digest milk and other dairy products, 7 percent of Swiss, and 8 percent of white Americans. In contrast, about 70 percent of black Americans are lactose intolerant, as well as 90 percent of Bantus, 85 percent of Japanese, 80 percent of Eskimos, 78 percent of Arabs, and 58 percent of Israeli Jews.

Despite the body's ability to adapt to long-term dairy consumption, the excessive intake of fat and cholesterol in milk, cheese, butter, ice cream, and similar foods has taken a heavy toll as the consumption of these foods has increased. The per capita intake of dairy food in the United States now stands at 350 pounds a year, including 72 gallons of milk. In the United States there is now one cow for every two people.

In composition, milk is 28 percent fat, cheese is 50 percent, butter is 95 percent, and yogurt is 15 percent. Fatty acids and cholesterol from these foods can build up around the organs and tissues, contributing to heart disease, cancer, and other degenerative conditions. Mentally and psychologically, dairy foods affect the brain and nervous system, contributing to dullness, passivity, and dependence. Studies show that people from ethnic groups that are lactose intolerant tend to have higher IQ's than those that are not. The fat from cow's milk also insulates and impedes the flow of electromagnetic energy through the body, diminishing sexual polarity and attraction between men and women.

The quality of milk and dairy food consumed today has also changed from the past. The milk itself is changed from its natural state through modern heating procedures, homogenization, sterilization, and addition of other ingredients such as vitamin D. In an effort to make them produce greater quantities of milk, modern dairy cows are fed a variety of hormones, antibodies, and other chemicals that further dilute the quality of the milk. Today 75 percent of all U.S. dairy cows are artificially inseminated and through superovulation and embryo transfer a cow can now give birth to a dozen calves a year instead of only one.

As a result, the dairy products available today are very different from those consumed by previous generations. Until modern times, most cultures limited their dairy products to fermented foods such as yogurt, kefir, or other foods containing enzymes and bacteria, allowing them to be broken down in the digestive process in the absence of lactase. Cultured products like yogurt are superior to other dairy foods. However, they still cannot be recommended for regular consumption because they are now not traditionally and naturally processed and cannot be properly assimilated by people with sedentary lifestyles. A fermented vegetable food such as miso, tempeh, natto, or tamari soy sauce is preferable if processed naturally and is an important part of a cancer-prevention diet.

In the past, animal milk (especially goat, sheep, or donkey milk) was used for infants whose mothers could not breastfeed, for certain medicinal purposes, or in small quantities with other dairy products for personal enjoyment on special occasions. The abuse of dairy food in the modern diet and its degenerating artificial quality are major factors in the rise of breast cancer, heart disease, and other serious illnesses. The quality of our daily food determines the quality of our blood. The quality of blood, in turn, determines the quality of mother's milk and the biological strength of the next generation.

MEDICAL EVIDENCE

• In the early eighteenth century, Scottish physician George Cheyne reported that a grain-based diet could prevent and relieve serious illnesses, including cancer. He asserted that any cancer that can be cut out, such as breast cancer, could by a "seed diet continued ever afterward, be made as easy to the patient and his life and health as long preserved, almost, as if he had never been afflicted with it." By seeds, Cheyne meant "rice, sago, barley, wheat, millet, and the like." Source: George Cheyne, M.D., *An Essay on Regimen* (London, 1740).

• In his medical writings, early nineteenth-century Prussian physician Christoph W. Hufeland, M.D. warned against giving babies cow's milk:

> Nothing is more injurious to the health than artificial suckling. I have almost always found that children brought up in this way were more or less disposed to the scrofulous disease [tuberculosis]. . . . Compare children that are nourished at the maternal breast with those that are artificially brought up, and you will see that, generally, while the former are fat, fresh looking, and healthy, the latter remain weak and languid, at least during the first year of their existence. . . . Marasmus, pulmony consumption, dropsy, cancer, caries, and malignant ulcers: such are the consecutive affections of scrofulous which generally terminate in death." Source: C.W. Hufeland, M.D., *A Treatise on the Scrofulous Disease* (Philadelphia, pp. 37-39, 90, 1829).

• "A real cancer may be taken out," Pierpont Bowker, a nineteenth-century authority on American Indian native medicine, wrote, "but this can never cure the disease in the person, for it is in every part more or less. To cure a real cancer, whether the common kind or what is called a rose cancer, the whole system must be first cleansed of canker. When this is done, there is nothing left to support what is called the cancer." For eliminating toxins from the breast, he recommended a poultice made of bread and milk in which various herbs were mixed. Source: Pierpont Bowker, *The Indian Vegetable Family Instructor* (Utica, N.Y., 1851).

• In an address before the Belgium Cancer Congress in 1923, Frederick L. Hoffman, cancer statistician for the Prudential Life Insurance Company, reported that cancer was unknown among the Indians of Bolivia and Peru. "I was unable to see a single case of malignant disease. All the physicians whom I interviewed on the subject were emphatically of the opinion that cancer of the breast among Indian women was never met with. Similar investigations of mine among the Navajo and Zuni Indians of Arizona and New Mexico have yielded identical results." Hoffman associated the rise of cancer in industrial society to overnutrition and the introduction of refined and artificial foods. Source: quoted in *Cancer* 1:215–17, 1924.

• In 1942 Albert Tannenbaum, M.D., cancer researcher at Michael Reese Hospital in Chicago, reported that mice on a caloric restricted diet had substantially less induced breast tumors, lung tumors, and sarcoma than mice on an unrestricted diet. Source: A. Tannenbaum, "The Genesis and Growth of Tumors II: Effects of Caloric Restriction Per Se," *Cancer Research* 2:460–67.

• In another experiment in 1942, Dr. Tannenbaum reported that mice on a high-fat diet had a significantly higher incidence of spontaneous breast cancer and induced skin tumors than mice on a low-fat diet. He noted also that tumors appeared about three months earlier in the high-fat group. Source: A. Tannenbaum, "The Genesis and Growth of Tumors III: Effects of a High-Fat Diet," *Cancer Research* 2:468–75.

• Sunlight or daylight appears to exert a protective effect against breast cancer. In studies between 1959 and 1961, Dr. Samuel Lee Gabby of Sherman Hospital in Elgin, Illinois, reported that in chemically induced tumor experiments of thirty pairs of mice, every female mouse except one kept in a room with pink fluorescent light developed breast cancer. All but six of those in a room lit with white fluorescent lights contracted cancer. Of eight pairs of controls in daylight cages, six females developed breast cancer two months later than the other mice and two remained healthy. Source: John Ott, *Light, Radiation, and You* (Old Greenwich, Conn.: Devin-Adair, p. 100, 1982).

• In regions where total and long-term breastfeeding is practiced, breast cancer is rare. In 1969 Canadian medical researcher Otto Schaefer, M.D. reported that over a fifteen-year period only one case of breast cancer was observed in a group of Eskimo whose population grew from 9,000 to 13,000. In populations of Eskimo where breast cancer was very low but on the increase, Dr. Schaefer cited a decrease in the duration of breastfeeding or its complete elimination as a contributing factor. A 1964 study of breast cancer patients at

Roswell Park Institute in New York found that breastfeeding for seventeen months decreased the risk of breast cancer. Women who had lactated for a total of thirty-six months had a much reduced risk. As for possibly transmitting some cancer-causing substance through mother's milk, two other recent studies showed no difference in the breast cancer incidence in daughters who were breastfed by mothers who later were found to have cancer. Source: Marian Tompson, president, La Leche League International, *The People's Doctor: A Medical Newsletter* 4(4):8, 1980.

• In 1973 researchers reported a high positive correlation with breast and colon cancer and total fat, animal protein, and simple sugar consumption but practically none with dietary fiber. Source: B.S. Drasar et al., "Environmental Factors and Cancer of the Colon and Breast," *British Journal of Cancer* 27:167–72.

• In a 1975 case-control study of seventy-seven breast cancer cases and seven controls, five categories of foods were associated with breast cancer: fried foods, fried potatoes, hard fat used for frying, nonmilk dairy products, and white bread. The researcher also reported that Seventh-Day Adventist women age thirty-five to fifty-four have 26 percent less breast cancer than the general population and women in the church over fifty-five have 30 percent less. The Seventh-Day Adventists, about 50 percent of whom are vegetarian, emphasize whole grains, vegetables, and fruit in their diet and avoid meat, poultry, fish, coffee, tea, alcohol, spices, and refined foods. Source: R.L. Phillips, "Role of Life-Style and Dietary Habits in Risk of Cancer among Seventh-Day Adventists," *Cancer Research* 35:3513–22.

• In 1975 an epidemiologist reported that there was a five- to tenfold difference in breast cancer mortality between countries with an average per capita low-fat diet and those with a high-fat diet. Source: K.K. Carroll, "Experimental Evidence of Dietary Factors and Hormone-Dependent Cancer," *Cancer Research* 35:3374–83.

• A 1976 study of the relationship of diet and breast cancer in forty-one countries found that a high intake of refined sugar was associated with increased incidence of the disease. Source: G. Hems, "The Contributions of Diet and Childbearing to Breast-Cancer Rates," *British Journal of Cancer* 37:974–82.

• Since 1949 the consumption of milk and milk products has increased 23 times in Japan, meat 13.7 times, eggs 12.9 times, and oil 7.8 times. While stomach cancer rates have declined, the incidence

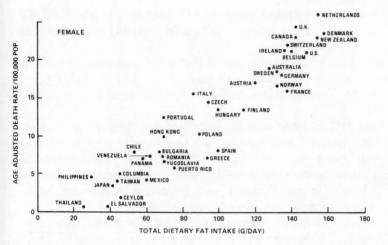

of breast and colon cancer have substantially increased. "Among all nutritional elements, dietary fat intake has shown the most striking increase in Japan in recent years," the epidemiological study concluded. Source: T. Hirayama, "Changing Patterns of Cancer in Japan with Special Reference to the Decrease in Stomach Cancer Mortality," in H.H. Hiatt et al. (ed.), *Origins of Human Cancer, Book A., Incidence of Cancer in Humans* (Cold Spring Harbor, N.Y.: Cold Spring Harbor Laboratory, pp. 55–75, 1977).

• A 1977 study reported a higher incidence of breast cancer in the unsuckled left breast of women in Hong Kong fishing villages who traditionally breastfed only with the right breast. The study of 2,372 Tanka women from 1958 to 1975 concluded that "in postmenopausal women who have breastfed unilaterally, the risk of cancer is significantly higher in the unsuckled breast and that breastfeeding may help to protect the suckled breast against cancer." Source: R. Ing et al., "Unilateral Breastfeeding and Breast Cancer," *Lancet* 2:124–27.

• In a 1978 test, significantly more breast tumors were observed in rats fed refined sugar than in those fed rice and other starches. "These results are consistent with epidemiological data showing that age-adjusted breast cancer mortality in humans is positively correlated with sugar intake and negatively correlated with intake of complex carbohydrates," the researchers concluded. Source: S.K. Hoehn and K.K. Carroll, "Effects of Dietary Carbohydrate on the Incidence of Mammary Tumors Induced in Rats by [DMBA]," *Nutrition and Cancer* 1:27–30.

• In 1979 researchers reported that dairy products as a class increased the risk of breast cancer. Source: S.P. Gaskill et al., "Breast Cancer Mortality and Diet in the United States," *Cancer Research* 39:3628–37.

• An MIT biologist reported in 1979 that studies of women medically screened for breast cancer and women who went unscreened showed both a lower incidence of breast cancer and substantially lower mortality from breast cancer in the unscreened group. Source: M.S. Fox, "On the Diagnosis and Treatment of Breast Cancer," *Journal of the American Medical Association* 241:489–94.

• Studies of breast cancer mortality in England and Wales from 1911 to 1975 linked the rise of the disease with consumption of fat, sugar, and animal protein one decade earlier. Source: G. Hems, "Association Between Breast-Cancer Mortality Rates, Child-Bearing, and Diet in the United Kingdom," *British Journal of Cancer* 41:429–37, 1980.

• In 1980 scientists reported that a diet high in soybeans reduced the incidence of breast cancer in laboratory experiments. The active ingredient in the soybeans was identified as protease inhibitors, also found in certain other beans and seeds. Source: W. Troll, "Blocking of Tumor Promotion by Protease Inhibitors," in J.H. Burchenal and H.F. Oettgen (eds.), *Cancer: Achievements, Challenges, and Prospects for the 1980s, Vol. 1* (New York: Grune and Stratton, pp. 549–55).

• In a case-control study of 577 cases and 826 control, researchers reported in 1981 that relative risk of breast cancer increased significantly with more frequent consumption of beef and other red meat, pork, and sweet desserts. Source: J.H. Lubin et al., "Breast Cancer Following High Dietary Fat and Protein Consumption," *American Journal of Epidemiology* 114:422.

• In 1981 researchers reported a direct association between intake of serum cholesterol and breast cancer. Source: A.R. Dyer et al., "Serum Cholesterol and Risk of Death from Cancer and Other Causes in Three Chicago Epidemiological Studies," *Journal of Chronic Diseases* 34:249–60.

• In 1982 scientists at the University of Western Ontario reported that the addition of soy protein in a person's diet could reduce serum cholesterol levels irrespective of other dietary considerations. In addition to animal studies, the researchers compared human volunteers who drank either cow's milk or soy milk and reported that "both cholesterol and triglyceride values dropped substantially during the soy period." Source: *Journal of the American Medical Association* 247:3045–46.

• Vegetarian women are less likely to develop breast cancer, researchers at New England Medical Center in Boston reported in 1981. The scientists found that vegetarian women process estrogen differently from other women and eliminate it more quickly from their body. The study involved forty-five pre- and postmenopausal women, about half of whom were vegetarian and half nonvegetarian. The women consumed about the same number of total calories. Although the vegetarian women took in only one third as much animal protein and animal fat, they excreted two to three times as much estrogen. High levels of estrogen have been associated with the development of breast cancer. "The difference in estrogen metabolism may explain the lower incidence of breast cancer in vegetarian women," the study concluded. Source: B.R. Goldin et al., "Effect of Diet on Excretion of Estrogens in Pre- and Postmenopausal Incidence of Breast Cancer in Vegetarian Women," *Cancer Research* 41:3771–73.

• A fifty-year study of diet and breast cancer mortality in England and Wales between 1928 and 1977 showed that at the onset of World War II breast cancer mortality markedly fell as consumption of sugar, meat, and fat declined and consumption of grains and vegetables increased. By 1954, consumption of these foodstuffs returned to prewar levels. Breast cancer mortality did not return to prewar levels until some fifteen years later, suggesting a lag time between the ingestion and appearance of the disease. Source: D.M. Ingram, "Trends in Diet and Breast Cancer Mortality in England and Wales, 1928-1977," *Nutrition and Cancer* 3(2):75–80, 1982.

• In laboratory experiments, a diet consisting of 20 percent polyunsaturated fat, such as that found in margarine, enhanced tumors more effectively than saturated fat, provided that it served as an adequate source of essential fatty acids. Source: *Diet, Nutrition, and Cancer* (Washington, D.C.: National Academy of Sciences, p. 5:19, 1982).

DIAGNOSIS

Ninety percent of breast cancer in the United States is diagnosed following discovery of a lump by the woman or her partner. Although 80 percent of lumps are classified as benign, doctors like to take a soft-tissue x-ray of the entire breast called a mammogram. If a malignancy is suspected, a biopsy will be taken to determine whether the growth is a cyst or a tumor. Hormone tests, x-rays of the chest and skeleton, bone-marrow aspiration, and scans of gallium, liver, and bone will generally follow. Until the mid-1970's mammography was widely offered as a preventive measure to detect cancer in the early stages. However, in 1976, Dr. John Bailar III, editor of the *Journal of the National Cancer Institute*, reported that breast x-rays could cause as many deaths through radiation as they could save through early detection. Since then, mammography has been curtailed and is now recommended by doctors usually only for women over fifty, women over thirty-five with cancer in one breast, and women forty to forty-nine whose mother or sister have had breast cancer.

In addition to self-examination of the breasts, Oriental medicine looks for signs of developing mammary disorders in the condition and complexion of the cheeks. As a result of parallel embryonic development, the cheeks reflect underlying changes in the chest region, including the lungs and breasts, and in the reproductive region.

Cheeks with well-developed firm flesh and a clean, clear skin color show sound respiratory and digestive functions, especially if there are no wrinkles or pimples in the area. Red or pink cheeks, except during vigorous exercise or when out in cold weather, show abnormal expansion of the blood capillaries, caused by heart and circulatory disorders due to the overconsumption of yin foods and drinks, including fruits, juices, sugar, and drugs. Milky-white cheeks are caused by the overconsumption of dairy products such as milk, cheese, cream, and yogurt. A pinkish shade mixed with the white indicates excessive intake of flour products and fruits. Both these colors indicate accumulation of fat and mucus in various regions of the body, including the breasts, lungs, intestines, and reproductive organs.

Fatty spots that are dark, red, or white in color on the cheeks are a sign of fat accumulation in either the lungs or breast and often accompany the beginning of cyst or tumor formation. Coffee and other stimulant, aromatic beverages may contribute to the appearance of this color on the cheeks. Pimples on the cheeks show the elimination of excessive fat and mucus caused by the intake of animal food, dairy products, and oils and fats. If these pimples are whitish in color, the main cause is milk and sugar. If yellowish, the cause is cheese, poultry, and eggs. A green shade on the cheeks shows that cancer is developing in the breasts, lungs, or large intestine.

Certain colors and marks appearing on the white of the eye also indicate abnormal conditions in the corresponding areas of the body. In the case of the breasts, a transparent or pale-white color in the upper outer region of the eye shows the presence of stagnated fat and mucus, which may be growing into a cyst or tumor. Cataracts also may indicate cyst formation. If these colorings or swellings occur in the right eye, the right breast is affected; if in the left eye, the left breast.

Green vessels appearing along the Heart Governor meridian or Long meridian from the wrist toward the elbow on the inside softer side of the arm also show the development of cancerous conditions in the breast or lung region. A similar condition is indicated by the appearance of green and dark colors, together with irregular swelling on the inside of the wrist.

DIETARY RECOMMENDATIONS

For breast cancer, all dairy food and all fatty, oily food, including meat, poultry, eggs, and other animal products, are to be eliminated. Sugar, honey, and other sweeteners as well as soft drinks and other foods and beverages treated with sugar are also to be avoided. Tropical fruits, fruit juices, and vegetables such as potato, yam, sweet potato, asparagus, tomato, and eggplant should not be consumed. Because they are excessively mucus-producing, all flour products are to be avoided except for occasional consumption of nonyeasted unleavened whole-wheat or rye bread. Chemicalized and artificially produced and treated foods and beverages are to be completely eliminated. Even unsaturated vegetable oil is to be completely avoided or minimized in cooking for a one- or two-month period. All ice-cold foods and drinks including ice cream should be avoided. Although they are not the cause of breast cancer, all stimulants, spices, coffee, alcohol, and aromatic, fragrant beverages and drugs should be avoided because they enhance tumor development.

The following general dietary guidelines are recommended for breast cancer:

• Fifty to sixty percent of daily consumption, by volume, should be whole-cereal grains. The most preferred are pressure-cooked medium or small-grain brown rice and, frequently, millet and barley. All other grains can be used occasionally including whole-wheat berries, barley, rye, and oats. Buckwheat groats may also be eaten from time to time, though corn may need to be used less than other grains. In addition to nonyeasted unleavened whole-wheat or rye bread, traditional breads and grain products such as chapati, matzo, tortillas, and corn arepas may be eaten from time to time. These flat breads should be made from cooked grains and mashed rather than processed from flour. Whole-wheat and buckwheat pasta or noodles may be used also on occasion for variety and a change of flavor.

• Five to ten percent soup, consisting of one to two bowls per day of miso soup or tamari soy sauce broth cooked with kombu, wakame, or other sea vegetables and with various land vegetables such as onions and carrots. Occasionally, a grain-based soup such as brown-rice soup with vegetables or barley soup with vegetables can be used as substitutes. In selecting miso, naturally processed miso, especially barley miso or hatcho miso, is preferred and it should have fermented for a long time, one-and-a-half to two years or more. Similarly, tamari soy sauce should also be naturally made and aged for a comparable period.

• Twenty to thirty percent vegetables, cooked in a variety of forms. When steaming or boiling, the water can be squeezed out of the vegetables by hand before serving. Root vegetables such as burdock, carrots, daikon, and jinenjo (long mountain potato), should be used almost daily. Round vegetables such as cabbages, onions, fall-season squashes and pumpkins, and hard or leafy vegetables such as watercress, broccoli, and dandelion are also recommended and can be prepared separately or together. To season these vegetables during cooking, use unrefined sea salt, tamari soy sauce, or miso in moderate volume. Pickled vegetables may be eaten in small volume, but they should be a type that is aged for a long time. Daily or frequent consumption of dried daikon and daikon leaves, pickled for a long time with rice bran (nuka) and unrefined sea salt, are recommended to help clean fatty substances from the blood. In the event that oil is desired, sautéed vegetables can be made with a small volume of sesame oil or, occasionally, corn oil. No raw salad is recommended for a short period, depending upon the person's condition, though a boiled salad that has cooked for one to two minutes may be consumed often. Oily salad dressings should not be used.

• Five percent small beans, such as azuki beans or lentils, may be used daily, cooked together with sea vegetables such as kombu or with onions and carrots. Chickpeas and black soy beans can be used infrequently, though it is preferable to avoid all large beans for an initial period of a few months. For seasoning, a small volume of unrefined sea salt or tamari soy sauce or miso can be used. Bean products, such as tempeh, natto, and dried or cooked tofu may be used occasionally but in moderate volume.

• Five percent or less sea vegetable dishes. All sorts of sea vegetables can be used and cooked in various styles, though hijiki and arame and very well cooked kombu are to be eaten more often.

The best condiments for women with breast cancer are gomashio (sesame salt), kelp or wakame powder, and umeboshi plum, and tekka, though all other regular macrobiotic condiments may be used. These condiments may be used daily on grains and vegetables, but the volume should be moderate to suit individual appetite and taste.

Finely chopped scallions mixed and heated with an equal volume of miso and a small portion of grated ginger are helpful to soften hardening of tissues and tumor. One or two teaspoons may be used each day on grain and vegetable dishes.

Fish and other animal food are to be avoided. However, in the event that animal food is craved, powdered dried, small fish can be used as a condiment for grains, soups, and vegetable dishes. Small pieces of nonfatty white-meat fish may be used when very strong cravings for animal food develop.

Sweets, desserts, fruits, and fruit juices are to be avoided. However, in the event of cravings, cooked or dried fruits that are locally grown and in season may be eaten in limited, small amounts and very infrequently.

Nuts and nut butters are to be avoided due to their high amount of fat and protein. Roasted seeds such as sunflower seeds and pumpkin seeds may be consumed occasionally as a snack.

Seasoning, such as unrefined sea salt, tamari soy sauce, and miso, as well as condiments, are to be used moderately in order to avoid unnecessary thirst. If you become particularly thirsty after the meal or in between meals, you should cut back on these seasonings and condiments until the normal level of thirst returns.

All beverages and other dietary practices can follow the general recommendations as outlined for cancer patients in the cooking section. In the event of hunger pains, which women sometimes get with this condition, one or two bowls of brown rice with half an umeboshi plum put inside and wrapped with toasted nori may be eaten.

The most important thing in connection with dietary practice is chewing very well, until all food becomes liquid in the mouth and well mixed with saliva. It is also important to avoid overeating and eating just before sleeping.

As explained in the introduction to Part II, cancer patients who have received or who are currently undergoing medical treatment may need to make further dietary modifications.

HOME CARES

• If the breast tumor is small and hard, a ginger compress may be applied daily, although this application should be avoided for a large tumor. For a large tumor, an application of clay can be helpful in some cases. Also, a white potato plaster mixed with mashed leafy green vegetables can be applied for a few hours following the application of a ginger compress for five to ten minutes. This potato-vegetable plaster should be made in paste form, adding 20 to 30 percent white flour, with possibly a little water to moisten if too dry. The application should be continued for three to four hours daily.

• A taro potato plaster applied for three to four hours on the area of the tumor and repeated every day may also be very beneficial. The taro plaster should be applied following a ginger compress for five to ten minutes to activate circulation. However, depending upon the case, this plaster may temporarily enlarge the tumor by withdrawing the excess mucus and fat from the inner part of the mammary tissues toward the surface of the skin. Eventually, the fatty mucus, sticky substances, and unclean blood that make up the tumor will drain out. Accordingly, the application of the taro plaster should be administered carefully and may not be proper for some cases. In the event the tumor has already burst and active drainage of toxins is occurring, clean vegetable oil can be applied on the area covered with a sanitized cotton cloth to prevent open tissues from directly contacting the clothing. Preferably, the administration of the taro plaster should be under the guidance of an experienced macrobiotic counselor or medical professional.

• In cases where the taro plaster results in too rapid a discharge, a lotus root plaster can be used instead. This consists of a 50/50 mixture of grated fresh lotus root and mashed cabbage or other green vegetable leaves, mixed thoroughly with 20 to 30 percent white flour to hold them together and 5 to 10 percent grated ginger. This plaster is applied directly on the skin, kept for three to four hours, and repeated daily for about two weeks.

• In cases where a breast has already been surgically removed and the surrounding lymph nodes, neck, and in some cases arm have become swollen, a buckwheat plaster can be applied following a brief ginger compress.

• In the event the lymph glands under the armpit and along the arm become swollen due to the cancer spreading from the breast through the lymph system, medical attention may be necessary. Again, qualified macrobiotic counselors or medical associates should be consulted. Massage is often helpful in reducing such swelling.

OTHER CONSIDERATIONS

• Breast-cancer patients are subject to depression and should do everything possible to maintain a cheerful and calm attitude. Smile, be optimistic, dance, sing, and enjoy each day for itself.

• Daily scrubbing of the whole body with a towel that has been immersed in hot gingerroot water helps to accelerate circulation of body fluids and energy. It will also help eliminate through the skin accumulated toxins caused by intake of excessive fat and protein.

• Avoid wearing wool and synthetic fabrics. At the minimum wear cotton underwear and sleep on cotton sheets and pillow cases.

• Avoid wearing metallic jewelry, including rings, bracelets, and necklaces. These pick up excess charges from the atmosphere and transmit them to the internal organs via the meridians running along the fingers and hands. It is fine, though, to wear a wedding ring.

• Avoid watching television for long stretches. Radiation weakens the chest area. Similarly, avoid other artificial sources of electromagnetic energy such as video terminals, smoke detectors, and hand-held electrical appliances.

• If possible, avoid birth-control pills or estrogen replacements. These are extremely weakening and can accelerate breast cancer.

• Breastfeed your baby if you are able. There is no danger of transmitting the disease to your child, and breastfeeding will have a protective effect on both mother and baby.

PERSONAL EXPERIENCE

Metatastic Breast Cancer

In October 1972, Phyllis W. Crabtree, a fifty-year-old home-maker, nursery school teacher, and grandmother from Philadelphia, had an operation for cancer in which her uterus, ovaries, and Fallo-pian tubes were removed. By January 1973, the tumor metastasized, and she had a modified radical mastectomy of the right breast.

In the hospital, her son Philip, who had studied macrobiotic cook-ing, brought her miso soup, brown rice, and bancha tea. The first food offered Phyllis by the hospital had been a bowl of Froot Loops.

Breast surgery was a very frightening experience for her. "One of the most terrifying is the signing of that paper which gives a doctor the right to cut out or off any part that he deems necessary," she observed afterward. "By the time I was admitted for the mastectomy, it was my fourth admission in ten weeks, my fourth signing, and this time I knew what they were going to take. For each operation, there was an initial trip for biopsy, an okay from the frozen section, and then a return trip for surgery when more lab work had been com-pleted. Another very simple hospital procedure that was sheer horror for me was the presurgical shave and shower. Watching the surgical nurse shave my chest from armpit to armpit and washing my breasts for what might have been the last time was a very emotional pro-cedure. Before the biopsy, as I washed (and the tears flowed almost as fast as the shower) I wondered if I would have none, one, or two the next day." Mrs. Crabtree was so distraught from the experience that she had to see a psychiatrist afterward to help her deal with her loss.

Over the next three years, she gradually began to implement macrobiotics with the support of her son, daughter, and husband. She cut out sugar from her diet, increased vegetables, and reduced her intake of red meat, dairy food, and martinis. In the summer of 1976, however, the newspapers and television were filled with stories about a connection between cancer and contraceptives and hormone medication. Mrs. Crabtree, who had taken these drugs, became depressed again and suspected that cancer was spreading to her liver.

Once again her son impressed upon her the need to follow the diet closely and to take full responsibility for her condition and recovery. In March 1977, she attended the East West Foundation cancer and diet conference in Boston and came to see me. "I listened and had an appointment with Michio Kushi," she recalled later. "One phrase from the classroom kept haunting me: 'There are no cancer victims, only cancer producers.' Michio recommended a healing diet and sent me off to eat far more strictly than ever before."

The next summer Mrs. Crabtree returned, and I told her that she was 60 percent healed and to continue eating carefully. By autumn of 1978, Phyllis had completed the five-year "cure" period for her original illness and outlived 85 percent of women who had had similar operations on uterus and breast.

"I'm grateful to macrobiotics for more than a cancer 'cure,'" she stated. "For myself, there has been an improvement in my aching back (caused by osteoporosis) and a urinary infection (both ailments of thirty years' duration). The migraine headaches are fewer in number and less in intensity and duration. Even my motion sickness has lessened.

"My husband has benefitted from the diet through weight control. Michio's lectures in Los Angeles many years ago were instrumental in returning Phil to us from his 'hippy' world. My daughter adopted a baby girl because she had been unable to conceive. She now has three daughters, two of them 'macrobiotically brewed.'"

Source: Phyllis W. Crabtree, "A Grandmother Heals Herself," *East West Journal*, November 1978, pp. 74–81.

14.

Female Cancers: Ovary, Endometrium, Cervix, and Vagina

FREQUENCY

Cancer of the reproductive organs is the second most common form of cancer in American women. Breast cancer, with which it is often associated, is first. In 1983 an estimated 22,500 women will die of cancers of the ovary, endometrium, cervix, vagina, and other reproductive organs, and 117,200 new cases will develop as well as 45,000 new cases of noninvasive cancer of the cervix.

Ovarian cancer, which will claim 11,500 lives, is rarely detected early and kills most patients in less than a year. There are many varieties of ovarian tumors, both benign and malignant, and precancerous conditions including dermoid cysts. Standard treatment for ovarian cancer is a *hysterectomy* (surgical removal of the uterus) and a *salpingo-oophorectomy* (removal of the ovary and Fallopian tubes). This operation may be done through the vagina or the abdomen, and the woman will no longer have menstrual periods or be able to conceive children. An *omentectomy* is also often performed as a preventive measure, and this operation involves removing a fold of abdominal membrane, which is often the site of metastases. Internal or external radiation treatment may follow surgery, and chemotherapy may be used for maintenance. The current survival rate for ovarian cancer is from 31 to 55 percent.

Cancer of the uterus, especially the endometrium, comprises 4 percent of all cancers in the United States and will account for 39,000 new cases in 1983 and 3,000 deaths. In some parts of the country it is growing at the rate of 10 percent a year. This dramatic rise, almost unparalleled in the history of cancer, has been associated with use of the birth-control pill by women of child-bearing age and estrogen replacement therapy in menopausal women over fifty. Usual treatment is a total abdominal hysterectomy. The ovaries, Fallopian tubes, and pelvic lymph nodes may also be taken out depending on the individual case. Radiation treatment and chemotherapy commonly follow, along with hormone therapy, especially large doses of progesterone. The remission rate is 66 percent.

Cancer of the cervix appears primarily in women over forty. However, it is on the increase in younger women, and cervical dysplasia and sometimes herpes type 2 virus are considered precancerous conditions. Cervical cancer can spread to other reproductive sites as well as the rectum, bladder, liver, lymph, and bones. It is treated with a hysterectomy, radium implants, or experimental chemotherapy. Cervical dysplasia is often treated with cryosurgery, a procedure in which nitrous oxide or other gas is used to freeze and kill affected cells. In 1983, about 7,000 American women will die of cervical cancer, and 16,000 new cases will develop. The five-year survival rate ranges from 10 to 85 percent.

Cancers of the vagina and vulva are rarer, accounting for about 1,000 deaths in 1983 and 4,400 new cases. They affected women mostly over fifty, but are increasingly found in younger women as well. Vaginal tumors tend to spread quickly to the pelvic lymph nodes, and vulvar tumors may spread to the vagina, lungs, liver, or bones. Depending on the stage and type, the patient may receive a hysterectomy, a vaginectomy (removal of the vagina), or a vulvectomy (removal of the vulva). Internal radiation implants and external pelvic irradiation may be used to supplement surgery. Survival rates range from 8 to 75 percent.

STRUCTURE

The ovaries are the primary organs of the female reproductive system. Each of these tiny paired organs is about the size of an almond and the production of eggs (ova) takes place in the follicles. A follicle consists of an ovum surrounded by one or several layers of follicle cells. At birth, the ovaries contain about 800,000 follicles. This number decreases until, at menopause, few, if any, follicles remain. When a follicle has reached maturity, it will either rupture and release its ovum or collapse and decompose. The former process is known as ovulation. The latter process is called atresia and involves the natural degeneration and discharge of follicles from the body during menstruation.

Following ovulation, the egg enters a fingerlike end of the Fallopian tube and begins its movement into the uterus. If intercourse has taken place, the egg has the possibility of being fertilized. The union of egg and sperm occurs in the fimbriated end of the uterine tube. If an ovum is fertilized, it begins to develop as it passes through the uterine tube and into the uterus. Implantation of the fertilized ovum in the uterus takes place after about seven to ten days. The uterus or womb averages two-and-a-half inches in length and weighs approximately fifty grams. It has a capacity of two to five cubic centimeters and is tightly constructed. During pregnancy it increases substantially and at full term reaches a length of about twenty inches. The uterus returns to its original condition following delivery.

The lining of the uterus, which is shed during menstruation and is regenerated after about two days, is called the endometrium. The neck of the uterus, connecting the womb with the vagina, is called the cervix. The chief organs of intercourse are the vagina and the vulva, consisting of the major and minor lips, and the clitoris.

CAUSE OF CANCER

Female sexual disorders have risen sharply in recent years. In 1979, approximately 700,000 American women had hysterectomies. At this rate, about half of the women in the country will have their uterus and ovaries removed by age sixty-five. The variety of sexual disorders ranges from menstrual cramps and irregularities to vaginal discharge, blocked Fallopian tubes, ovarian cysts, fibroid tumors, and cancer. To understand the origin and development of these illnesses, we must examine the menstrual cycle.

The cycle of menstruation correlates with the process of ovulation. During the first half of the menstrual cycle, between the woman's period and ovulation, the hormone estrogen reaches its peak. During the second half of the menstrual cycle, between ovulation and onset of the period, the hormone progesterone predominates. The length of time taken for each stage in the cycle is largely dependent on the types of food that a woman eats. If a woman eats primarily whole grains and cooked vegetables, menstruation usually takes only three days. However, among women who eat a diet high in meat, sugar, and dairy products, five or six days is the norm. The next phase, in which the endometrium regenerates itself, usually takes two days.

However, with proper eating, this can be accomplished in only one day. The following stage, in which the follicle matures, lasts about eight days, and ovulation should occur in the part of the cycle that is exactly opposite to the onset of menstruation or, ideally, fourteen days. In healthy women, conception usually arises at this time or four to five days after ovulation. During this phase, the yellow endocrine body (corpus leteum) found in the ovary in the site of the ruptured follicle matures and secretes progesterone. This hormone influences the changes that take place in the uterine wall during the second half of the menstrual cycle. The follicle and corpus luteum eventually decompose during this phase if not fertilized and are discharged during menstruation.

If a woman is eating properly, her menstrual cycle should correlate with the monthly lunar cycle, or about twenty-eight days. During the full moon, the atmosphere becomes brighter and charged with energy. A woman who regularly eats grains, cooked vegetables, and other yang foods and is physically active will usually menstruate at this time. The condition of the atmosphere will cause her to become more energized, necessitating the discharge during her period. During the new moon, the atmosphere is darker or more yin. Women who menstruate at this time are usually consuming a more expansive diet. After eating properly for some period a woman begins to menstruate at the time of either the full or new moon, indicating that her condition is in harmony with the natural atmospheric and lunar cycle.

During the first half of the menstrual cycle, women quickly regain balance and can readily follow a more centered diet of whole grains, cooked vegetables, and seasonal fresh fruit. Immediately prior to ovulation, fertility is expressed with general feelings of joy, contentment, and bliss. The woman usually feels wonderful, exudes cheerfulness and confidence, and her eating remains centered during the few days of ovulation.

During the second half of the cycle, as menstruation approaches, some women experience dissatisfaction, irritability, and constant hunger. Overcooked foods, animal food, and other heavier substances may become unappealing and if taken in too great a quantity frequently lead to excessive intake of sweets, fruits, salad, and liquid. In such cases, just prior to menstruation, some women may experience swelling of the breasts and a general bloated feeling. The woman may continue to crave strong foods in the yin category and to feel impatient and melancholy.

In order to have a smooth menstrual cycle, it is important for the woman to adjust her diet during the two halves of her month. During the first two weeks, between menstruation and ovulation, she should eat plenty of dark, leafy, green vegetables along with whole grains and other more substantial foods to which she will be naturally attracted. During the last two weeks, between ovulation and menstruation, she will feel more comfortable if she reduces her intake of overcooked foods and avoids animal food altogether. Otherwise they will produce an increased craving for sweets, fruit, juices, salads, and lighter foods. To prevent this compulsion from arising, the woman can eat more lightly cooked vegetables at this time along with lighter seasonings and less salt. Special dishes, such as mochi, turnip or radish tops, or amasake, are very helpful and will reduce cravings for more extreme foods.

An irregular menstrual cycle results if the diet is imbalanced too much in one direction or the other. For example, if it totals less than twenty-eight days, this usually indicates an overly yang condition from eating excessive animal and overly energizing foods. A cycle longer than average, up to thirty-two or thirty-five days, shows that a woman may well be consuming too many foods in the yin category such as sweets, fruits, and dairy food. Both conditions can be corrected by eating a more central diet of grains and vegetables.

Menstrual cramps are usually caused by an excessive intake of animal products, especially meat, fish, eggs, and dairy food, in combination with too many expansive foods such as sugar, soft drinks, refined flour, and chemically processed foods. Cramps can be eliminated in two to three months on a balanced standard macrobiotic diet.

Excessive menstrual flow can result from overconsuming either too many foods from the yin or yang category. In the case of too many contractive foods, including animal foods rich in protein and fat, the blood thickens and the flow lasts longer. This is often accompanied by an unpleasant odor. When too many expansive foods, including foods that slow down the body metabolism, are consumed, the blood becomes thinner than normal, and menstruation is prolonged. When a woman eats a more balanced diet, menstruation will be of shorter duration and the flow will be lighter.

Biologically, women need not eat any animal food, except occasional consumption, if desired, of very light white fish or shellfish. Imbalanced diet can give rise to headaches, depression, and emotional outbursts prior to menstruation. This condition has recently been recognized by medical science under the name Premenstrual Syndrome. It can be corrected by centering the diet, especially avoiding extremes of meat and sugar and chemicalized food.

Deposits of fat and mucus, coming largely from animal foods, dairy foods, sugar, and refined flour products, often accumulate in the inner organs if an imbalanced way of eating continues over several years. In women this buildup tends to concentrate in the breasts and in the uterus, the ovaries, the Fallopian tubes, and the vagina. The solidification of mucus or fat around these organs can result in the development of cysts. Those which occur in the comparatively tight ovaries are saturated in quality, or yang, whereas those in the more expanded vagina or vulva contain more grease and mucus— their quality is yin. Most cysts are soft when they begin to form, but with the continuation of an improper diet they harden and often calcify. This type of cyst is something like a stone and is very difficult to dissolve. Some varieties of cysts contain fat and protein and can become extremely hard, in which case they are called dermoid cysts. Tumors represent the final stage in this process as the body attempts to localize the continuing influx of unhealthy nutrients by creating blockages and obstructions in various organs and sites of the body. The accumulation of fat and mucus can also block the Fallopian tubes, preventing the passage of egg and sperm and resulting in the inability to conceive.

The overconsumption of foods that create cysts and tumors in the reproductive organs include varied combinations of milk, cheese, ice cream, and other dairy products; sugar, soft drinks, chocolate, and other sweeteners; fruit and fruit juices; nut butters; greasy and oily foods; refined flour and pastries such as croissants, doughnuts, and sweet rolls; hamburger and other animal foods. Once again, serious reproductive illnesses may be relieved by eliminating extreme foods and centering the diet on whole grains, beans, vegetables, sea vegetables, and small volumes of fruit and seeds.

Recently some cancer specialists have linked the spread of herpes type 2 virus with cancer of the cervix. This type of herpes can be considered a precancerous condition, but it is not caused by a virus introduced from the outside. Herpes is the effect of poor eating, especially foods high in fat and sugar. A multitude of viruses and other microorganisms live in symbiosis with the human organism and usually will not give rise to disease unless the blood quality is weakened. If the blood quality is strong, the body's immune system will neutralize and destroy any harmful bacteria, viruses, or other organisms. The current epidemic of herpes is the result of degenerating blood quality. Widespread consumption of synthetic and artificial foods, on top of meat and sugar, have created a weakened condition in which harmful viruses can thrive. People who eat a balanced diet and over time have strengthened their blood and immune system need have no fear of getting infected with herpes.

MEDICAL EVIDENCE

• In 1674 an English physician named Wiseman associated cancer with the effects of faulty nutrition on the blood and sexual organs. "This disease might arise from an error in diet, a great acrimony in the meats and drinks meeting with a fault in the first concoction, which, not being afterwards corrected in the intestines, suffered the acrimonious matter to ascend into the blood; where, if it found vent either in the menstrua in women, or by the hemorrhoids or urine in men, the mischief might have been prevented." Source: Frederick Hoffman, *Cancer and Diet* (Baltimore: Williams & Wilkins, p. 6, 1937).

• In 1896 Robert Bell, M.D., senior staff member at the Glasgow Hospital for Women adopted a nutritional approach to tumors of the uterus and breast after twenty years as a cancer surgeon. "I had been taught that this [surgery] was the only method by which malignant disease could be successfully treated, and, at the time, believed this to be true. But failure after failure following each other, without a single break, inclined me to alter my opinion. . . . The disease invariably recurred with renewed virulence, suffering was intensified, and the life of the patient shortened. . . . That cancer is a curable disease, if its local development is recognized in its early stage, and if rational dietetic and therapeutic measures are adopted and rigidly adhered to, there can be no doubt whatever." Source: Robert Bell, M.D., *Ten Years' Record of the Treatment of Cancer Without Operation* (London: Dean & Son, pp. 6, 14–15, 1906).

• As early as 1938, when it was synthesized, laboratory tests associated DES (diethylstilbestrol) with breast cancer. From 1945 to 1970 the drug was widely used to prevent miscarriage, control menstrual disorders and estrogen deficiencies, serve as a "morning after" birth control pill, and act as a chemotherapeutic agent for prostate cancer in men and for breast cancer in postmenopausal women. In 1954 DES was approved by the U.S. Department of Agriculture as a feed additive for poultry, cattle, and hogs, and by 1970, 75 percent of all beef in the United States had been fattened with DES. In the early 1970s epidemiological studies associated the use of DES during pregnancy with an increase in vaginal and cervical cancer among the daughters of DES users, primarily between the ages of ten and thirty. DES was discontinued in 1979. Sources: Samuel S. Epstein, M.D., *The Politics of Cancer* (New York: Doubleday, pp. 214–33, 1979) and *Diet, Nutrition, and Cancer* (Washington, D.C.: National Academy of Sciences, 14:13–14, 1982).

• In 1974 epidemiological data associated ovarian cancer with a high-fat diet. Source: C.H. Lingeman, "Etiology of Cancer in the Human Ovary," *Journal of the National Cancer Institute* 53:1603–18.

• In 1975 researchers reported a direct correlation between per capita intake of total fat and incidence of cancer of the uterus and mortality from ovarian cancer. They also linked total protein consumption with endometrial cancer and total protein and fruit consumption with cervical cancer. Source: B. Armstrong and R. Doll, "Environmental Factors and Cancer Incidence and Mortality in Different Countries with Special Reference to Dietary Practices," *International Journal of Cancer* 15:617–31.

• Seventh-Day Adventist women in California ages thirty-five to fifty-four have 84 percent less cervical cancer and 12 percent less ovarian cancer than the national average, according to a 1975 epidemiological study. Female church members over fifty-five have 36 percent less cervical cancer and 47 percent less ovarian cancer. Together both age groups have 40 percent less uterine tumors of other kinds. The Seventh-Day Adventists, about half of whom are vegetarian, eat 25 percent less fat and 50 percent more fiber, especially whole grains, vegetables, and fruit, than the general population. Source: R.L. Phillips, "Role of Life-Styles and Dietary Habits in Risk of Cancer among Seventh-Day Adventists," *Cancer Research* 35:3513–22.

• "Worldwide use of birth control pills, in spite of conclusive evidence of carcinoginicity of estrogens in experimental animals," warned Samuel S. Epstein, M.D., "constitutes the largest uncontrolled experiment in human carcinogenesis ever undertaken." The cancer specialist cited studies estimating that oral contraceptives could cause 10,000 fatalities a year, especially from ovarian cancer. Source: Samuel S. Epstein, M.D., *The Politics of Cancer* (New York: Doubleday, p. 222, 1979).

• Endometrial cancer increased sharply during the early 1970's.

Researchers associated this with excessive use of synthetic estrogens by women at the time of menopause. In 1976, following publicity about the hazards of oral contraceptives and synthetic hormones, the use of estrogens partially diminished and endometrial cancer rates began to fall. Source: H. Jick et al., "The Epidemic of Endometrial Cancer," *American Journal of Public Health* 70:264–67, 1980.

• A 1981 epidemiological study in Hawaii found a direct association between ethnic patterns of total fat consumption (including animal fat, saturated fat, and unsaturated fat) and uterine cancer. Source: L.N. Kolonel et al., "Nutrient Intakes in Relation to Cancer Incidence in Hawaii," *British Journal of Cancer* 44:332–39.

• Writing in an American Cancer Society journal for clinicians in 1982, David Schottenfeld, M.D., chief of epidemiology and director of cancer control of Memorial Sloan-Kettering Cancer Center in New York, asserted that "some evidence suggests that the risk of uterine cervical dysplasia and carcinoma in situ may be increased by the long-term use of oral contraceptives." He stated that among women using Oracon®, the risk of endometrial cancer was 7.3 times that of non-users. There is also a risk for liver cancer among users of oral contraceptives, though recent studies show a lowered risk for ovarian cancer in pill users. Discussing iatrogenesis, or doctor-caused disease, he concluded, "The risk-benefit evaluation of a drug should take into account the likely outcome of the disease if untreated, and whether or not safer alternative therapies are available." Source: David Schottenfeld, M.D., "Cancer Risks of Medical Treatment," *Ca—A Cancer Journal for Clinicians* 32:258–79.

DIAGNOSIS

Ovarian cancer is generally diagnosed by gynecologists on the basis of a pelvic examination, a Pap smear, and a parancentesis or cul-de-sac aspiration in which fluid from between the vagina and rectum is drained out by needle for examination under a microscope. A needle biopsy will be taken if a malignancy is suspected, and metastases will be detected through a mammogram, GI series, or intravenous pyelogram (IVP). Uterine cancer is commonly observed following a pelvic examination and a D and C (dilatation and curettage) in which a small amount of tissue is scraped from the inside of the uterus. Metastases will be checked with x-rays to the chest, IVP, bone and liver scans, and endoscopy of the lower colon and bladder. Cervical, vaginal, and vulver cancers are diagnosed with a pelvic examination, a Pap smear, and a colposcopy, in which a viewing scope transmits a magnified area of the sex organs to a television monitor.

The condition of the reproductive system can be observed directly without technological intervention or potentially harmful x-rays. If the woman has a vaginal discharge, for example, its color can help locate the site and extent of the swelling. If the discharge is yellowish in color, a cyst is developing. A white discharge is less serious, but usually leads to development of a soft type of cyst unless the woman changes her way of eating. A green discharge signifies tumorous growth, especially if the color has been occurring for any length of time.

Vaginal discharges, ovarian cysts, and fibroid tumors are frequently indicated by a yellow coating in the lower part of the eye-whites. Dark spots in the eye-white indicate ovarian cysts or tumors or kidney stones.

The eyelashes also correspond with reproductive functions. Eyelashes that curve outward show degeneration of the sex organs due to consumption of excessive yin foods, especially fruits, juices, and dairy products during early childhood. Eyelashes that curve inward indicate excess intake of strong foods in the yang category including eggs and meat. In this case, there may be menstrual cramps or lack of menstruation due to contraction of the ovaries. Menstrual cramps are also indicated when a woman smiles by the presence of a horizontal line or ridge appearing between the upper lip and nose.

Split fingernails and abnormal colors on the fingertips, resulting from a chaotic way of eating, indicate malfunctions in the reproductive system as well. If one thumbnail or thumb tip shows these conditions and the other is normal, it indicates that the ovary corresponding to the abnormal side is malfunctioning.

Pimples in the center of the cheeks with a fatty appearance may reflect the formation of cysts in the ovarian region.

Along the bladder meridian, a green shade appearing around either ankle on the outside of the leg indicates developing cancer in the uterus or bladder. Also, a fatty swelling along the ankle region indicates mucus and fat accumulation in the uterine region and may be a sign of a precancerous condition.

DIETARY RECOMMENDATIONS

Cancer in the ovarian, uterine, cervical, and vaginal areas is largely caused by overconsumption of food rich in protein and rich in fat. It appears that the cancer is accelerated by the intake of synthetic chemicals, including various kinds of drugs and hormone substances, as well as artificial birth-control methods and other unnatural regulation of reproductive and menstrual functions. Accordingly, all these things should be avoided. Foods to be discontinued are all animal food rich in protein and fat such as meat, poultry, eggs, and dairy food, as well as fatty and oily fish and seafood. Sugar, sugar-treated foods, and other sweeteners, including artificial ones, also should be avoided. Flour products such as white bread, pancakes, and cookies tend to form mucus and fat and should not be eaten. Food and beverages that possess stimulant, aromatic, and fragrant characteristics, including seasonings such as curry, mustard, and pepper, coffee, alcohol, soft drinks, and herb teas should also be avoided. Oils, even unsaturated vegetable oils, should be minimized. All chemicalized foods and beverages are not to be ingested, while those of more organic and natural quality are recommended.

Following are general guidelines for daily food consumption:

• Fifty to sixty percent whole-cereal grains, including brown rice, whole wheat, oats, millet, rye, barley, corn, and buckwheat groats. Among them, brown rice is to be the primary food, barley and millet secondary foods, and the other grains used occasionally. Unyeasted whole-wheat or rye bread may be occasionally consumed as well as whole-wheat and buckwheat noodles and pasta. All the above cereal grains and their products are to be cooked without oil.

• Five to ten percent soup. Miso or tamari soy sauce can be used as seasoning for soup in which sea and land vegetables can be cooked. Occasionally, grain soup may be made. One to two bowls should be consumed daily.

• Twenty to thirty percent vegetables cooked in various styles, including steaming and boiling. However, sautéing and frying should be minimized because it is important to use as little oil as possible during the initial period. Kinds of vegetables can be varied—some root vegetables, some leafy, some round—but potato, sweet potato, yam, tomato, eggplant, and other vegetables that historically originated in the tropics even though now grown in temperate zones are to be strictly avoided. Raw, fresh salad is to be minimized. Except for homemade pickles, it is preferable to limit all raw vegetables for some period.

• Five to ten percent beans and bean products. Smaller beans such as azuki beans, lentils, and chickpeas are preferred over large beans. They can be cooked with sea vegetables such as kombu or hijiki or with vegetables such as carrots, onions, or squash. Tempeh, natto, or tofu (cooked) can be used occasionally.

• Five percent or less sea vegetables, cooked in various styles. All sea vegetables rather than just one or two kinds should be used regularly. They may be cooked with vegetables or served as a separate side dish and lightly seasoned with miso, tamari soy sauce, or sea salt.

All animal food, even fish and seafood, is to be avoided if possible. However, in the event that some animal food is craved, a moderate amount of nonfatty, white-meat fish may be eaten. This should be served with a volume of cooked, hard, leafy vegetables that is several times larger than the amount of fish prepared, and garnished with grated daikon or radish or a small amount of grated ginger. For seasoning, miso or tamari soy sauce may be used moderately.

Fruits and fruit juices are to be avoided, though cooked or dried nontropical fruits may be taken in small amounts, if craved.

Nuts and nut butters are to be avoided because of their high fat content. However, roasted sesame seeds, sunflower seeds, and pumpkin seeds may be consumed occasionally in small volume as a snack.

In the event of cravings for sweets, sweet brown rice and its product, mochi, may be prepared more often as well as cooked carrots, pumpkin, squashes, and other naturally sweet vegetables. If an even sweeter taste is craved, barley malt or rice syrup and other cereal-based natural sweeteners can be used in moderate volume.

A sour taste can be provided by sauerkraut, homemade pickles, and rice vinegar, though they should be used only occasionally and in moderate volume.

All seasonings, whether salty, sweet, or sour, are to be moderate.

All oily or greasy cooking methods, including deep frying, are to be avoided for some period until the condition improves. Salad dressings, mayonnaise (dairy or soy), and other oily dressings and spreads are to be avoided.

There are several special foods and beverages that are particularly beneficial for the female reproductive condition. Drinking one or two cups of sea vegetable juice every day is recommended. Simply boil the sea vegetable in water for ten minutes and consume the liquid. Arame is especially helpful.

In the event of a hard cyst or tumor, a small portion of dried shiitake mushrooms may be consumed every day cooked in soup or with vegetables. Prepare by cooking with daikon and seasoning moderately with miso or tamari soy sauce. They may also be cooked with wintermelon (obtainable in Chinese or Oriental grocery stores) and seasoned with miso.

For some cases of blocked Fallopian tubes or obstructions in other passages of the reproductive area, one to two cups of grated daikon, cooked with nori sea vegetable, seasoned with tamari soy sauce or miso, can be eaten daily.

Beverages for daily consumption include bancha twig or bancha stem tea, roasted brown rice tea, roasted barley tea, cereal grain coffee, and other nonaromatic, nonstimulating herbal teas. Among these, properly prepared Mu tea is highly recommended if consumed for a few-months period or occasionally. Mu is a medicinal tea made from either nine or sixteen different herbs that serve to warm the body and strengthen weak female organs.

Chewing thoroughly until all food substances become liquid is essential, as is avoiding overconsumption of food and not eating for three hours preceding sleep. All other dietary practice may follow the general recommendations for cancer prevention.

As explained in the introduction to Part II, cancer patients who have received or who are currently undergoing medical treatment may need to make further dietary modifications.

HOME CARES

• In the event of frequent vaginal discharges, a hip bath will facilitate the elimination of accumulated fat and mucus. Ideally, the water for the hip bath should contain dried leafy greens such as daikon or turnip greens. To prepare this bath, hang several dozen bunches of these leaves to dry, either near a window or outside, but not under direct sunlight. The leaves will first turn yellow and then brown, at which time they are suitable for use. Boil two or three bunches of dried leaves for each evening's bath for ten to twenty minutes in several quarts of water to which a handful of sea salt or kombu sea vegetable can be added. The water will turn brownish in color. Then, run hot water in the bathtub, add the mixture along with another handful of sea salt, and get in. The water should cover your hips. Wrap a thick cotton towel around your upper body to avoid chills and to absorb perspiration. As the water begins to cool, add more hot water, and stay in the tub for ten to fifteen minutes.

If dried leaves are not available for this bath, use sea vegetables, especially arame. If these cannot be obtained or are too expensive, add two handfuls of sea salt to the bathwater and proceed as above.

In the bath, your lower body will become very red as circulation in that area increases, and the stagnated fat and mucus inside the sex organs start to loosen. Immediately following the hip bath, douche with a preparation made with one teaspoon of sea salt, two teaspoons of rice vinegar or lemon juice, and one quart of warm bancha tea. This hip bath and douche can be taken every evening or every other evening for five to ten days and thereafter once every five days or once a week, until mucus and fatty substances are generally eliminated from the uterus and vaginal regions.

• In the case of a cyst, tumor (including fibroid tumor), or cancerous condition, it is helpful to apply a taro potato plaster for three to four hours on the lower abdominal region. This should be preceded by a ginger compress for five to ten minutes to warm the area and accelerate circulation. The taro application may be repeated every day for two to four weeks until substantial improvement is made.

• In the case of pain, one half hour of palm healing is helpful. This is done simply by placing one hand on a piece of cotton over the affected area, synchronizing the breath, keeping a peaceful mind, and allowing the natural energy of the environment to flow through the hand. Palm healing is more effective when a second person performs the healing, but it can be done alone. To relieve pain, it is also helpful in some cases to apply a paste of mashed green leafy vegetables mixed with flour for one to two hours, after warming the area with a hot towel. This green leafy plaster should be kept warm during the application by placing roasted sea salt wrapped with cotton cloth above the plaster. It is also helpful to apply a very hot compress, for example, a ginger compress, repeatedly on the base of the spine.

• Scrubbing the whole body daily with a towel, dipped in hot ginger water and squeezed out, is very helpful for circulation of blood and energy and thus improvement in the overall condition.

OTHER CONSIDERATIONS

• Avoid artificial methods of regulating your period, especially birth control pills, estrogens, and tubal ligation, which severs the flow of electromagnetic energy through the body. As your eating improves, your menstrual cycle will become more regular and attuned to the lunar cycle, and you can gradually begin natural birth-control methods.

• Avoid abortion and Caesarean section if possible. Study natural methods of delivery and, if you are in good health, consider home birth with the assistance of a midwife or other experienced medical person. Breastfeeding will help protect you and your child against future illnesses, including cancer.

• Avoid synthetic underwear and stockings, artificial tampons, chemical douches or toiletries, talcum powder, and other synthetic products that may be irritating or harmful to the reproductive system.

• During the menstrual period, a woman's excess is discharged through the skin as well as through the menstrual flow. It is recommended that a woman not take cold showers or wash her hair with cold water, since both of these tend to draw this excess away from its normal course of discharge. To clean yourself, use a wet towel or sponge.

• Deep relaxation exercises, including Do-in or shiatsu acupressure massage, around the lower back prior to menstruation, can help reduce physical and emotional discomfort. Active physical exercises are also important for healthy living.

PERSONAL EXPERIENCES

Uterine Tumor

In 1947 film star Gloria Swanson learned that she had a tumor in her uterus. She went to three gynecologists, and each one recommended an immediate hysterectomy. Finally she went to see a specialist who was considered to be the top woman's doctor in the country. "After examining me," she later recalled in an article for *East West Journal*, "he didn't say exactly what the first three had, but he did say, 'Well, you know this has to come out by Christmas'— which was about five months away."

Instead, Miss Swanson went to California to see Dr. Bieler, a physician who treated illness with diet. He said to her, "Now, Gloria, what is the function of a protein?" She said, "It's a cell builder, Dr. Bieler." He asked her, "Are you fully grown?" She said, "Dr. Bieler, don't pull my leg. You know I'm forty-seven." He said, "Well, maybe you're a ditch digger. Or are you a tennis pro? A football player?" She said, "What are you trying to tell me?"

Dr. Bieler went on to remind Gloria Swanson that she had had a hard time with the birth of her child in 1920. He also reminded her that cancer doesn't develop overnight but can sometimes take twenty years to develop.

"Have you been eating a lot of protein?" he asked her. "Well, I guess I have," she replied. "Well, now, what are you going to do about that, if it's a cell builder?" he inquired. "Do you really think I can starve this to death?" she said. The doctor smiled and said, "You get enough protein; you don't need all that animal protein." Gloria responded, "All right. As of this moment I shall not eat any more animal protein. How long do you think it will take?" The physician replied, "I don't know: a year, two years, maybe three."

For the next two years, despite a heavy travel schedule and demanding routine, Gloria carried around her own food, consisting primarily of whole grains and vegetables and a little bit of fruit. Two-and-a-half years had elapsed by the time she went back to see the famous specialist. "I had a feeling the tumor was gone," she wrote. "He hadn't heard from me since the time he told me what was going to happen around Christmastime (that would have been a nice Christmas present for somebody—a pathologist, I guess). I hopped up on his table, and he started hunting. Oh, it was fascinating to watch his face. I said, 'It isn't there, is it, Doctor?' 'No'—reluctantly. I said, 'Don't you want to know what I did?' 'What do you mean, what you did?' 'Well,' I said, 'I went on a diet.'"

The doctor threw his head back and laughed. "He thought it was very funny," she continued. "A diet: ha-ha-ha. I said, 'It was a non-animal protein diet, Doctor.' He laughed even harder. I said, 'Well, you can laugh; I don't think it's a laughing matter. I'm still a woman, and what's more, I'm very happy about it. But I'm not laughing about it, and I don't think you should laugh either. I'd hoped you might learn something, because I have. And I don't really think you ought to send me a bill.' And I hopped off and went home, and he never did."

In the more than thirty years since, Gloria has been extremely active in promoting natural foods and macrobiotics. Several years ago she and her husband, Bill Dufty, author of *Sugar Blues*, joined my wife Aveline and me on a visit and speaking tour of Japan. "You're responsible for your own health," Gloria tells people who ask her how she has maintained her health and beauty for over eighty years. "It's quite true. There's nobody who can chew your food for you. And so if you really want to be well, you have to do it yourself." Source: Gloria Swanson, "I'm Still a Woman," *East West Journal*, March 1977, pp. 34–35.

Dermoid Tumor

In the spring of 1977, Audrey Isakson of Kennebunkport, Maine, began to have very frequent menstrual periods and considerable back pain. "My doctor advised me to get into the hospital immediately and have surgery," she recounted after a large tumor was discovered on her right ovary. "But I decided to first try to heal myself through macrobiotics." She had just read Gloria Swanson's article in *East West Journal* and resolved to relieve her own uterine condition before submitting to surgery.

In August she attended the East West Foundation's summer program at Amherst College and in September visited Ed Esko, a macrobiotic consultant in Boston. In addition to the Cancer-Prevention Diet, he recommended that she apply taro potato plasters over the afflicted region and take regular daikon hip baths. In a short time Audrey's back pain subsided, and her menstrual periods started to become normal again.

"I went to the doctor six weeks after I had first seen her, and she examined me," she related. "The orange-size growth was gone." "How can you explain that it went away?" she asked her doctor. "I can't," the woman responded. Audrey then told her about the nutritional approach she had tried. "I'm rather skeptical," the doctor told her. "I really don't believe those kinds of things. But it seems to have worked for you." A final medical checkup four months later confirmed that "my ovary had returned to its normal size." Source: "Dermoid Tumor," *Cancer and Diet* (Brookline, Mass.: East West Foundation, 1980, p. 70).

Uterine Cancer

In December 1970, Janice Rokowski was five months pregnant. As part of a prenatal examination, she took a Pap test, which indicated the twenty-six-year-old woman had uterine cancer. Doctors confirmed the malignancy and told her that she had only six months to live. They suggested an immediate cone biopsy, a surgical procedure that might cause an abortion to the baby.

Janice refused to have the biopsy and within four days had moved from her home in Minneapolis to a macrobiotic study house in Boston. She had already been eating natural foods, but during her pregnancy had widened her diet to include sugar, refined and canned foods, dairy products, and meat three times a week in addition to grains and vegetables. At the study house, she eliminated meat, sugar, and refined foods from her diet and increased the amount of whole grains, beans, fermented soy products, land and sea vegetables, and nuts and seeds. Once a week she ate fish and an unsweetened cooked fruit dessert.

After following the Cancer-Prevention Diet for three weeks, chewing her food very well, and exercising, she had another Pap smear and there was no indication of cancer. Janice had no difficulties in the ensuing pregnancy or delivery, and her baby was entirely normal and healthy. "I feel that the good quality food I ate and the activity I engaged in brought about the change in the condition of my uterus in that short amount of time," she concluded. Source: "Uterine Cancer," A *Dietary Approach to Cancer* (Boston: East West Foundation, 1977, p. 25).

Cervical Cancer

In 1969, twenty-seven-year-old Donna Gail of New Haven, Connecticut learned that she had cancer on the surface of her cervix. Several Pap smears, two biopsies, and a conization, in which several layers of tissue around the cervix were scraped, at Yale New Haven Community Hospital confirmed the diagnosis.

Prior to that time she had not paid much attention to her diet, and her favorite foods had been frozen sweets (including ice cream, cake, and candy bars), beef, macaroni, salt, tomato sauce, and cheese. She also drank about twenty cups of coffee a day. Concerned about her weight and health, Donna altered her diet considerably following discovery of the cancerous condition. She reduced the volume of her food consumption in general and reduced animal foods, including dairy food, by about a third. She reduced her intake of refined flour, sugar, and sweets by 75 percent and tried to cut out all processed and artificial food.

In 1972 she learned about macrobiotics and came to hear me at a lecture in Rhode Island. The next day she decided to make whole grains the center of her diet and eliminated meat and dairy products entirely as well as strong sweets and raw food. "My diet became more balanced," she explained the change. "I now had a principle to follow. That was very important, because I had never had any dietary principle, nor had I understood the idea of balance."

In 1975, after a period of difficulty in her life, her eating habits became irregular and the cervical cancer returned. The gynecologist told her, "We have to do a biopsy. I am almost 100 percent sure you have cancer, and you need to have your reproductive organs removed." Donna returned the next day expecting him to tell her the biopsy had been positive. "No, you absolutely do not have cancer," the doctor reported. "You have an irritation. However, I still highly recommend that you have all of your organs removed as a preventive measure."

Donna refused and came to see me again for a consultation. I told her that she was consuming too many flour products and that even whole-wheat bread and baked products could contribute mucus to her system. Grains are preferably eaten in whole form rather than as flour. Donna reduced her consumption of flour and flour products, and the irritation in her cervix went away.

A variety of other ailments also cleared up as her understanding of macrobiotics and practice of the Cancer-Prevention Diet improved. She experienced reserves of energy for the first time in years, and her fainting spells stopped. Before, her menstrual period had also been debilitatingly painful. After two months on the Cancer-Prevention Diet, all pain disappeared. The flow had lightened and decreased from seven to five days. She had no more bloating before her period or soreness in her breasts. A scalp condition from which she suffered since childhood vanished, and her hemorrhoids went away.

There were other unexpected benefits as her way of life became more harmonious. "One of the most important changes I have been able to make since becoming macrobiotic," Donna relayed, "involves my relationship with my father. Up until two years ago, I hadn't spoken with him since I was twelve years old. Now we communicate regularly and have discovered a great mutual respect and caring for one another."

Donna is now a licensed practical nurse (LPN). She has worked as a nutritional consultant on both the East and West coasts, and her own experience overcoming cancer has greatly benefited others. Source: "Cervical Cancer," *The Cancer Prevention Diet* (Brookline, Mass.: East West Foundation, 1981, pp. 84–86).

Fibroid Tumor

Since childhood Diane Silver had been constantly ill. She first had pneumonia at age two, and her tonsils and adenoids were removed at the age of four. Beginning in 1957 she suffered from severe painful cystitis, and for the next fourteen years was treated every few months with sulfa. Pneumonia returned periodically for which she received antibiotics. Diane had a painful diaphragmatic hernia and had to sleep sitting up. She had premenstrual tension, edema, and severe menstrual cramps. In 1960 doctors removed a large mole growing on her forehead and told her she might have malignant melanoma. In 1969 a large fibroid tumor was surgically removed from her uterus. In 1971 a tumor was found in a lymph node on her neck, and she was diagnosed as having thyroid cancer. During the next few years she had bumps on her back and breasts that turned out to be benign. The fibroid tumor, however, returned and her Pap tests were irregular. By the fall of 1975 her endocrinologist told Diane that she would have to take sulfa drugs for the rest of her life. Tests indicated the cancer had spread to her kidney.

One day in October 1975, while bedridden with pneumonia, Diane received a phone call that changed her life. It was from a young man named Alan Ginsberg, who introduced himself as a friend of a friend in New York. "When he heard my gasping and coughing he remarked, 'You sound sick,'" Diane said, recalling the conversation. "'Yes, I have pneumonia,' I rasped. 'What are you eating?' he said. 'Well, in all my thirty-eight years of life, no physician had ever asked what I was eating.'

"I told Alan I was eating some cottage cheese, salad, lots of grapefruit and orange juice 'because I need fluids.' He asked me if I had considered that there were nine to twelve grapefruits in the two or three glasses of juice I was having every day; that grapefruits grow in hot climates—'That this is November and you're in Toronto in the winter and it's getting cold, and furthermore, cottage cheese and all dairy foods create mucus in the body, and you don't need any more mucus!' Was he some kind of nut, I wondered? Or was he making sense?"

Alan asked her if she had any whole grains in the house. She had only oatmeal, and he advised her to eat just oatmeal, with no milk or sugar on it, for several days and he would call back. Diane was very skeptical, but after a few days of just oatmeal she was out of bed, feeling better, and ready to listen to what Alan had to say. He called back, explained to her the principles of macrobiotics and sent her some books to read. After a few months on the diet, Diane was strong enough to begin to exercise and take short walks.

At the end of December 1975, I gave a lecture in Toronto and Diane came to see me. "Mr. Kushi reaffirmed for me everything Alan had said," she noted in reviewing her case. "He amazed me because he diagnosed all my conditions simply by looking at my face and feeling my arm. Mr. Kushi said that I was still cancerous and gave me a list of foods to eat and those to avoid."

When Diane subsequently gave up taking birth-control pills, she said: "My doctor assured me I would be back for a hysterectomy very shortly because the fibroid tumors would grow wildly without hormonal control. The following year at my regular check-up, he reported that they had disappeared—and that I was in better shape than I had been for years." Diane's Pap smear registered normal, her diaphragmatic hernia caused no further trouble, and her menstrual periods came without pain, swelling, or tension. Other longstanding problems also vanished, including pneumonia, the varicose veins in her legs, and the lumps and bumps on her back and breasts.

"Last winter I took up cross-country skiing and ice skating again," Diane reported in 1978. "I used to feel chilled all winter. Now I find pleasure at being outdoors in the cold. My attitude and my body have changed drastically; my entire life has changed for the better." In the six years since her recovery, Diane has become active in the East West Center in Toronto, teaching macrobiotic cooking and a more natural way of life to others. Source: "Thyroid Cancer, Fibroid Tumors," *Cancer and Diet* (Brookline, Mass.: East West Foundation, 1980, pp. 72–73).

Endometriosis

In the early 1970's, nineteen-year-old Tonia Gagne was diagnosed as having endometriosis, a disease that results from an implantation of tissue within the walls of the uterus and around the ovaries and intestines. She had just had a baby, which she gave up for adoption, and soon after began to have a profuse vaginal discharge and agonizing cramps. Following two months in the hospital, she had her left ovary and Fallopian tube surgically removed. Doctors put her on hormonal therapy and prescribed Enovid-10. As a result of taking this pill three times a day for nine months, her hair began to fall out and her mental state, already fragile, deteriorated.

In 1973 Tonia went to live at the Zen Center in San Francisco, and meditation helped center her life. A friend introduced her to macrobiotics and the principles of ecological cooking. Nevertheless, Tonia, whose ancestry was partly Puerto Rican, was still attracted to some of the tropical food on which she grew up. "One of the things I loved was fried bananas," she said, looking back on this time in her life. "When I was told that if I wanted to practice macrobiotics correctly, I would have to give up fried bananas, I said, 'Oh no, not that.'" She included some brown rice, miso soup, and vegetables in her diet but continued to eat dairy food, sugar, and fried bananas. She went off Enovid-10, but her health continued to worsen.

In April 1976, Tonia returned to New England, and doctors at South Boston Community Center told her that the endometriosis had come back. Medical tests showed that she also had uterine cysts, and her right ovary had swollen to the size of a tennis ball. The doctors told her they would have to operate and she would never be able to have children again.

Tonia decided against the operation and moved into a macrobiotic study house where trained cooks prepared a special diet for her condition. Within three months on balanced food and no fried bananas, the cyst had disappeared. Over the next year her health improved, but the vaginal discharge persisted, and she still suffered from occasional cramps. In August 1977, Tonia and her new husband came to see me at the East West Foundation's summer program in Amherst.

"I sat down with Michio and he looked at my left hand and my left foot," she noted afterward. "He looked into my eyes and examined my face and then he said to me, 'You have no left ovary, right? Also, right ovary not so good, right? Also, tumor in your descending colon.' Then he looked at me and said, 'Maybe you have cancer.'"

I took out a piece of paper and drew a diagram describing the exact proportions of food she should be eating. I told her to eat 60 percent whole-cereal grains, the rest cooked vegetables, miso soup, various condiments, and to avoid all animal products, especially dairy food and meat. I told her to eliminate all oil, flour products, and fruits from her diet until her condition improved and to take regular hip baths in daikon leaves and to apply a plaster of taro potato over her reproductive organs to loosen the accumulation of fat and mucus.

"Within two weeks after I followed that diet," Tonia reported, "the pain subsided. I had a feeling of elation. My energy came back and a lot of worry was gone."

During the next two years, Tonia had to eat very strictly. Even the slightest deviation, such as an occasional peanutbutter cookie or a carob brownie, would bring back the pain, cramps, and other symptoms of endometriosis. Gradually, however, she began to enjoy macrobiotic cooking and adjusted to living in a temperate climate without eating bananas and other tropical foods. About seven months after she began to practice the diet correctly, she became pregnant. Six weeks after giving birth to her son, Taran, she underwent a full examination by her physician. Medical tests showed no sign of endometriosis.

"Now I find myself much happier and more fulfilled," Tonia concluded several years after fully restoring her health. "Macrobiotics isn't any kind of religion or belief system. I had thought that macrobiotics would take the fun out of my life, but instead, I have learned to have more fun. I've learned balance. My life (and sense of enjoyment) is much simpler and much more fulfilling than I have ever before felt."

In January 1981, Tonia gave birth to a second child by natural childbirth at her home and experienced no complications. For a woman who was told she would never have children again, Tonia has become a living example of faith in the healing powers of nature. A balanced diet is the birthright of us all. Sources: "Endometriosis and Tumor in the Colon," *The Cancer Prevention Diet* (Brookline, Mass.: East West Foundation, 1981, pp. 90–91) and Tom Monte, "Journey to Motherhood: Tonia's Triumph Over Illness and Infertility," *East West Journal*, March 1982, pp. 44–48.

15.

Cancer of the Large Intestine

FREQUENCY

Cancer of the large intestine, including the colon and rectum, is the second most common cancer in the United States (lung being number one for men and breast for women). It is also known as colorectal cancer, bowel cancer, and cancer of the gut. In 1983 an estimated 58,100 Americans will die of this disease, and about 126,000 new cases will develop. Rectal cancer is slightly more prevalent in men, colon cancer more frequent in women, and each type is on the increase in both sexes. About 54 percent of tumors appear in the rectum, 23 percent in the sigmoid colon, 13 percent in the ascending or right colon, 8 percent in the transverse colon, 3 percent in the descending colon, and 1 percent in the anus. Bowel cancer is much less common in the Far East. In Japan the rate is about one-fourth the American incidence.

Current medical treatment calls for surgical removal of part or all of the large intestine. After the tumor and some healthy adjacent tissue are taken out, the ends of the remaining part of the colon are sewn together. If this is not possible, a colostomy is performed in which an opening is made in the skin and a disposable plastic bag is worn to collect feces. Radiation and chemotherapy may be administered after surgery in an attempt to control metastases. Cancer of the large intestine often spreads to the lungs or liver and, in women, the ovaries. Forty-four percent of patients who have surgery for colon or rectal cancer can expect to live five years or more. This is one of the higher survival rates achieved by modern cancer therapy. However, unless the diet is changed, tumors tend to recur in the intestinal tract or elsewhere, occasioning further surgery.

STRUCTURE

The large intestine meets the small intestine at the cecum, turns upward (ascending colon), crosses the abdomen (transverse colon), winds down (descending colon), makes an S-shaped turn (sigmoid colon), and extends straight (rectum) to the anus. Altogether, the entire bowel tract is about five feet long. Like other organs, the large intestine can be classified according to its relative degree of expansion and contraction, or yin and yang. In structure, the large intestine is yin—long, soft, expanded, smooth. In contrast, its complementary opposite, the lungs, are more yang—small, firm, compact, textured.

The major functions of the large intestine are 1) to absorb water, vitamins, and minerals through its mucus-lined tissue to be sent to the liver for distribution through the body, and 2) to eliminate waste and excessive nutrients from the body including iron, magnesium, calcium, and phosphates. The large intestine's functions are complementary to the lungs, which 1) regulate delivery of oxygen to the heart for distribution in the bloodstream, and 2) regulate elimination of carbon dioxide and other gaseous wastes from the body. Interestingly, the total number of cases of cancer of the large intestine and cancer of the lung are almost the same: 120,000 and 122,000, respectively. Without drawing too much from this correlation, this close incidence may suggest an underlying relationship between the origin and development of these two forms of cancer. Oriental medicine has traditionally treated them as a pair of organs that are antagonistic and complementary to each other.

CAUSE OF CANCER

People living in modern society suffer from a multitude of intestinal disorders. These include diarrhea, constipation, gas, enteritis, colitis, hernia, appendicitis, obesity, hemorrhoids, diverticular disease, and spastic or irritable colon. In general, these conditions arise from overeating, inadequate chewing of poor-quality food, overworking, and not enough exercise. The colon becomes further abused because of irregular patterns of eating, especially snacking between meals and eating before bedtime, which puts an increased burden on the inner organs.

A sedentary lifestyle, including long hours watching television or the habit of riding in cars for short distances instead of walking, is another major factor contributing to intestinal ailments. In traditional societies, where intestinal disorders and cancer of the colon are rare, people are much more orderly and active. They eat only two or three times a day, rarely eat between meals or before going to sleep, and approach their daily activity as creative participants rather than as passive spectators.

The traditional diet, which has protected hundreds of human generations from cancer and other degenerative diseases, is high in what today we call fiber or roughage. Fiber includes the insoluable cellulose found in the cell walls of cereal grains, vegetables, and fruit; the endosperm of seeds; and the lignins or substances that constitute the woody pulp of growing plants. Whole grains are the best source of fiber, containing about four to five times as much as a similar volume of vegetables and about fifteen to twenty times as much as fruit. In the large intestine, fiber works like a sponge to absorb water, bile acids, and other waste products, giving bulk to the feces and propelling them quickly through the system. Fiber also serves to modify cholesterol metabolism, bind trace metals, and neutralize various irritants, residues, and toxins that accumulate in the intestinal lining. In addition, there are several hundred different kind of bacteria in the colon that synthesize enzymes and vitamins, especially the B-complexes. A regular diet of fibrous whole grains and vegetables is necessary for the proper functioning of these bacteria.

The consumption of meat, dairy products, and other animal foods, on the other hand, weakens the digestive tract and can lead to various colonic disorders. Unlike grains and vegetables, which do not usually putrefy before they are eaten, animal protein starts to decompose as soon as the animal is killed. This process is offset by refrigeration or the addition of preservatives in the form of spices or chemicals. But putrefaction resumes as soon as the animal protein is cooked and eaten, and by the time it reaches the colon, decay has set in. The harmful bacteria from this decay tend to accumulate in the large intestine.

In addition to the synthesizing yang group of bacteria in the colon, there is a yin group of bacteria, which decomposes the remaining food particles into elementary compounds. These bacteria can break down a small amount of animal fat and protein in the colon, but the volume of these foods ingested by many people today cannot be properly metabolized. As a result, excess ammonia and bile acids begin to accumulate in the bowel tract. Along with the harmful bacteria produced by the putrefaction of animal food, these substances give rise to mutations in the lining of the large intestine, injure and kill cells, and lower the body's natural immunity to infection.

The shape, size, color, texture, and frequency of the bowel movement indicate the specific condition of the large intestine and overall health of the individual. People consuming a traditional or macrobiotic diet high in whole grains usually pass from thirteen to seventeen ounces of solid waste a day. Those consuming a high-fat, high-protein diet discharge only three to four ounces a day. On the whole-grain diet, food takes about thirty hours to travel from the mouth through the gastrointestinal tract. On the modern diet, transit time averages two to three days and in elderly people can take up to two weeks. Nearly 100 percent of the foods in humanity's traditional diet contain fiber, and this way of eating produces a bowel movement that is large and long, light in color, soft in consistency, and floats in water. Only 11 percent of the calories from the modern diet come from foods with fiber, and the bowel movement tends to be small, compact, dark in color, hard in consistency, and sinks in water. Lack of fiber in the diet slows down the movement of feces and allows the buildup of harmful bacteria. Furthermore, the muscles of the large intestine must work harder to propel small, compact wastes. As pressure builds, small sacs erupt in the lining of the colon called diverticula. These pockets, in turn, can become inflamed as harmful bacteria and waste material become trapped.

Cancer of the large intestine is generally preceded by spastic colon, colitis, or diverticulosis and the growth of polyps. Though usually classified as benign nodules by modern medicine, polyps should be viewed as a precancerous condition. Polyps, or abnormal growths in the mucosa of the colon, represent a defensive measure on the part of the large intestine to limit the passage of harmful material. When the colon can no longer protect itself with benign resistance, full-fledged obstructions in the form of cancerous tumors result. Of course, these blockages may be cut out by surgery. But unless daily diet, the source of the disease, is changed, cancer will spread to other organs and eventually the patient will die.

Nearly 75 percent of intestinal cancer in the United States occurs in the rectum and sigmoid or lower colon—the compact yang end of the gut. This suggests overconsumption of meat, eggs, salty cheeses, poultry, and other extreme yang foods as major causative factors. However, the intestines can also become loose and sluggish from excessive intake of sugar, alcohol, refined flour, and other extreme yin substances, resulting in cancer of the ascending colon. Tumors in the transverse or descending colon result from a combination of extreme yin and yang foods and beverages.

Over the last decade there has been increased scientific interest in the relationship between diet and colon cancer. Among the major forms of cancer, colon and breast cancer are now generally associated with a high-fat, high-protein diet by epidemiologists and clinical researchers. Still, the progressive development of intestinal sickness is not widely understood. Modern medicine continues to employ a variety of laxatives, enemas, and colonics to speed up elimination, relieve constipation, and reduce pain. In the long run, these medications only further expand and weaken an already overactive bowel tract. Additional complications then develop requiring a still stronger application of temporary, chemical antidotes. We must begin to look at the other end of the digestive system for a permanent solution to intestinal disease. A balanced diet centered around whole grains offers lasting relief from colonic ills and the promise of improved health and vitality in the future.

MEDICAL EVIDENCE

• In 1809 Dr. William Lambe published a book associating cancer with a diet high in meat and other animal products. He reported that tumors in the digestive system could be progressively reduced and eliminated by a diet centered on plant foods. "We may conclude that it is the property of this regimen, and, in particular, of the vegetable diet, to transfer diseased action from the *viscera* to the exterior parts of the body—from the central parts of the system to the periphery. . . ." Source: Dr. William Lambe, *Effects of a Peculiar Regimen in Scirrhous Tumors and Cancerous Ulcers* (London: J. Mawman, 1809).

• In the mid-nineteenth century Ellen White, prophet and leader of the Adventist movement, encouraged her followers to give up meat, rich casseroles, and pastries and eat plain food, prepared in the simplest manner, according to climate and season. "Those who eat flesh are but eating grains and vegetables second-hand, for the animal receives from these things the nutrition that produces growth. The life that was in the grains and vegetables passes into the eater. We receive it by eating the flesh of the animal. How much better to get it direct, by eating the food that God provided for our use. . . . People are continually eating flesh that is filled with tuberculous and cancerous [substances]." Source: Ellen White, *Ministry of Healing* (Mt. View, Calif.: Pacific Press Publishing Association, p. 313, 1905).

• At the beginning of the twentieth century, British cancer specialist and Fellow of the Royal College of Surgeons W. Roger Williams linked the rise of cancer in Western society to excess protein, especially animal protein, and asserted that cancer was a disease of the whole body, not just separate organs. In his 519-page book, *The Natural History of Cancer*, he asserted:

Tumour formation has too commonly been regarded as an isolated pathological entity, having no connection with other biological processes. Yet between tumour formation and morphological variation in general there is, I believe, real affinity; and in ultimate analysis both may be regarded as the outcome of the cumulative effects of changed conditions of existence. Of these conditions the most important seems to me to be changed environment and excess of food. . . . Malignant tumours in mankind and animals consist mainly of albuminous or protein substances; and it seems not unreasonable to suppose that they may be the outcome of excess of these substances in the body, and especially of such of them as serve for nuclear pabulum. When excessive quantities of such highly stimulating forms of nutriment are ingested, by beings whose cellular metabolism is defective, I believe there may thus be excited in those parts of the body where vital processes are most active, such excessive and disorderly proliferation as may eventuate in cancer. . . . It has been clearly established, that cancer is of most frequent occurrence among the well-to-do, highly nourished communities of occidental Europe; and, within the limits of these communities, as I have proved, the disease is commonest among the well-to-do groups. Source: W. Roger Williams, M.D., *The Natural History of Cancer* (New York: William Wood and Co., pp. 12–13, 1908).

• During World War I, Mikkel Hindhede, M.D., Superintendent of the State Institute of Food Research, persuaded the Danish government to shift its agricultural priorities from raising grain for livestock to grain for direct human consumption. Accordingly, in the face of a foreign blockage, the Danes ate primarily barley, whole-rye bread, green vegetables, potatoes, milk, and some butter. In the nation's capital, the death rate from all causes, including cancer, fell 34 percent during 1917 to 1918. "It was a low protein experiment on a large scale, about 3 million subjects being available," Hindhede reported to his medical colleagues: ". . . People entered no complaints; there were no digestive troubles, but we are accustomed to the use of whole bread and we knew how to make such bread of good quality." Sources: M. Hindhede, "The Effects of Food Restriction During War on Mortality in Copenhagen," *Journal of the American Medical Association* 74:381–82, 1920.

• In 1932 an English medical writer linked cancer with diet and an artificial way of life, recommending brown rice and other whole foods for relieving gastrointestinal tumors. "Brown breads, standard bread or whole-meal bread or unpolished rice are also helpful by furnishing coarse particles for that stimulation of the bowels, so desireable for their movement." Source: John Cope, *Cancer: Civilization: Degeneration* (London, 1932).

• After serving as a surgeon for the British in Africa from 1941 to 1964, Denis P. Burkitt, M.D. concluded that cancer and other degenerative diseases were rare and in some cases virtually unknown among traditional societies. Over the course of thirteen years, the internationally renowned cancer specialist (after whom Burkitt's lymphoma is named) reported that in one South African hospital with 2,000 beds only six patients were observed with polyps, a condition of the colon that sometimes precedes cancer. He attributed the "replacement of carbohydrate foods such as bread and other cereals by fat (and animal fat in particular)" with the rise of cancer and other degenerative diseases during the last century. Burkitt also cited studies showing that forty to fifty years ago, the incidence of colon cancer among Afro-Americans was less than whites but higher than among rural Africans today. In recent years, as American blacks began to eat less grains, especially cornmeal, and more fat and protein, their rate of intestinal cancer rose to that of whites. Source: Denis P. Burkitt, M.D., *Eat Right—To Stay Healthy and Enjoy Life More* (New York: Arco, pp. 11, 66–71, 1979).

• In the early 1960's, Dr. Maud Tresillian Fere, a physician living in New Zealand, reported curing herself of colon cancer by adopting a whole-grain diet that excluded meat, fish, cheese, sugar, stimulants, spices, and refined salt. She theorized that cancer and other degenerative diseases resulted from excess acidity or alkalinity. "In good health our blood and lymph are slightly alkaline, as also are our bodies. . . . It is no good having a bit of one's body cut out, as in a cancer operation, if the irritant poison is in one's whole body. One must eat the right food in the right proportion and so purify the bloodstream, thus rendering the operation unnecessary." Source: Dr. Maud Tresillian Fere, *Does Diet Cure Cancer?* (Northamptonshire, England: Thorsons, pp. 18–21, 1971).

• In 1961 surgeon Donald Collins, M.D. reported that five of his long-time patients had cured themselves of rectal cancer by eating an organically grown diet. He noted that each of the five patients lived for a further twenty-one to thirty-two years, and medical tests showed they died from causes other than cancer. "The only constant factor in the lives of these five persons was the fact that they all ate home-raised organically grown foods that were free from chemical preservatives and insect repellant sprays." Source: D.C. Collins, M.D., "Anti-Malignancy Factors Apparently Present in Organically Grown Foods," *American Journal of Proctology* 12:36–37.

• In 1968 a major epidemiological study indicated that dietary habits and environmental influences are the chief determinants of the world's varying cancer rates and not genetic factors as some scientists had believed. Data showed that in the course of three generations, Japanese migrants in the United States contracted colon cancer at the same rates as the general American population. In contrast, the regular colon cancer rate in Japan remained about one fourth the American incidence. Source: W. Haenszel and M. Kurihara, "Studies of Japanese Migrants," *Journal of the National Cancer Institute* 40:43–68.

• In 1969 scientists reported a high correlation between animal protein consumption and colon cancer incidence. Source: O. Gregor et al., "Gastrointestinal Cancer and Nutrition," *Gut* 10:1031–34.

• In 1973 British researchers found a high positive correlation with colon and breast cancer and total fat and protein consumption. Source: B.S. Drasar and D. Irving, "Environmental Factors and Cancer of the Colon and Breast," *British Journal of Cancer* 27:167–72.

• In 1973 British scientists reported that bran and fiber in the diet inhibited the production of bile salts by intestinal bacteria in the colon. The researchers contrasted this with white flour and sugar and hypothesized that the refining of foods might be a cause of cancer of the large intestine. Source: E.W. Pomare and K.W. Heaton, "Alteration of Bile Salt Metabolism by Dietary Fibre," *British Medical Journal* 4:262–64.

• In 1974 researchers for the National Cancer Institute linked colon cancer with high beef consumption. "The evidence suggests that meat, particularly beef, is a food associated with malignancy of the large bowel." Source: J.W. Berg and M.A. Howell, "The Geographic Pathology of Bowel Cancer," *Cancer* 34:807–14.

• A 1975 study found that laboratory animals fed a diet consisting of 35 percent beef fat experienced a significant increase in intestinal tumors. Source: N.D. Nigro et al., "Effect of Dietary Beef Fat on Intestinal Tumor Formation by Azoxymethane in Rats," *Journal of the National Cancer Institute* 54:439–42.

• In 1975 Harvard Medical School researchers reported that Boston-area macrobiotic people eating a diet of whole grains, beans, fresh vegetables, sea vegetables, and fermented soy products had significantly lower cholesterol and triglyceride levels and lower blood pressure than a control group from the Framingham Heart Study eating the standard American diet. The average serum cholesterol in the macrobiotic group was 126 milligrams per deciliter versus 184 for controls. Analysis further showed that consumption of dairy foods and eggs significantly raised cholesterol and fat levels in those eating macrobiotically, although fish was consumed as much as dairy and eggs combined. "The low plasma lipid levels in the vegetarians," the researchers concluded, "resemble those reported for populations in nonindustrialized societies," where heart disease, cancer, and other degenerative illnesses are uncommon. Source: F.M. Sacks et al., "Plasma Lipids and Lipoproteins in Vegetarians and Controls," *New England Journal of Medicine* 292:1148–51.

• In 1975 an epidemiological study associated cancer of the large intestine among women in twenty-three countries with either increased meat consumption or lowered consumption of cereal grains. Source: J. Cairns, "The Cancer Problem," *Scientific American* 233 (11):64.

• Epidemiological studies in 1977 reported the strongest correlation between cancer of the large intestine and per capita consumption of eggs, followed by beef, sugar, beer, and pork. Source: E.G. Knox, "Foods and Diseases," *British Journal of Preventive Social Medicine* 31:71–80.

• In 1977 an Indian cancer researcher asserted that the virtual

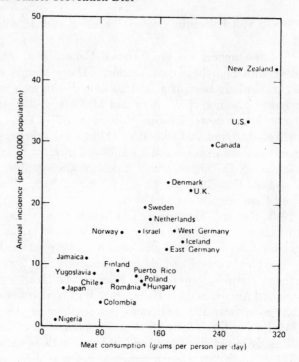

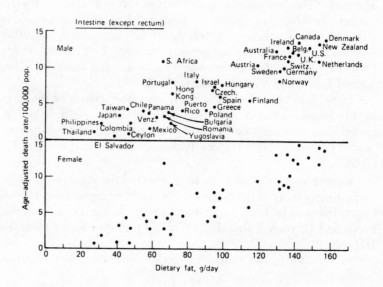

absence of colon cancer among Punjabis in northern India appeared to be due to their high-fiber diet. The Punjabis' diet consists primarily of whole-grain chapatis, thick dal made with lentils, vegetable curry, and a small amount of fermented milk products. In South India, where colon cancer is prevalent, the staple is polished white rice and considerably more fat, oil, and spices are used in cooking. The researcher further concluded that thorough chewing seemed to lower the risk of cancer, "The proper chewing of meals ensuring that mucous-rich saliva mixed with the food seemed to be protective factors." Source: S.L. Malhotra, "Dietary Factors in a Study of Cancer Colon from Cancer Registery, with Special Reference to the Role of Saliva, Milk and Fermented Milk Products, and Vegetable Fibre," *Medical Hypotheses* 3:122–26.

• In 1977 researchers associated consumption of dietary fat and age-adjusted mortality from cancer of the colon in forty-one countries. Source: E.L. Wynder and B.S. Reddy, "Diet and Cancer of the Colon," in Myron Winick (ed.), *Nutrition and Cancer* (New York: John Wiley, p. 57).

• A 1978 case-control study in New York reported that a decreased risk of colon cancer was associated with frequent ingestion of vegetables, especially cabbage, brussels sprouts, and broccoli. Source: S. Graham et al., "Diet in the Epidemiology of Cancer of the Colon and Rectum," *Journal of the National Cancer Institute* 61:709–14.

• In 1980 scientists reported an increased risk of both colon and rectal cancer from elevated consumption of calories, total fat, total protein, saturated fat, oleic acid, and cholesterol. The highest risk was found for saturated fat consumption and there was evidence of a dose-response relationship. Source: M. Jain et al., "A Case-Control Study of Diet and Colo-Rectal Cancer," *International Journal of Cancer* 26:757–68.

• In a 1981 study of twenty-one macrobiotic individuals, Harvard medical researchers reported that the addition of 250 grams of beef per day for four weeks to their regular diet of whole grains and vegetables raised serum cholesterol levels 19 percent. Systolic blood pressure also rose significantly. After returning to a low-fat diet, cholesterol and blood pressure values returned to previous levels. Source: F.M. Sacks et al., "Effects of Ingestion of Meat on Plasma

Cholesterol of Vegetarians," *Journal of the American Medical Association* 246:640–44.

• A preliminary 1981 report implicated refined sugar in the development of induced colon tumors in rats. Test animals given a 1.6 percent glucose solution developed approximately twice the number of tumors than controls. Source: D.M. Ingram and W.M. Castleden, "Glucose Increases Experimentally Induced Colorectal Cancer," *Nutrition and Cancer* 2:150–52.

DIAGNOSIS

In a doctor's office or hospital, cancer of the large intestine is usually diagnosed through a rectal examination; blood, urine, and stool tests; x-rays; a proctosigmoidoscopy, in which a rigid tube is inserted through the rectum to provide a view of the lower colon; or a colonoscopy, in which the tube is inserted and air is forced in to expand the complete colon for viewing.

Traditional Oriental medicine analyzes the condition of the bowel tract with simple external means rather than complex internal ones. In facial diagnosis, the lower lip corresponds to the large intestine, and by observing its condition we can take preventive or remedial dietary action to counter intestinal disorders, including bowel cancer. A swollen lower lip signifies a swollen, yin condition of the large intestine. In modern society, up to 75 percent of the population have swollen lower lips, indicating irregular bowel movements and enteritis or inflammation of the intestinal tract. Usually a swollen lower lip indicates constipation from a combination of excessive yin and yang foods. However, if the lip is wet, diarrhea is indicated. An extremely contracted, yang lower lip shows overconsumption of meat and other protein. The virtual absence or receding of the lower lip shows a tendency toward cancer of the sigmoid colon or rectum.

The different colorations of the lower lip further show specific disorders: white indicates fatty mucous deposits in the colon; pale shows weak metabolism of nutrients and anemia; bright red indicates expansion and hyperactivity of the blood capillaries and tissue; yellow around the edges of the lips shows hardening of fatty deposits in the large intestine and blockages in the liver and gallbladder; blue or purple shows stagnation of feces and blood in the colon; and a green shade around the mouth probably indicates colon cancer.

These discolorations may also occur around areas along the meridian of the large intestine especially on the area around the base of the thumb on the inside of the hand. A blue or green color in this region may indicate developing intestinal cancer. Also, the fleshy part of the outside of the hand between the thumb and index finger often takes on a green or bluish hue in the case of colon cancer. If this coloring appears on the left hand, the descending colon is affected. If on the right hand, the ascending colon is diseased.

The condition of the colon is also revealed in the forehead. The right part of the forehead shows the ascending colon, the upper forehead the transverse colon, and the left part the descending colon. Swellings, colorations, patches, pimples, or spots indicate where fat deposits, ulcers, or cancerous growths are developing in the colon.

General skin color also offers clues to intestinal disorders. A purplish shading, from the consumption of extremely yin foods and beverages, or a brown shade, from excessive yang animal food and yin tropical vegetables and fruits, or yellow, white, hard fatty skin from the consumption of excessive eggs, poultry, cheese, and other dairy foods are early warning signs of overactive intestines and general digestive troubles.

DIETARY RECOMMENDATIONS

For cancers of the large intestine—the ascending, transverse, and descending colon and the rectum—it is advisable to eliminate all animal food including meat, poultry, eggs, all dairy food, and even fish and seafood. Furthermore, any greasy, oily, or fatty foods and beverages are to be avoided. Sugar, sugar-treated food and beverages, refined flour, soft drinks, tropical fruits and vegetables, various nuts and nut butters, spices, stimulants, and aromatic food and drinks are also to be discontinued. Dietary guidelines for daily consumption, by volume, are generally as follows:

• Fifty to sixty percent of every meal should be whole-cereal grains, especially pressure-cooked short-grain or medium-grain brown rice. In the event that rice is not available, pressure-cooked whole oats or barley may be substituted. These two grains, as well as all other grains, can occasionally be used for variety or in combination with brown rice. However, for a contracted condition such as colorectal cancer, buckwheat should be limited in use because it is the most contractive of the grains. Flour products, even unrefined whole-wheat bread, chapati, pancakes, or cookies, should be totally avoided or limited in volume for a period of a few months. Whole-grain pasta and noodles also should not be used more than a couple times a week in small volume.

• Five to ten percent soup. One to two bowls of miso soup, especially that made with barley miso and cooked with kombu or wakame and with hard, leafy vegetables, are recommended daily. Occasionally, grain soup can be eaten. Tamari broth soup may be used to replace miso soup a few times a week. Brown rice, barley, and other cooked grains may also be added to these soups occasionally.

• Twenty to thirty percent vegetables, cooked in various styles, mainly steamed, boiled, and occasionally sautéed. For cancer of the ascending colon, lighter and quicker cooking, which preserves freshness and crispness, is preferred over longer cooking with a strong, salty taste. Leafy vegetables are preferable to root vegetables for this cancer, though root vegetables should also be used occasionally. For cancer of the transverse colon, leafy vegetables and round vegetables such as cabbages, onions, and pumpkins and squashes may be used almost equally. The cooking style should be medium, neither too short nor too long. For cancer of the descending colon and rectum, round and root vegetables should receive more emphasis than leafy vegetables, though the latter are also necessary. For any of these conditions, seasoning with unrefined sea salt, tamari soy sauce, and miso or condiments is to be moderate. If desired, a boiled or a fresh salad may often be eaten in moderate volume. Sautéed vegetables made with unrefined sesame or corn oil can also be frequently consumed.

• Five to ten percent beans and bean products. Smaller beans such as azuki, lentils, and chickpeas are preferred to larger beans. They should be cooked with either 10 to 20 percent kombu, onions and carrots, or acorn or butternut squash. Tempeh, natto, tofu (dried or cooked), and other soybean products may be used in moderate volume. However, beans and bean products should not be consumed in large volume.

• Five percent or less cooked sea vegetables. Any variety may be taken as a small side dish once a day. The kinds of sea vegetables should be alternated, though hijiki and arame are preferred. Seasoning may be with a little volume of tamari soy sauce and occasionally rice vinegar.

As a condiment, a small amount of miso sautéed in sesame oil with the same volume of chopped scallions can be used daily on grains. One teaspoon of sautéed whole dandelions is also helpful for cancer of the large intestine.

For relieving tumors, a small dish of shiitake mushrooms cooked with kombu, seasoned with miso while cooking, is helpful. One tablespoon may be consumed daily.

A dish of dried, shredded daikon soaked in water and cooked with kombu and seasoned with either miso or tamari soy sauce is also helpful for colon cancers if consumed daily or several times a week.

A small amount of pickled vegetables may also be frequently consumed. Rice bran (nuka) pickles are the most suitable. Umeboshi plums are also helpful for aiding digestion and may be eaten or used in cooking regularly.

For colon cancer, fruits should be completely avoided. However, a small volume of cooked temperate-climate fruit may be consumed occasionally, if craved. Natural sweeteners, if desired, should be grain-based ones such as barley malt or rice syrup. They should be consumed only in small volume.

All foods should be well chewed until they liquefy in the mouth and are thoroughly mixed with saliva. It is also important neither to overeat in general nor to eat two to three hours before sleeping.

The general dietary guidelines for relieving cancer can be followed in all other respects, including beverages.

As explained in the introduction to Part II, cancer patients who have received or who are currently undergoing medical treatment may need to make further dietary modifications.

HOME CARES

• Cancer patients and many physicians are concerned that weight loss is not beneficial and thus a tendency arises to overconsume, especially food rich in protein and fat. Actually, this practice serves to enhance the cancerous condition, especially in the case of the large intestine. Having an energetic and tireless condition is more of a barometer to health than maintaining previous weight.

• For a short period—seven to fourteen days—persons with

large-intestinal cancer may eat only pressure-cooked brown rice served with either umeboshi plum or gomashio (sesame salt) and with toasted nori. The rice and condiments should be chewed very, very well. In making gomashio, the proportion of roasted sea salt to crushed sesame seeds should be from one to twelve to one to four-teen. Along with the brown rice, one to two cups of miso soup and one or two dishes of cooked vegetables may be consumed every day. This limited rice diet is very beneficial to cleansing and revitalizing the intestinal tract. However, it should not be continued longer than two weeks without proper supervision of a qualified macrobiotic counselor or medical professional.

• For intestinal and rectal tumors, a taro potato plaster may be applied for three to four hours following administration of a ginger compress for five to ten minutes. This plaster may be repeated daily.

• In the event of swelling in the abdominal region, repeated ap-plication of a buckwheat plaster can help absorb excessive liquid. The buckwheat plaster should be kept warm while being applied.

• In the event of pain, a ginger compress applied for about ten to fifteen minutes, and a plaster of mashed green leafy vegetables mixed with 20 to 30 percent white flour in order to make a paste, is helpful. The vegetable plaster should be preceded by a ginger compress. Gentle massage and acupuncture treatment may also help relieve pain and bowel-tract stagnation.

• In the event of appetite loss, genuine brown-rice cream can be consumed with a piece of umeboshi plum and a small amount of gomashio or tekka.

• In the event that part of the descending colon or rectum has become narrowed or blocked by tumorous growth, the bowel channel may be widened or opened by one of the following special measures:

1. Drink two to three cups per day of liquid made from boiling spring water with shiitake dried mushrooms, grated daikon, a small portion of grated ginger, with a slight taste of tamari soy sauce. (Grated lotus root may be used instead of either shiitake mushrooms or grated daikon.)

2. Drink two to three cups per day of boiled water in which dried tangerine or orange peel has cooked. The same liquid can be used for an enema if needed.

3. Drink miso soup, two to three cups daily, cooked with sliced daikon or radish; garlic or ginger; and onion or scallion.

4. Eat a dish of cooked agar-agar (kanten) seasoned with apple juice or barley malt together with grated ginger a couple of times per day.

• To eliminate intestinal gas, all food should be chewed very well. It is also helpful to eat less, even skipping breakfast for a period of a few weeks.

• Avoid exposing the abdominal region to cold air or consuming cold beverages, which have a paralyzing effect on the intestines. Keeping the abdominal region warm is essential for restoring smooth digestive functions. For that purpose, a small volume of scallions or garlic cooked in miso soup or in bancha tea, consumed daily or several times a week, is also helpful.

• Daily scrubbing of the whole body, including the intestinal region, with a very hot towel that has been immersed in gingerroot water is helpful. This will activate circulation of the blood and general energy, promoting better digestion.

OTHER CONSIDERATIONS

• Nonexhausting, daily exercise is important for improving appetite and digestion.

• Avoid direct contact of the skin with synthetic clothing. Use cotton material for undergarments and sleepwear.

• Those who suffer with intestinal cancer, as in the case of lung cancer, tend to be depressed, sad, and melancholy. It is important to keep a positive, optimistic happy mood. Good breathing exercises are very helpful not only for lung metabolism, but also for the smooth functioning of the large intestine.

PERSONAL EXPERIENCE

Colon Cancer

In 1969 Mrs. Terezia Matyas underwent a cancer operation in her native Hungary to remove part of her large intestine. Doctors performed a colostomy, creating a small sac on her left side for discharging her bowels. The operation allowed her to live several years, but by the summer of 1974 the cancer had reappeared in the colon and spread to the stomach and uterus, resulting in constant bleeding.

Doctors declared Mrs. Matyas terminally ill and transferred her to a sanitorium to die. Her husband had died of cancer the previous year.

Meanwhile, in Chicago, her son Charles Matyas, a life-insurance salesman, received a telegram from his sister Erzsebet, the chief lab technician in the hospital where their mother was operated on. Charles had recently learned of the case of Professor Jean Kohler, who had relieved himself of pancreatic cancer on the macrobiotic diet; he wired his sister to take their mother home and he would send some food that would help relieve her condition. "Looking at the problem through medical eyes, I do not think a brown-rice diet will help at all," the sister replied. Nonetheless, she agreed to try out the nutritional approach and took the mother home.

The first shipment of brown rice and bancha tea arrived on September 19, 1974, and the next day Mrs. Matyas began the new diet. On her son's instructions, she devoted one to one-and-a-half hours to eating each bowl of rice, chewing thoroughly. By September 28, a little more than a week later, the constant bleeding had stopped, and her bowel movements had become normal. During this time, she took medication only once, for a noise in her ear. Two weeks later she began eating cooked vegetables and miso soup along with the rice, and all pain disappeared. She grew well enough to get up from her bed and walk around the block for an hour after each meal.

"The greatest and most pleasant surprise came when my mother walked about three miles to the hospital on November 12," her son later recorded. "It was also a surprise to the doctors who could not operate on my mother because of the mass of cancer and who also predicted her death in one month. The result of her walking to the hospital was that on the fourteenth of November she underwent a complete checkup. To the bewilderment of the doctors, they could not even find a trace of the cancer."

Mrs. Matyas' health gradually returned to normal, and the next spring and summer she worked happily in her garden growing vegetables, soybeans, azuki beans, and flowers. However, in July, feeling that she had fully recovered, she gradually began deviating from the standard macrobiotic guidelines. Although she didn't eat meat or milk, she began using too much oil and fish. With no other people in her area or community involved in macrobiotics to support her, she did not have proper cooking lessons or a counselor to check up periodically on her condition. On one of my European tours that summer, I tried to set up some seminars for doctors in Hungary and to visit Mrs. Matyas but was officially turned down by government authorities.

In December 1975, Mrs. Matyas returned to the hospital and had a blood transfusion for hemorrhaging from the uterus. On and off through the spring, her condition fluctuated. Finally, in June 1976, after receiving another blood transfusion, she returned to the hospital because of swelling in the ankles. The doctors assumed that her cancer had returned and gave her a cobalt treatment.

The daughter, Erzsebet, protested, declaring that the symptoms indicated a kidney disorder, but the doctors disregarded her advice and gave the mother another cobalt treatment and intravenous chemotherapy. That night Mrs. Matyas died.

In Chicago, Charles was very distraught to learn of his mother's death and wired for medical records. Erzsebet discovered that except for one blood test the mother's medical records had all disappeared from the hospital and could not be located. Fortunately, she had seen the original autopsy report, which stated that Terezia Matyas' last illness had been the result of a severe kidney infection. Medical tests revealed no trace of cancer, but there was scarred tissue where the cancer had been. Sources: *Case History Report*, Vol. 1, No. 1 (Boston: East West Foundation, 1975, pp. 26–27); Jean and Mary Alice Kohler, *Healing Miracles from Macrobiotics* (West Nyack, N.Y.: Parker, pp. 251–54, 1979).

Colon Cancer with Metastases to the Liver

In September 1977, Neil Scott, then forty-nine, an inmate in the state prison in Huntsville, Texas, first complained of bowel incontinence. In December 1978, surgeons at John Sealy Hospital in Galveston diagnosed cancer of the cecum and removed part of his intestine. The doctors gave Scott only ninety days to live and put him on chemotherapy.

Not yet ready to die, Scott sought an alternative, and from acquaintances heard about a natural foods approach to cancer. Three weeks after surgery he gave up meat, dairy food, and poultry and began eating asparagus, carrots, peanut butter, brown bread, and other foods available, as well as vitamin C tablets. Prison food was generally poor in quality, and regulations forbade prisoners from receiving food from the outside. Still, Scott persisted, and he became the first cancer patient in Huntsville in seventeen years to outlive his prognosis. In March 1980, he stopped chemotherapy, and in June he obtained a complete remission.

However, by fall of 1980 the prison kitchen cut back its supply of carrots and other fresh vegetables. Scott felt the cancer return and feared the illness had spread to his liver. In July 1981, after experimenting with a variety of nonstandard approaches including vitamin therapy, immunological methods, and Laetrile, he wrote Alex Jack, editor of *East West Journal*, for nutritional advice. Jack and Frank Salvati, who corresponds with prisoners for the East West Foundation, introduced Scott to macrobiotics. Though unable to obtain whole grains in prison, Scott shifted the emphasis of his diet from fresh vegetables and fruits to bran cereals, other breakfast cereals low in sugar, white rice, and cooked vegetables. By the end of 1981, as Scott began to implement this approach, x-rays confirmed the spread of cancer to his liver. Prison doctors told him he had only six months to live.

Meanwhile, through legal means and interviews with the media, Scott waged a campaign for dietary and medical reform at the prison. In January 1982, Texas Department of Corrections officials transferred Scott from the prison hospital's cancer ward to the main cell block and asked him to return to a work detail. The press was no longer allowed to see him.

Within this environment, Scott persevered and continued corresponding with Jack and Salvati almost daily on the progress of his condition. To counterbalance the lack of nourishing food, he performed yoga and other exercises and engaged in visualization. In March 1982, Scott was taken to the oncology unit of John Sealy Hospital. Since he had refused chemotherapy, doctors feared the worst. To their surprise, a liver-spleen scan showed no sign of cancer. All Scott's blood tests, including the carcinoembryonic antigen test, were normal.

In a subsequent letter describing his remission, Scott wrote:

Since metastases to the liver was diagnosed almost four months ago I have, in following the invaluable macrobiotic way, been able to make dietary modifications which have apparently cleared my liver of suspicion. During the period between the last two scans I eliminated all fruit, decreased ascorbic acid to one gram per day, and increased grain cereals to 70 percent of total diet with vegetables, both fresh and canned, comprising the balance. I had been using too much yin food.

I have also increased time spent in visualization and imagery. My liver continues to prance around Los Angeles county with its glorious handle-bar moustache waving in the soft ocean breeze. Maybe I'm a nut, but am having one hell of a lot of fun with my liver. I have increased exercise regimen, the yoga, and others. One group of exercises in particular which appeared in articles in the January and February 1982 *East West Journals* with photos are working particularly well. I visualize while doing them. "The Monkey" number [a traditional Taoist exercise] designed especially for the liver is a hot one. I can see the cancer cells leaving town when I bend over and press the elbows into the body.

"Cancer is not the indestructable enemy of life which almost everyone seems to believe," Scott wrote in another letter. "It is relatively easy to cure, given proper food and courage." Sources: David Brisson, "Prison Food Is Killing Me: Neil Scott vs. the Sovereign State of Texas," *East West Journal*, June 1982 (pp. 36–40); personal letter to Alex Jack, March 25, 1982, including oncology report from John Sealy Hospital dated March 23, 1982.

16.

Leukemia

FREQUENCY

Leukemia, a form of cancer affecting the blood, will claim an estimated 16,100 lives in the United States in 1983, and 23,900 new cases will arise. Leukemia is the leading cause of death, after accidents, for children under fifteen and among cancers heads the mortality rate for ages fifteen to thirty-four. Leukemia affects males slightly more than females. Characterized by the uncontrolled production of white-blood cells, leukemia is classified into acute and chronic types. The acute variety tends to grow rapidly, affects children more commonly, and spreads to the liver, spleen, and lymph nodes. Patients with acute leukemia are very susceptible to anemia, secondary infections, and hemorrhaging and may die from these complications. Chronic leukemia develops more slowly and usually affects those in the middle to older age brackets. The four most common forms of leukemia are: 1) *Acute lymphocytic* or *lymphoblastic* (ALL), the most prevalent cancer among children, characterized by diminished granulocytes, the white-blood cells that resist infection; 2) *Acute myelocytic* (AML), the most prevalent leukemia among adults over forty, characterized by a decrease in platelet production; 3) *Chronic myelocytic* or *granulocytic* (CML), an illness accompanied by an abnormal chromosome and affecting young and middle-aged adults; and 4) *Chronic lymphocytic* (CLL), a disease that affects primarily the elderly and usually involves malfunction of the spleen.

Modern medicine treats leukemias of all types principally with chemotherapy. Surgery or irradiation by roentgen rays or radioactive phosphorous may also be used if the lymph system is affected or other organs are enlarged. Fresh blood transfusions or bone-marrow transplants are sometimes given in order to provide a fresh source of red-blood cells, which scientists believe are produced in the bone marrow. In hospitals, leukemia patients will often be isolated in such devices as the Life Island, a bed enclosed with a plastic canopy designed to provide an environment free of microorganisms. Children's cancer clinics claim an overall 50 percent survival rate for childhood leukemias, although there are often recurrences of the disease. For all forms of leukemia, 14 to 15 percent of patients live five years or longer following medical treatment.

STRUCTURE

Our slightly salty bloodstream is a replica of the ancient sea in which biological life developed during most of its evolutionary history. The blood consists of liquid in the form of plasma and formed elements consisting of red-blood cells, white-blood cells, and platelets. The tighter and more compact red-blood cells are yang in structure, while the larger, more expanded white-blood cells are yin. The platelets, an important factor in blood clotting, are smaller than red-blood cells and because of their contractive ability and size are classified as extremely yang. The plasma comprises about 55 percent of the blood by volume, while the various formed elements, which are suspended in the plasma, constitute the remaining 45 percent.

Our bodies contain about 35-trillion red-blood cells. Each of these tiny disc-shaped cells is about 7.7 microns in diameter and about 1.9 microns thick. Men have about 5 million per cubic millimeter, and women about 4.5 million per cubic millimeter. The number of red-blood cells is dependent on a variety of circumstances, including age, altitude, temperature, and level of activity or rest. For example, as we grow older, the number decreases from the 6 million per cubic millimeter that we had at birth.

Hemoglobin comprises between 60 and 80 percent of the red-blood cell and consists of hematin, a more condensed form of protein containing iron, and a simpler, larger protein. Hematin attracts oxygen in the lungs and transports it to the cells of the body. Then, as the oxygen-depleted blood returns through the veins, it attracts and transports carbon dioxide back to the lungs, where it is exhaled. This process is essential for life, and the efficiency with which it is accomplished directly influences our health. In a normal adult, about

20-million red-blood cells are destroyed every minute, and new red-blood cells are continuously formed to replace them. The total volume of hemoglobin in the body is about one kilogram, twenty grams of which are destroyed and rebuilt every day.

The human body contains far fewer white-blood cells than red-blood cells—about 6,000 per cubic millimeter. They are usually larger than red-blood cells, possess a nucleus, and have the power of movement similar to that of an amoeba. White-blood cells are attracted to bacteria entering the body, which they envelop and devour. They also gather around inflamed external injuries.

CAUSE OF CANCER

Normal blood is slightly alkaline, with a pH between 7.3 and 7.45, thus giving rise to its mildly salty taste. A pH of less than 7 is acid, while more than 7 is alkaline. If the pH of the blood dips below its normally weak alkaline level and becomes acidic, acidosis arises. Acidity is classified as a yin condition. When the pH factor of the blood moves into the high pH range, the more yang condition of alkalosis occurs. Daily diet is the principal determinant of the blood's relative alkalinity or acidity. More expansive, yin foods and beverages such as sugar, coffee, fruits, juices, milk, and alcohol thin the blood and make it more acid. Contractive foods, including salt, are overly alkaline and constrict the circulatory system. The body compensates for poor-quality blood by several mechanisms. For example, when we exhale, excess acids are discharged along with carbon dioxide, and the kidneys continuously filter excess acids from the food and discharge them through urination. Also our blood contains a variety of buffers, such as sodium bicarbonate, which serve to neutralize acids. In this way the blood can maintain a weak alkaline condition despite regular consumption of extreme foods and beverages.

Under certain circumstances, however, blood equilibrium cannot be maintained, and serious disorders, such as leukemia, result. In blood cancer, the number of red-blood cells decreases, while the number of white-blood cells increases dramatically. In some cases, leukemia patients may have as many as 1 million white-blood cells per cubic millimeter instead of the normal 5,000 to 6,000.

In a normal healthy subject, food reaches the small intestine in the form of chyme, a homogenous liquid that is ready to be absorbed into the bloodstream. The small intestine is akin to a jungle. The villi resemble a forest of hair with millions of bacteria and viruses furthering transmutation by digesting food, changing its quality with their enzymes, and discharging it. Animal foods, strong acids such as sugar and fruits, medications, drugs, and chemicalized food kill these bacteria and cause indigestion, reduce blood production, and create the foundation for serious illness. In properly functioning intestines, molecules of jellified food attach themselves to the ends of the hairs, or villi, become intestinal tissues, and contribute to the production of blood. White-blood cells are larger and more flexible than red-blood cells and can be classified as yin. They tend to be produced by consumption of expansive foods such as sugar, while red-blood cells are created by more yang substances. Leukemia, a condition characterized by too many white-blood cells, is caused by overconsumption of yin foods, while scurvy, an excess of red-blood cells, is a sign of an overly yang diet.

Scurvy, of course, is no longer a problem because eighteenth-century British sailors learned how to balance their extremely yang diet of salt pork with very yin citrus food. However, leukemia is a modern scourge, and modern medicine has been unable to discover its origin or cure. The rise of leukemia among children and young people has accompanied the explosion of yin foods and beverages manufactured and commonly eaten since World War II. These include snack, party, and dessert foods made with sugar, honey, chocolate, and other sweets; candy and chewing gum; soft drinks, diet colas, and artificial beverages; white bread, rolls, pretzels, and other refined flour products; oranges, bananas, pineapples, and other tropical fruits; french-fried potatoes and potato chips; milk, cottage cheese, ice cream, milkshakes, and yogurt. Many children today eat a diet with a largely sweet taste that is soft in texture, large in size, and refined or processed in quality. Such a diet will produce an extremely thin quality of blood. Leukemia is also on the rise among Western vegetarians, especially those who eat large amounts of dairy products, fruit, raw foods, curried foods, aromatic herbs, and vitamin pills. Many of these substances are native and natural to tropical or subtropical environments. However, when they become a major part of the diet in temperate climates, serious illnesses will occur.

The increased incidence of leukemia since World War II has often been attributed to nuclear radiation. Estimates of total U.S. cancer deaths from atomic fallout and nuclear power plant emissions over the next generation range from several thousand to a million or more.

Epidemiological studies show that residents living near nuclear sites or workers handling nuclear materials have higher cancer rates than other people. While nuclear radiation is dangerous and should be avoided whenever possible, the underlying way of eating governs the degree of susceptibility to cancer in any given instance.

In 1945, for example, there were a small number of people following a macrobiotic diet who lived in Hiroshima and Nagasaki at the time of the first atomic explosions. Among those who survived the initial blast, the individuals who ate macrobiotically were able to function normally and help many other survivors overcome radiation sickness, a form of leukemia, by eating brown rice, well-cooked vegetables, miso soup, sea vegetables, pickled plums, and natural sea salt. From the symptoms of atomic disease, they realized that radiation was extremely expansive or yin, and that the blood could be strengthened or yangized with counterbalancing opposite factors such as a salt-rich grain and cooked-vegetable diet.

In traditional Oriental medicine, the hair on the head corresponds with the hairlike villi of the small intestine. When people's hair began to fall out after the bombings, it indicated trouble in the intestine and severely curtailed blood production. In the decades since the first atomic bombings, scientists have confirmed that miso and sea vegetables contain substances in addition to salt that can help protect the body from radiation by binding and discharging radioactive elements.

At the social level, various government agencies have proposed that nuclear waste materials be stored in salt mines or deposits in order to neutralize their deadly emissions. This is an example of how yin and yang are used in the modern world, although scientists do not understand the underlying principle of balance—namely, macrobiotic philosophy—involved.

There are many other sources of artificial radiation in modern society in addition to nuclear energy. Color television, computer and video terminals, xerox machines, air conditioners, smoke detectors, garage-door openers, supermarket checkout scanners, and numerous other appliances and devices contribute to our rapidly growing electronic environment. Some of this radiation is low level, such as that emitted by an electric hairdryer. Some radiation is stronger, such as that from microwave ovens. Day by day, all artificial electromagnetic stimuli have a cumulative effect on health and vitality.

A healthy human body has a marvelous capacity to adjust to its environment, even a radioactive or transistorized one. People following the standard macrobiotic way of eating need have no fear of leukemia or other serious illnesses. Of course, in an emergency situation, such as the accident at Three Mile Island, a more limited diet should be followed. However, at current world radiation levels, people still eating the modern refined diet have a much lower tolerance for radioactivity and are at risk of developing leukemia and other cancers. Reversing the biological degeneration of modern society is the key to curing atomic sickness and other forms of cancer. Return to a more natural way of farming, eating, and daily life will make nuclear energy unnecessary and contribute to lasting health and enduring peace.

MEDICAL EVIDENCE

• J. MacKenzie, an eighteenth-century Scot, who lived from about 1680 to 1761, maintained that health and longevity depended primarily on daily nourishment and opposed artificial means of prolonging life, including blood transfusions.

He who would thoroughly understand this subject, must not only know what qualities every sort of food is endowed with from nature, but also what new qualities it received from art [cooking], in the various ways of dressing it . . . and it is of great moment to a man's health, whether his common bread be white or brown, well or ill baked. Every physician should endeavor to understand the nature and constitution of different persons, with respect to what they eat and drink; and should not only make himself acquainted with the various complaints which arise from various sorts of ailment, but should also know why they happen to some, and not to others. . . . The transfusion of young blood into old veins, tho' performed with the utmost precaution and dexterity, will [n]ever avail to bestow strength and vigour on the bulk of mankind. . . .
Source: J. MacKenzie, *The History of Health and the Art of Preserving It* (Edinburgh: William Gordon, 1759).

• At the end of the nineteenth century, a New York physician asserted that all diseases could be traced back to an abnormal condition of the blood and an imbalance of alkalines and acids generated by the circulation of vital energy. "It ought to surprise no one," wrote Dr. Edward Foote, "when I say that many derangements of the blood arise from the use of improper food." Refuting the germ theory of disease and biochemical means to combat illness, Dr. Foote stated that natural vegetable medicines are "far more efficacious and harmless, as antidotes for human infirmities, than . . . can possibly be made in the laboratory of the most skilful chemist." Source: Edward B. Foote, M.D., *Plain Home Talk About the Human System* (New York: Murray Hill, 1891).

• Nuclear radiation has been associated with various cancers, especially leukemia, in scientific studies since the 1940's. Among those most affected have been Japanese survivors of the atomic bomb, U.S. servicemen who helped in the cleanup of Hiroshima and Nagasaki, U.S. soldiers who viewed the A-bomb tests in Nevada in the 1950's, schoolchildren in Utah living downwind of the Nevada tests, workers at shipyards handling nuclear-powered vessels, workers at nuclear labs and fabricating areas, and people who live near nuclear power plants. Source: Harvey Wasserman and Norman Solomon, *Killing Our Own* (New York: Delta, 1982).

• In 1944 mice on a 60 percent caloric restricted diet registered substantially less induced and spontaneous leukemias than mice fed at pleasure. The incidence of blood cancer in a high leukemia strain of mice fell from 65 to 10 percent and length of life was considerably prolonged. Source: J.A. Saxton, Jr. et al., "Observations on the Inhibition of Development of Spontaneous Leukemias in Mice by Underfeeding," *Cancer Research* 4:401–09.

• In 1947 researchers reported that a high-protein diet enhanced leukemia induced in mice. Source: J. White et al., "Effects of Diets Deficient in Certain Amino Acids on the Induction of Leukemia in DBA Mice," *Journal of the National Cancer Institute* 7:199–202.

• In 1964 scientists at the Gastro-Intestinal Research Laboratory at McGill University in Montreal, Canada, reported that a substance derived from the sea vegetable kelp could reduce by 50 to 80 percent the amount of radioactive strontium absorbed through the intestine. Stanley Skoryna, M.D. said that in animal experiments sodium alginate obtained from brown algae permitted calcium to be normally absorbed through the intestinal wall while binding most of the strontium. The sodium alginate and strontium were subsequently excreted from the body. The experiments were designed to devise a method to counteract the effects of nuclear fallout and radiation. Source: S.C. Skoryna et al., "Studies on Inhibition of Intestinal Absorption of Radioactive Strontium," *Canadian Medical Association Journal* 91: 285–88.

• In 1969 medical studies linked two common corn-soil pesticides to leukemia in test animals and humans. Tests showed that chlordane and heptachlor were concentrated in the food chain and appeared in the majority of the nation's dairy products, meat, poultry, and fish. The pesticides were phased out of production in the late 1970's by order of the Environmental Protection Agency, but their residues persist. Source: Samuel S. Epstein, M.D., *The Politics of Cancer* (New York: Doubleday, pp. 271–81, 1979).

• In 1972 a Japanese scientist reported that leukemia in chickens could be reversed by feeding them a mixture of whole grains and salt. The experiment was conducted by Keiichi Morishita, M.D., technical chief for the Tokyo Red Cross Blood Center and vice president of the New Blood Association. Source: K. Morishita, M.D., *The Hidden Truth of Cancer* (San Francisco: George Ohsawa Macrobiotic Foundation, 1972).

• Seventh-Day Adventist women in California have 44 percent less leukemias than the general population and men have 30 percent less, according to a 1975 study. The members of this religious group tend to consume whole grains, vegetables, fruit, and nuts and avoid meat, poultry, rich and refined foods, coffee, tea, hot condiments, spices, and alcohol. Source: R.L. Phillips, "Role of Life-Style and Dietary Habits in Risk of Cancer among Seventh-Day Adventists," *Cancer Research* 35:3513–22.

DIAGNOSIS

Blood tests and bone-marrow samples are used by doctors to diagnose leukemia. A bone-marrow aspiration and biopsy will also be taken if a malignancy is suspected. Chest x-rays, lymphangiogram, liver, spleen, and bone scans, CAT scan of the head, and a lumbar puncture may also be administered.

Oriental medicine diagnoses the quality of the blood by a variety of simple, safe visual techniques. A white color on the lips indicates a deficiency of hemoglobin, abnormal constriction of the blood capillaries, or stagnation and slowness of blood circulation in general. Anemia, leukemia, and similar blood conditions can produce this lip color.

A whitish color in the pink area inside the lower eyelid also indicates a weakened condition caused by excessive intake of either extreme yin or yang foods. This color also often accompanies leukemia.

Whitish fingernails further indicate underactive blood circulation, low hemoglobin, general anemia, and a tendency toward leukemia or other forms of cancer. Normally healthy people do not have this whitish color in the nails except when the fingers are stretched.

DIETARY RECOMMENDATIONS

The major cause of leukemia is the longtime, continuous consumption of foods and beverages in the extreme yin category including sugar, sugar-treated foods and drinks, ice cream, chocolate, carob, honey, soft drinks and soda, tropical fruits, fruit juices, oily and greasy foods, dairy foods, especially butter, milk, and cream, and many chemicals contained in foods, beverages, and supplements. All of these should be avoided in daily eating. However, the consumption of these items is often accompanied by the intake of foods from the extreme yang category including meat, poultry, eggs, and cheese in order to achieve a rough counterbalance. Accordingly, all these animal foods are also to be avoided, with the exception of fish and seafood, which can be consumed occasionally in moderate volume. Although they are not the direct cause, the following enhance leukemic conditions and should also be discontinued: ice-cold food and drinks, hot, stimulant and aromatic spices, various herbs and herb drinks that have stimulant effects, and vegetables that historically originated in the tropics including potato, tomato, and eggplant.

The nutritional recommendations for early childhood leukemia are included in "Baby Food Suggestions" in Part III. Following are daily dietary guidelines, by volume, for the prevention and relief of leukemia in older children or adults:

• Fifty to sixty percent whole-cereal grains. All pressure-cooked cereal grains are recommended, though brown rice and barley are most suitable as daily staples. They can be cooked often in the form of soup together with vegetables and a small volume of sea vegetables. Whole-grain bread can also be used occasionally if unyeasted. Whole-wheat or buckwheat pasta and noodles may also be used a few times a week.

• Five to ten percent soup. Miso or tamari soy sauce soup cooked with sea vegetables such as wakame or kombu, together with vegetables such as carrots and onions are to be the staple soups. Both miso and tamari soy sauce should be a type that has fermented naturally for one-and-a-half years or longer. Barley miso or hatcho miso is preferable to other types of miso. Together with sea vegetables and vegetables, soup can be made occasionally with whole grains such as brown rice, barley, millet, or buckwheat. Less frequently, a small portion of white-meat fish or small dried fish can also be cooked into the soup with vegetables, sea vegetables, and/or grains. Two to three times a week, vegetables may be lightly sautéed with a small volume of sesame oil or corn oil before cooking them in the soup.

• Twenty to thirty percent vegetables. Except for potato, tomato, eggplant, and other vegetables originally native to the tropics, vegetables can be prepared in a variety of cooking styles. In general, leafy vegetables, round, hard vegetables grown near the surface of the earth, and root vegetables can be used in about equal volume, i.e., one third of each type for daily consumption. During cooking, they can be seasoned moderately with sea salt, tamari soy sauce, or miso. Unrefined vegetable oil, especially sesame or corn oil, may be used for sautéing vegetables several times a week, though oil should not be overconsumed. Fresh raw salads are to be avoided except a few times a week and can be replaced by boiled salads and homemade pickled vegetables.

• Five to ten percent beans and their natural products. Smaller beans such as azuki beans, lentils, chickpeas, and black beans can be used often, cooked with such sea vegetables as kombu, fall-season, hard, sweet squash, or small volumes of onions and carrots. Bean products such as tempeh, natto, and tofu can be cooked and used for occasional change.

• Five percent or less sea vegetables. All cooked, edible sea vegetables are recommended as a natural mineral source, especially a small dish of hijiki or arame a few times a week. Sea vegetables can be cooked with other vegetables or sautéed with a small volume of sesame oil after softening them by soaking and boiling lightly in water.

Although the main cause of leukemia is the overconsumption of extreme yin foods over a long period of time, seasonings such as miso, tamari soy sauce, and sea salt, as well as salty condiments, which have yang contracting effects, should not be overused.

In the event that animal food is desired, a small portion of cooked white-meat fish can be prepared with a garnish of grated daikon or radish. To balance and detoxify the undesirable animal qualities of the fish, two to three times as much leafy vegetables, lightly cooked, should be consumed.

Fruits and fruit juices are to be avoided, but if craved, cooked or dried temperate-climate fruits can be used in small volume occasionally. Fall-season pumpkin, squash, carrots, chestnuts, and other naturally sweet foods, as well as cereal-grain-based sweeteners such as barley malt and rice syrup, may be used to satisfy a further desire for a sweet taste.

A natural sour taste can be satisfied with the use of pickled vegetables such as sauerkraut and with rice vinegar.

Nuts and nut butters are primarily to be avoided, though lightly roasted seeds such as pumpkin seeds, sunflower seeds, and sesame seeds may be used for an occasional snack.

Leukemia patients may also consume some supplemental dishes, which, taken in small volume, can strengthen blood quality. These dishes include:

1. Shio-kombu (salty kombu)—sliced sheets of kombu (about one-half-inch square), cooked in a mixture of one-half tamari soy sauce and one-half water, and boiled down until the liquid becomes completely absorbed by the kombu (usually two to four hours). Consume several pieces daily with cereal grain dishes.

2. Kimpira—burdock roots and carrots shredded into small pieces, sautéed together with sesame oil, and seasoned with tamari soy sauce or miso. Consume several times a week as a small supplemental dish.

3. Carp and burdock soup (koi koku)—whole carp cooked with shredded burdock roots, seasoned with miso and a little grated ginger. This soup may be used as the soup dish a few times a week for a period of several weeks. See the recipe in Part III.

Overeating and excessive drinking are to be avoided. Chewing very well, mixing food substances with saliva, is very important for improving this condition. Also avoid the consumption of food three hours prior to sleeping.

All other dietary recommendations, including those for regular beverage intake and use of condiments, can follow the general guidelines for cancer patients provided in the recipe section.

As explained in the introduction to Part II, cancer patients who have received or who are currently undergoing medical treatment may need to make further dietary modifications.

HOME CARES

• Scrubbing the whole body including the abdominal region and the spinal region with a hot towel that has been immersed in ginger-root water is very helpful for better circulation of blood, lymph, and other body fluids, as well as for activating physical and mental energies.

• Swelling of the spleen and abdominal regions sometimes accompanies leukemia and is caused by overeating in general, especially protein, and excessive intake of beverages, seasonings, and condiments. In such cases, food consumption should be simplified for a period of several days up to ten days. During this period, daily consumption may consist of pressure-cooked brown rice and barley, one to two cups of miso soup, a small dish of half-dried daikon and daikon leaves pickled for a long period (over two months) with sea salt and rice bran, a dish of vegetables such as onions, carrots, and cabbage sautéed with sesame oil, and several cups of bancha twig tea. However, this simplified diet should not be continued for longer than ten days unless under supervision of an experienced macrobiotic counselor or medical associate.

• In the event of appetite loss, two to three bowls of genuine brown-rice cream can be served daily with a condiment of either gomashio (sesame salt), umeboshi plum, or tekka. This rice cream may also be used occasionally as part of the regular whole-grain diet.

OTHER CONSIDERATIONS

• General physical exercise and deep breathing exercises are recommended, especially outside in the fresh air. Shiatsu massage and other treatments to relax and loosen any physical and psychological stagnations and hardenings are also very helpful.

• Maintaining clean, fresh air inside the home is important, and for this purpose green plants can be placed in each room. Indoor air circulation can also be maintained by frequently opening the windows.

• Wearing cotton underwear and avoiding synthetic fabrics are helpful for better skin metabolism and facilitate energy flow through the body.

• Avoid exposure to artificial electromagnetic radiation. Keep common hand-held appliances to a minimum. If you have a choice, work and live in areas away from nuclear installations.

PERSONAL EXPERIENCE

Radiation Sickness

At the time of the world's first plutonium atomic bombing on August 9, 1945, Tatsuichiro Akizuki, M.D. was director of the Department of Internal Medicine at St. Francis's Hospital in Nagasaki, Japan. In his book, Dr. Akizuki explained how he was able to save numerous survivors of the blast from radiation sickness and cancer of the blood:

On August 9, 1945, the atomic bomb was dropped on Nagasaki. Lethal atomic radiation spread over the razed city. For many it was an agonizing death. For a few it was a miracle. Not one coworker in the hospital suffered or died from radiation. The hospital was located only one mile from the center of the blast. My assistant and I helped many victims who suffered the effects of the bomb. In the hospital there was a large stock of miso and tamari. We also kept plenty of rice and wakame (seaweed used for soup stock or in miso soup). I had fed my co-workers brown rice and miso soup for some time before the bombing. None of them suffered from atomic radiation. I believe this is because they had been eating miso soup. . . .

On the tenth of August at 8 A.M., the Uragami Hospital was still burning. It was truly a miracle that there was not a single death in the hospital. I took up again the treatments of the maladies at 9 A.M., praying to God as I could not believe what happened. The supply of medicine was low. The hospital attendants prepared as usual a meal consisting of brown rice, miso soup with Hokkaido pumpkin and wakame, two times per day, at 11 A.M. and 5 P.M. They distributed the trays of brown rice to our grim neighbors and to the wounded.

At this period the scientific Americans declared that the center of the explosion area would be uninhabitable for the next seventy-five years. We disregarded this horrible declaration and continued, in straw sandals, to go around the city of Nagasaki the next day after the explosions to visit the sick in their homes.

The third day: at the clinic the number of injured grew; they were affected with bleeding of the gums, diarrhea, hemorrhages with no signs of any considerable wounds. The patients usually said: "It is because I have breathed a toxic gas that I bleed." One notices these violet bloody spots under the skin and in the membranes. Is it dysentery or purpura? The fact is very curious that the persons affected by these symptoms are not burned. It happened in the shade at the moment of the explosion. Now we know the symptoms were in reality those of the first stage of radioactive contamination. . . .

I resolved to try my method—using miso soup, unpolished brown rice, and salt. Sugar is poison to the blood. Obstinately I persuaded the people around me, again and again. I myself was more or less eccentric. I had no knowledge of the new biophysics or atom-biology; no books, no treatise, on atomic disease yet . . . I had no idea what kind of ray the atomic detonation might produce. I made a diagnosis and reasoned thus far: it may be radium, Roentgen ray, or gamma ray, which probably destroys hematogenic tissue, and marrow tissue of the human body. . . .

I gave the cooks and staff strict orders that they should make unpolished whole-grain rice balls, adding some salt to them, make salty thick miso soup at each meal, and never use sugar. When they didn't follow my order, I scolded them without mercy: "Never take sugar, no sweets, sugar will destroy blood."

My mineral method made it possible for me to remain alive and go on working vigorously as a doctor. The radioactivity may not have been a fatal dose but ever since, Brother Iwanaga, Reverend Noguchi, Chief Nurse Miss Murai, I, and other staff members and in-patients kept on living on the lethal ashes of the bombed ruins. It was thanks to this salt mineral method that all of us could work away for people day after day, overcoming fatigue or symptoms of atomic disease, and survived the disaster free from severe symptoms of radioactivity.

In addition to the testimony of Dr. Akizuki, there are additional accounts by survivors of Nagasaki and Hiroshima who healed themselves of radiation sickness, keloid tumors, and other serious effects of the bombing. Source: T. Akizuki, M.D., *Documentary of A-Bombed Nagasaki* (Nagasaki: Nagasaki Printing Co., 1977); Ida Honoroff, "A Report to the Consumer," May 1978; Hideo Ohmori, "Report from Japan," *A Nutritional Approach to Cancer* (Boston: East West Foundation, 1977, pp. 28–32).

17.

Liver Cancer

FREQUENCY

An estimated 10,000 Americans will die of liver cancer in 1983. Another 13,300 new cases will develop, almost evenly divided between men and women. Accounting for about two percent of primary cancers in this country, the liver is a common site of metastases from other parts of the digestive system, the breast, and the lungs. There is a higher incidence of liver cancer in Asia. In China liver cancer is one of the top three cancers, and it is also high in the Philippines, Hong Kong, and Papua New Guinea.

Hepatomas, tumors involving the epithelial lining of both lobes of the liver, and *cholingiocarcinomas,* which begin in the bile ducts and spread to the liver itself, account for half of all liver cancers in the United States. Other varieties include *hemangiosarcomas* or mixed tumors of sarcoma cells and dilated blood vessels; *mixed sarcomas,* which spread to other parts of the liver and lymph nodes in the vicinity of the lung and brain; *hepatoblastomas,* rare granular tumors found in children; and *adenocarcinomas,* glandular tumors that develop in the bile ducts.

Most liver cancer patients die from liver failure within six months of diagnosis. Only one percent currently survive five years or more. Current medical treatment usually calls for a total hepatic lobectomy, a surgical operation in which the tumor and part or all of the healthy tissue in one lobe around it are removed. For inoperable cancers, a chemotherapy technique called hepatic artery infusion is offered. This procedure calls for placing a catheter directly into blood vessels going to the liver in order to concentrate drugs in that organ.

STRUCTURE

The liver is situated in the right side of the abdominal cavity above the intestines and adjacent to the stomach, gallbladder, and pancreas. About the same size as the brain, it weighs approximately three pounds and governs many of the body's digestive, circulatory, and excretory functions. Its many operations include filtering toxins from the blood; making and transporting bile; controlling blood sugar levels; converting carbohydrates, fat, and protein into one another; and manufacturing hormones and enzymes. In traditional Oriental medicine, the liver is known as the body's general because of its commanding functions. Using a contemporary metaphor, we may liken it to the body's Environmental Protection Agency, which monitors the quality of the internal environment and neutralizes any harmful substances. A person cannot live without a liver. However, even if 80 percent of the organ is removed, it will continue to function and the missing section often grows back.

CAUSE OF CANCER

When leaving the heart, part of the blood passes to the digestive organs where oxygen is supplied to the tissues and food that has been absorbed is picked up. Rather than circulating directly through the body, this metabolized material from the intestines and stomach goes directly to the liver. There it is cleansed of impurities before being sent into the bloodstream. A healthy liver can filter a relatively large and continuous amount of toxic substances that enter the body. For instance, the liver can neutralize about one third of an ounce of alcohol per hour. However, after years of imbalanced food and beverage intake, the liver may grow swollen or hard and lose its natural ability to function.

As a compact, active, and central body organ, the liver is yang in structure and thus particularly affected by overconsumption of beef, pork, poultry, eggs, dairy products, salt, and other strong yang foods. Though liver disorders tend to have a yang origin, the symptoms can be accelerated by expansive, yin substances such as alcohol, foods high in fat and oils, flour products, sugar, tropical fruits and vegetables, raw food, and stimulants.

A look at fat metabolism is helpful at this point to understand the mechanism of degenerative disease and tumor formation, including liver cancer, at the cellular level. Lipids are the family name for fats, oils, and fatlike substances including fatty acids, cholesterol, and lipoproteins. Fats are solid at room temperature, while oils are fluid. Solid lipids tend to contain more saturated fatty acids. Fatty acids are long chains of carbon and hydrogen atoms including an oxygen molecule at one end. Saturated fatty acids are bonded or saturated to hydrogen atoms. Unsaturated fatty acids lack at least one pair of hydrogen atoms. Polyunsaturated fatty acids are those in which more than one pair is missing.

Fatty acids are the building blocks of fats, just as simple sugars are the fundamental units of carbohydrates. In order to help digest fats, which are insoluble in water and form large globules, the liver secretes bile, a yellowish liquid stored in the gallbladder. In the intestine, bile serves to emulsify fats and enables them to be broken down into fatty acids and glycerol by digestive enzymes.

Lipids are essential to digestion but can be harmful to the body, especially saturated acids like stearic acid, found in animal tissues, which coats the red-blood cells, blocks the capillaries, and deprives the heart of oxygen. One of the main constituents of lipids is cholesterol, a naturally occurring substance in the body which contributes to the maintenance of cell walls, serves as a precursor of bile acids and vitamin D and also a precursor of some hormones. Cholesterol is not found in plant foods but is contained in all animal products, especially meat, egg yolks, and dairy products. Since cholesterol is insoluble in the blood, it attaches itself to a protein that is soluble in order to be transported through the body. This combination is called a lipoprotein. However, excess cholesterol in the bloodstream tends to be deposited in artery walls and as plaque eventually causes constriction of the arteries and reduces the flow of blood. Normally, fat is absorbed by the lymph and enters the bloodstream near the heart. However, if excess lipids accumulate in the body, eventually some will become deposited in the liver. Such stored fat, primarily from meat and dairy products, is usually the chief source of liver disorders culminating in the development of liver cancer.

Because of increased public awareness of the connection between cholesterol, saturated fat, and heart disease, many people have switched to unsaturated fats and oils, including vegetable cooking oils, mayonnaise, margarine, salad dressings, and artificial creamers and spreads. However, unsaturated fats serve to redistribute cholesterol from the blood to the tissues and combine with oxygen to form free radicals. These are unstable and highly reactive substances that can interact with proteins and cause the loss of elasticity in tissue and general weakening of cells. Medical studies show that polyunsaturated lipids actually accelerate tumor development more than saturated fats and oils.

Whole grains also contain polyunsaturated fats, but these are naturally balanced by the right proportion of vitamin E and selenium, which are usually lost in the refining process. Similarly, unrefined cooking oils (in which the vitamin E remains) are a balanced product and, if used in moderate amounts, will contribute to proper metabolism.

The liver also regulates the amount of sugar in the blood. It turns any excess sugar into a starch called glycogen, which is stored in the liver. When blood sugar levels are low, the liver converts glycogen back into sugar and sends it into the blood to nourish body cells. If we consume our principal food as complex carbohydrates such as whole grains, these starches will be broken down into sugar molecules slowly and be properly absorbed in the intestines and sent to the liver. But if we take much of our diet in the form of simple carbohydrates such as refined grains, fruit, sucrose, or honey, decomposition occurs primarily in the stomach, resulting in the release of strong acids and the rapid transfer of sugar to the liver in large quantities. If there is too much sugar already stored as glycogen or if the liver is weak from chronic abuse, excess sugar will get into the bloodstream and contribute to the eventual weakening of the organism.

Cancer of the liver is the culmination of chronic liver illness and may be preceded by hepatitis, jaundice, or cirrhosis. As we have seen, though essentially a yang disease, liver cancer is accelerated by extreme yin substances including alcohol, sugar, refined flour, and foods containing chemical additives, preservatives, or pesticides. It is interesting to observe that the incidence of hepatoma has risen sharply over the last thirty years. From 1907 to 1954, only sixty-seven cases were known in medical literature. During this period the Mayo Clinic had diagnosed only four cases. Hepatoma, a form of liver cancer affecting the epithelial tissue, appears to be linked with the tremendous explosion of yin foodstuffs following World War II. These include ice cream, soda pop, citrus fruits, ice-cold drinks, processed and artificial foods, white bread, and a wide range of prescription and nonprescription drugs such as aspirin, birth-control pills, and marijuana. Now each year several thousand Americans develop hepatomas.

MEDICAL EVIDENCE

• In the sixteenth century, Renaissance anatomist Gabriel Fallopius, who described the ovary and after whom the Fallopian tubes are named, associated malignant tumors with imbalanced diet and improper liver functioning. "The efficient cause of cancer, however, is a flux of atrabiliary humor, for only in the spleen and the liver can this tumor arise from congestion because it is there that this humor is generated . . . the cause of the flux is a faulty mixture of the humors due to bad food. . . ." Among the foods mentioned as possible causes of cancer were beef and salty and bitter foods. Source: L.J. Rather, *The Genesis of Cancer: A Study in the History of Ideas* (Baltimore: Johns Hopkins University Press, p. 17, 1978).

• In 1928 in Bielefeld, Germany, Max Gerson, M.D. reported relieving a case of cancer of the bile ducts with a whole-grain-based diet that excluded meat, white flour, alcohol, coffee, tea, spices, tobacco, and medications. Dr. Gerson went on to devote his life to the nutritional approach to cancer, and in 1941 fled Nazi Germany to set up a cancer clinic in New York. Several years later he testified before a U.S. Congressional committee and called for a return to the traditional diet in order to reverse the rising cancer rate. Summing up his twenty-five years of cancer research and treatment, he wrote, "Cancer is not a local but a general disease, caused chiefly by the poisoning of our foodstuffs prepared by modern farming and [the] food industry." In treating cancer patients, he saw detoxification of the liver as the key to stimulating the body's natural immunity. "In the near future," he predicted, "hospitals and cancer clinics for chronic degenerative disease will be more or less forced to use fruits and vegetables grown by organic gardening methods. . . ." Source: Max Gerson, M.D., *A Cancer Therapy: Results of Fifty Cases* (Del Mar, Calif.: Totality Books, 1958).

• In 1945 Dr. Albert Tannenbaum reported that spontaneous hepatomas in male mice were affected by both caloric restriction and a high-fat diet. Mice on a low-fat diet registered 9 percent liver tumors in contrast to 35 percent on a high-fat diet. Source: A. Tannenbaum, "The Dependence of Tumor Formation on the Composition of the Calorie-Restricted Diet as Well as on the Degree of Restriction," *Cancer Research* 5:616–25.

• In 1949 Dr. Tannenbaum and Herbert Silverstone reported to the National Cancer Institute that spontaneous liver tumors in mice were accelerated by increasing the protein in their diet. Mice on a diet high in casein, a protein found in milk and dairy products, registered 61 percent tumors compared to 11 percent malignancies in mice fed a grain-based diet. Source: A. Tannenbaum and H. Silverstone, "Effects of Varying the Proportion of Protein (Casein) in the Diet," *Cancer Research* 9:162–73.

• In 1955 physiologist Kasper Blond described the progressive development of diseases in the digestive tract, culminating in liver cancer, as interrelated rather than isolated phenomena, and characterized cancer as an illness resulting from incorrect nutrition, especially overconsumption of animal protein. "The whole syndrome of metabolic disorders which we call oesophagitis, gastritis, duodenitis, gastric and duodenal ulcer, cholecystitis, cholangitis, pancreatitis, proctitis, and others are considered only stages of a dynamic process, starting with liver failure and portal hypertension, and resulting in cirrhosis of the liver tissue and in cancer." Source: Kasper Blond, M.D., *The Liver and Cancer* (Bristol: England: John Wright & Sons, p. 136, 1955).

• Chlordane and heptachlor, related chemical pesticides, caused liver cancer, aplastic anemia, and leukemia in 1969 laboratory tests. Used primarily as corn-soil insecticides, chemical residues from these substances move up the food chain and are found in a majority of American dairy products, meat, poultry, and fish. In 1974 the Environmental Protection Agency suspended their use for most crops, but they are still used in termite control and on pineapples, strawberries, and Florida citrus fruits. In 1982, in Honolulu, heptachlor sprayed on pineapples turned up in the city's milk and ice cream supply and in the breastmilk of nursing mothers. As a result, the island of Oahu recalled its entire supply of milk. Sources: Samuel S. Epstein, M.D., *The Politics of Cancer* (New York: Doubleday, pp. 271–81, 1979) and *Boston Globe*, April 8, 1982.

• In 1972 Japanese researchers reported that wakame, a common sea vegetable eaten in Asia, suppressed the reabsorption of cholesterol in the liver and intestine in laboratory experiments. Other studies showed that hijiki, another sea vegetable, and shiitake mushroom also lowered serum cholesterol and improved fat metabolism. Source: N. Iritani and S. Nogi, "Effects of Spinach and Wakame on Cholesterol Turnover in the Rat," *Atherosclerosis* 15:87–92.

• In 1975 researchers reported a correlation between liver cancer incidence and per capita intake of potatoes in more than twenty countries. Source: B. Armstrong and R. Doll, "Environmental Factors and Cancer Incidence and Mortality in Different Countries, with Special Reference to Dietary Practices," *International Journal of Cancer* 15:617–31.

• In 1976 scientists reported more than 250 cases of liver cancer or other tumors in women using oral contraceptives. Studies indicated the risk of developing liver adenomas increased fivefold after five years of pill use and twenty-fivefold after nine years of use. Source: H.A. Edmondson et al., "Liver-Cell Adenomas Associated with Use of Oral Contraceptives," *New England Journal of Medicine* 294:470–72.

• In 1978 studies showed that test animals fed 20 percent of their caloric intake as sucrose developed liver cancer. The mice's diet contained the same proportion of sugar consumed by the average Briton. Source: B. Hunter et al., *Tumorgenicity and Carcinogenicity with Xylitol in Long-Term Dietary Adjustments in Mice* (Huntingdon, England: Huntingdon Research Centre).

• Excessive alcohol consumption, especially among smokers, can lead to cancers of the mouth, esophagus, throat, larynx, and liver, according to the director of the National Cancer Institute. Source: Arthur Upton, M.D., "Hearing Before the Subcommittee on Nutrition of the Committee on Agriculture, Nutrition, and Forestry of the U.S. Senate," Ninety-sixth Congress, Oct. 2, 1979.

• Azo dyes, a category of artificial colorings used in foods and cosmetics, have been linked with tumors in test animals, especially liver cancer. Processed foodstuffs that contain Azo dyes include Life Savers, caramels, filled chocolates, and other penny candies; soft drinks, artificial fruit drinks, ades; jellies, jams, marmalades; stewed fruit sauces, fruit gelatins, fruit yogurts; ice cream; pie fillings, puddings, caramel custard; whips, dessert sauces; crackers, cheese puffs, chips, cake and cookie mixes, waffle and pancake mixes; refined macaroni and spaghetti; mayonnaise, salad dressings; catsup, mustard; and some packaged and canned soups. The cancer tests were originally conducted on rabbits in 1906 and on rodents in 1924 and 1934.

Source: Ruth Winter, *Cancer-Causing Agents: A Preventive Guide* (New York: Crown, 1979).

• Mormons, who generally eat a well balanced diet high in whole grains, vegetables, and fruit, moderate in meat, and low in stimulants and tobacco have about 45 percent less liver cancer than other Americans, according to a 1980 epidemiological study. Source: J.E. Engstrom, "Health and Dietary Practices and Cancer Mortality among California Mormons," in J. Cairns et al. (ed.), *Cancer Incidence in Defined Populations, Banbury Report 4* (Cold Spring Harbor, N.Y.: Cold Spring Harbor Laboratory, pp. 69–90).

• In 1980 researchers reported that mice exposed to extract of black pepper developed significantly more tumors, especially of the liver, lung, and skin, than controls. The incidence in pepper-treated mice was 77 percent versus 11 percent for controls. The authors noted that U.S. per capita human consumption of pepper is 280 milligrams per day and suggested that this was the first experiment to study the possible link between the spice and cancer. Source: J.M. Concon et al., "Black Pepper [*Piper Nigram*] Evidence of Carcinogenicity," *Nutrition and Cancer* 1(3):22–26.

• Trichloroethylene (TCE), a chemical used in decaffinated coffee, has been linked with liver cancer in mice. The substance is also used in obstetrical anesthesia. In 1982 its replacement, methylene chloride, was discovered to cause cancer in laboratory animals. Sources: Thomas H. Corbett, M.D., *Cancer and Chemicals* (Chicago: Nelson-Hall, p. 182, 1977) and *Community Nutrition Institute Newsletter*, July 15, 1982.

• Toxaphene, the most widely used insecticide in the United States, causes significant increases of liver cancer in animals in National Cancer Institute tests. It is used on a variety of crops, including corn, wheat, soybeans, peanuts, lettuce, and tomatoes and on livestock. Residue of the chemical has seeped into many American lakes, rivers, and waterways, accumulating in the flesh of fish, oysters, shrimp, and other seafood. In 1982 the Environmental Protection Agency banned the pesticide for most common uses. Source: *Boston Globe*, Oct. 19, 1982.

DIAGNOSIS

Modern medicine employs a variety of technological methods to diagnose liver cancer. These include blood tests, x-rays, tomograms, CAT scan, liver scan, angiogram, and radiologic catheter invasion. If a tumor is suspected, a needle biopsy will follow these tests. An exploratory laparotomy, in which the abdominal wall is surgically opened to examine the inner organs, may also be performed to determine whether the tumor is primary or has metastasized from another area. Currently about 74 percent of liver cancers have spread from local to regional areas by the time they are detected.

The condition of the liver can be simply, safely, and accurately diagnosed by traditional Oriental medicine. The potential development of liver troubles, including cancer, can be spotted well ahead of time, allowing preventive or corrective dietary action to be taken. To begin with, the liver's relative condition can be noted by trying to place the fingers under the ribcage on the right side. If you feel pain here or are unable to place your fingers deeply under the ribs, your liver is swollen. You should be able to insert four fingers without feeling pain or tense resistance.

For more precise diagnosis, carefully observe the central region of the forehead immediately above the nose and between the eyebrows. This area corresponds to the liver in traditional Oriental physiognomy. Vertical lines or wrinkles appearing here are a sign of mucus and fat accumulating in the liver and the expansion or hardening of the organ. The deeper and longer the wrinkles, the more serious the condition. If only one or two lines show, the liver is harder and more rigid as a result of too much salt, animal food, and other yang substances as well as overconsumption of food. On the other hand, if the skin around the lines has puffed up, the cause is too much yin such as alcohol, sugar, drugs, fatty, oily food, and processed or artificial foods.

Pimples in this region above the nose show hard fat deposits in the liver or stone formation in the gallbladder due to excess intake of animal fat, including dairy products. Dry, flaky skin in this area, extending sometimes to the region over the eyebrows, indicates an overconsumption of fats and oils from either animal or vegetable sources together with flour products and a lack of adequate whole grains and cooked vegetables. If this area has white or yellow patches as well as vertical lines, development of a cyst or tumor in the liver or formation of a stone in the gallbladder is very likely.

The texture and coloring of the skin further show the condition of the inner organs. In the case of liver troubles, an oily skin condition suggests disorders in the liver, gallbladder, and general digestive system due to an overconsumption of oily foods from either animal or vegetable sources. Yellow shadings on the eyes, lips, hands, feet, or other areas of the skin show disorders of the bile function due to excessive yang food intake including meat, eggs, seafood, poultry, and salt. A blue-gray color, especially on the cheeks, indicates chronic liver hardening caused by yang animal foods aggravated by sugar, alcohol, stimulants, or other extreme yin. Tumor formation in general is indicated by green colorations on the skin. In the case of liver cancer, this hue often shows up along some area of the liver meridian, especially in the part that runs from inside the first toe up along the inside of the leg to the area below the knee. Also a green color appearing on the fourth toe and its area extending to the front of the foot below the ankle bone suggests developing liver cancer, duodenal ulcer, or gallstones.

DIETARY RECOMMENDATIONS

Liver cancer is mainly caused by overconsumption of animal food, especially that high in protein and fat, as well as by overconsumption of sugar, sugar-treated foods, stimulants, aromatic food and drink, alcohol, and various chemical additives. All these foods and beverages are to be avoided. Refined flour and flour products, even though of vegetable quality, are to be eliminated in order to prevent mucus formation. Vegetable oils are also to be limited, though most of them are unsaturated in quality, except for the occasional use of unrefined sesame oil, corn oil, and other good-quality oil. As a whole, overconsumption of food and drink—even though of healthy, natural, unchemicalized quality—is to be avoided. Any foods that make the body colder, including fruit juice, soft drinks, icy beverages, and ice cream, are also to be avoided. Refrain too from overuse of salt and salty food, as well as overcooking vegetables. All vegetables of tropical origin, even though they are now grown in temperate zones, including potato, sweet potato, yam, tomato, eggplant, and avocado, are to be discontinued. Tropical fruits and juices too are to be avoided as well as spices such as mustard, pepper, and curry; all stimulant seasonings and drinks including mint, peppermint, and other herb teas; all alcoholic beverages; and coffee and black tea.

The following are general guidelines, by volume of food, for daily consumption:

• Fifty to sixty percent whole-cereal grains. All whole-cereal grains are recommended, though brown rice and barley are especially advisable for daily consumption. The others can be used occasionally, except for buckwheat and buckwheat products, which should be avoided for a period of several months. Grains should be pressure-cooked with water and a pinch of sea salt. Baked flour products such as bread, pancakes, and cookies are to be avoided, though un-leavened nonyeasted whole-wheat or whole-rye bread may be con-sumed occasionally, if desired. While buckwheat groats and pasta are to be avoided initially, whole-wheat pasta or noodles may be used, if desired, a couple times a week.

• Five to ten percent soup. Daily consumption of one to two bowls of miso soup, lightly cooked with sea vegetables such as wakame or kombu and with green or white leafy vegetables, is rec-ommended. Miso can be replaced occasionally with tamari soy sauce, both of which are to be used lightly and should have been fermented naturally one-and-a-half years or longer. Occasionally, barley or oat soup can be used with sea vegetables and vegetables. Other grains may also be added to soup from time to time.

• Twenty to thirty percent vegetables. The majority of vegetables are to be lightly cooked green or white leafy vegetables. A minor volume of vegetables may be root varieties. These vegetables can be cooked in many different styles, including steaming and boiling. The use of oil for sautéing and frying is to be avoided. However, a couple of times a week, a small dish of vegetables sautéed with sesame or corn oil may be used, if craved. A small dish of fresh salad may be taken two to three times per week, if desired. Vegetable dishes may be seasoned with sea salt, tamari soy sauce, or miso, though they should be used moderately, avoiding a strong salty taste. Occasion-ally, boiled salad or fresh salad may be seasoned with brown-rice vinegar or umeboshi vinegar for a sour taste.

• Five to ten percent beans and bean products. It is best to use smaller beans such as azuki beans, lentils, and chickpeas for regular dishes. They can be cooked with a small volume of wakame or kombu sea vegetables, fall-season squash, chestnuts, or onions and carrots. Bean products such as tempeh, natto or tofu (cooked, not raw) may replace beans or can occasionally be used together with vegetables in moderate volume. Beans and bean products are to be consumed reg-ularly, but not necessarily every day.

• Five percent or less sea vegetables. Besides the sea vegetables used in soup, in some vegetable dishes, and in bean dishes, two to three times per week lightly cooked arame, nori, or wakame can be consumed as a side dish. They may be seasoned with a light taste of tamari soy sauce and/or rice vinegar, in small volume. Sea vegetables may also be used together with boiled salad or fresh salad.

All animal food, including fish and seafood, is primarily to be avoided. However, if craved, nonfatty, white-meat fish or immobile-type shellfish such as clams and oysters can be used in miso soup with vegetables and sea vegetables to make a fish and vegetable soup. Mobile shellfish such as shrimp and lobsters are to be avoided because of their high cholesterol content.

Fruits and fruit juices are best avoided, though cooked and dried fruits such as apples, cherries, strawberries, or other berries may be used in small portions, if craved. In the event that fresh fruit is desired, the volume should be moderate and intake infrequent. Only temperate-climate fruits, locally grown and in season, should be consumed.

If sweets are craved, cooked vegetables that are naturally sweet such as fall-season squash, cabbages, or carrots are preferred to special sweeteners. However, barley malt, rice syrup, and other cereal-grain-based sweeteners can occasionally be used in small volume.

Nuts and nut butters should primarily be avoided, though roasted seeds such as sesame, pumpkin, and sunflower may be used occasionally as a snack.

All regular macrobiotic condiments may be used. However, it is important that salt not be overconsumed, and it may need to be minimized in some cases.

For liver-cancer, a special daily drink of one or two cups of boiled shiitake mushroom can help relieve internal tension and improve the liver. This tea is made by soaking a dried shiitake mushroom, cut in quarters, in spring water and cooking with one to two teaspoons of grated daikon and one teaspoon of tamari soy sauce added for seasoning. Shiitake mushroom and fresh daikon may also be cooked frequently in miso soup or as a part of vegetable dishes and consumed several times per week. Shiitake is useful for helping to dissolve excessive animal fats in the body.

Overconsumption of food and beverages is strictly to be avoided. Chewing food very well, until all substances liquefy in the mouth, is essential for the improvement of health. Eating before sleeping should also be avoided for three hours beforehand. Other dietary practices, including daily beverage consumption, can follow the standard guidelines for cancer prevention in the recipe section.

As explained in the introduction to Part II, cancer patients who have received or who are currently undergoing medical treatment may need to make further dietary modifications.

HOME CARES

• A taro potato plaster can be applied on the liver region, front and back, for three to four hours or overnight, immediately after administering a hot ginger compress on the same area for five to ten minutes. These compresses will ease the tumor or hardening of the liver and improve the overall condition.

• Scrubbing the whole body with a very hot towel soaked in water containing grated gingerroot is helpful for promoting better circulation.

• Pains in the liver, front or back, including some areas along the spine, can be eased by the taro potato plaster, preceded by a ginger compress, as described above.

• In the event that appetite declines or is lost, genuine brown-rice cream can be consumed with a small volume of condiments such as gomashio (sesame salt), tekka, or umeboshi plum. Lightly seasoned miso soup with scallions and nori cooked in it can also be served. As appetite returns, regular dishes can gradually be added. A dish of raw fresh salad or temperate-climate fruit in season, in moderate volume, may also help restore the appetite.

OTHER CONSIDERATIONS

• Daily physical exercise that does not produce exhaustion is recommended. Ten to fifteen minutes of daily breathing exercises, especially emphasizing long exhalation, are also beneficial. These physical and breathing exercises contribute to relaxing tensions in the body and mind as well as harmonizing physical metabolism.

• Keeping air quality clean and fresh is important for maintenance of general health. For that purpose, green leafy plants can be placed in the house and the windows periodically opened to allow circulation of fresh air.

• For underwear, pillows, and bedsheets, cotton is preferable to synthetic fabrics.

• Exposure to artificial electromagnetic radiation from watching television, especially color television, for long periods, and to white fluorescent light should be avoided.

PERSONAL EXPERIENCE

Liver Cancer

In spring of 1979, sixty-two-year-old Hilda Sorhagen experienced a tenderness in her liver area, nausea, diarrhea, and constipation. Her color turned brownish-yellow, and her friends asked her if she had been to Florida because she appeared so dark. For several years she had been ailing and suffered from poor digestion, fatigue, and nervousness. Some years before, her husband died, and she faced mounting pressures from looking over his business and the demands of raising three teenagers. "I had seen so many doctors for one thing or another without improvement nor a positive diagnosis," she recalled of this period. "It was always 'go for x-rays' or 'see a specialist.' When I did go, I knew no more than before. They found nothing and blamed it on tension."

When her children grew up, she turned over the family business to the son and entered a yoga ashram in Pennsylvania. The community followed an Indian-style vegetarian diet high in dairy foods, spices, sweets, and raw fruit.

When preliminary medical tests failed to find anything, Hilda came to see me in April 1979, and I evaluated her condition as cancerous. Subsequent examination by her family physician confirmed a hardening of the lower part of her liver, and CEA blood tests were elevated in the cancerous range. However, because of her previous unsatisfactory experience with medical diagnosis, she refused x-rays and decided to begin the Cancer-Prevention Diet. Although her sister died from liver cancer two years previously, her doctors and children were not convinced that she had a malignancy and opposed her decision.

Taking a week off from her yoga work, Hilda came to Boston and took some introductory classes in medicinal cooking, visual diagnosis, and shiatsu massage at the East West Foundation. Upon her return, she found that since all the food in the ashram was prepared in a community kitchen, she could no longer fulfill her commitments to the ashram to her satisfaction. Locating an apartment nearby, she

resolved to live and cook by herself. Her children were not supportive of her approach, and she did not want to burden others with
taking care of her. Yet often she was so weak that she could not get
out of bed but "somehow managed to drag myself into the kitchen to
put up a pot of brown rice."

Looking back, she noted:

The first sign of improvement was change in energy which was
immediately noticeable. I felt stronger, I wanted to be more active. I remembered feeling that I wanted to walk up the hill to the
meditation room whereas before I could barely get in the car to
drive, even though it was only 1,500 yards away. I wanted to walk,
and when I had made it to the top I met one of the ashram members. He was surprised to see me so early in the morning. I felt
such a victory and gratitude that I wept with joy. There was a time
when I thought I would never be able to walk that path again.

In the summer of 1980 her condition had improved considerably,
and Hilda stayed in several macrobiotic study centers in Philadelphia
to develop her cooking further. I saw her again during this period and
observed that the tumor had disappeared.

Commenting upon her previous way of eating, she recalled,
"Michio told me to stop eating raw fruit. I argued that fruit was
healthy and one meal a day consisted of fruit only. I pleaded, 'Not
even an apple?' and he just looked at me. Now I understand why he
looked at me the way I now look at my students when they ask the
same question."

In addition to yoga, Hilda is now teaching cooking, and her relationship with her children has changed, and they have grown very
close. "I have more energy now than my children," she reported in
the autumn of 1982. "This lifestyle has helped me to speed up my
spiritual evolution and I have become a more loving person. I will
continue to live a macrobiotic way of life because I love the food, and
it has saved my life."

In the fall of 1981 a group at the ashram decided to experiment
with the macrobiotic diet for six weeks. The results were so remark-
able that Guru Amrit Desai, the community's spiritual leader, asked
the entire 150-member group to adopt the macrobiotic way of eating.
He described the approach as *sattvic* or balanced, pure, and cleans-

ing according to the traditional dietary ideals set forth in the Bhagavad Gita and other Hindu scriptures.

As grains, beans, sea vegetables, and fermented foods became the
focus of meal planning, the ashram cooks replaced cheese, eggs,
spices, and honey, which had been used extensively in the past.
Jeffrey Magdow, M.D., a staff physician at the community's Kripalu
Center for Holistic Health, reported about six months after the transition: "In addition to my own personal experience of many benefits
through the practice of this diet, I have seen stabilized energy patterns, improved elimination, and a heightened awareness of the
effects of foods on mental and physical well-being. . . ." Sources: Personal communication from Hilda Sorhagen, and Alex Jack and Karin
Stephan, "Whole-Grain Ashram," *East West Journal*, July 1982, pp.
8–9.

18.

Lung Cancer

FREQUENCY

In the last few decades, lung cancer has risen more sharply in the United States than any other form of cancer. Today it is the leading cause of cancer deaths in American men. From 1950 to 1977 incidence in women more than tripled from four per 100,000 to fifteen. Three out of four lung cancer patients are men, usually between the ages of forty and seventy. Altogether lung cancer will kill an estimated 117,000 Americans in 1983, and 135,000 new cases will develop. In other parts of the world, incidence differs widely. In Scotland, for instance, it is about twice as high as in America. In Portugal, lung cancer occurs only one eighth as frequently.

Lung cancers commonly spread to or from the liver, brain, or bone. Ninety percent of cases consist of four types: 1) *epidermoid carcinomas*, which are located centrally and spread by invasion to nearby tissues, 2) *adenocarcinomas*, which usually affect only one lobe of the lung but spread to other sites, 3) *large-cell carcinomas*, which are similar to adenocarcinomas, and 4) *oat-cell carcinomas*, which are fast growing. Early detection of lung cancer is not common, and 50 percent of tumors are considered inoperable. Surgery followed by radiation treatment is favored by the medical profession for the first three types. This may take the form of a lobectomy, involving removal of a lobe, or a pneumonectomy, removal of the entire lung. Oat-cell carcinoma is treated with chemotherapy. Drugs may also be given to those with the other forms of tumors to control pain. Eight percent of men and 13 percent of women with lung cancer currently survive five years or more. Chemotherapy for oat-cell carcinoma may produce regression lasting one to two years.

STRUCTURE

The lungs are twin respiratory organs situated along with the heart in the thoracic cavity. They are conical in shape and divided into five lobes. There are three on the right side and two on the left. The lobes are further subdivided into bronchi and alveoli. The alveoli consist of thousands of tiny air sacs. During breathing, oxygen enters the lungs and is picked up by the blood. The surface of the alveoli contains an array of blood vessels that total about 100 square yards. Oxygenated blood goes to the heart where it is pumped through the arteries to the cells. In the body's cells, oxygen combines with metabolized sugar or fat to produce energy, leaving behind carbon dioxide and water as byproducts. The carbon dioxide is picked up by the blood and carried to the lungs where it is breathed out. The lungs are also a major site for receiving electromagnetic energy from the surrounding environment and for stimulating certain digestive processes, especially the eliminatory function of the large intestine.

CAUSE OF CANCER

Modern medicine has focused considerable attention on lung cancer because of its steady increase. Cigarette smoking has been cited as the major cause, and epidemiologists say up to 80 or 90 percent of lung tumors could be prevented by eliminating tobacco. Other researchers have noted an association between lung cancer and increased pollution in the environment or workplace. In Houston, for example, lung cancer deaths increased by 53 percent during the 1970's. This seemed to correspond with a boom of petrochemical plants and refineries in the area. Lung cancer is also higher among asbestos workers, copper miners, and those who work with lead and zinc. In the last several years, the role of diet in protecting against lung cancer has received increased attention. Several medical studies show that people who regularly consume carrots and dark green or yellow vegetables containing beta-carotene, a precursor to vitamin A, have lower lung cancer rates than other people.

Each of these hypotheses is related to understanding the spread of lung cancer. However, the underlying cause of the disease is not smoking, pollution, or a temporary vitamin deficiency, but rather a long-time imbalance in the entire daily way of eating. Situated in the middle region of the body, the lungs are relatively balanced in structure, combining both expanded (yin) and contracted (yang) features. Respiratory disorders, including lung tumors, result from the excessive intake of extreme foods from both the yin and yang categories, including meat, eggs, poultry, dairy products, refined flour, sugar, fats and oils, fruits and juices, alcohol, stimulants, chemicals, and drugs.

As we have seen in the progressive development of disease, excess intake of acid, mucus-forming, and fatty foods eventually accumulates in various parts of the body, including the sinuses, inner ear, breasts, lungs, and kidney and reproductive organs. In the case of the lungs, aside from the obvious symptoms of coughing and chest congestion, mucus often fills the air sacs, and breathing becomes more difficult. Occasionally, a coat of mucus in the bronchi can be loosened and discharged by coughing, but once the sacs are surrounded it becomes more firmly lodged and can remain there for a long period. Then, if air pollutants or cigarette smoke enters the lungs, their heavy components, especially various carbon compounds, are attracted to and remain in this sticky environment. In severe cases, these deposits can give rise to tumors. However, the underlying cause of this condition is the accumulation of sticky fat and mucus in the alveoli and in the blood and capillaries surrounding them.

The subject of tobacco and its role in cancer is best understood in relation to daily diet. For centuries the North American Indians have smoked tobacco without developing cancer and have utilized the plant for many medicinal purposes. One of the main differences between the Indians' use of tobacco and our own is that they ate a balanced diet high in corn and other cereal grains, wild grasses, locally grown or foraged vegetables, fresh seasonal fruit, seeds, and a small to moderate amount of fresh game. Current studies suggest that in societies where a traditional way of eating is still followed and where smoking is widespread there is no clear correlation between smoking and lung cancer.

The quality of modern tobacco is also a contributing factor in the increase of respiratory illnesses. The original Indian tobacco was grown naturally without phosphate fertilizers or artificial pesticides and was air dried. Modern flue-cured tobacco is subjected to heavy amounts of chemicals during cultivation, and the drying process is speeded up from about three months to six days. Commercial cigarettes also often contain 5 to 20 percent sugar by weight, as well as humectants to retain moisture and other synthetic additives to enhance flavor and taste. In countries where tobacco is not flue-cured or mixed with sugar, such as in the Soviet Union, China, and Taiwan, medical studies generally indicate no significant correlation between smoking and lung cancer. Laboratory studies also show that mice on a low-fat diet will not get lung cancer from smoking but when put on a high-fat diet will develop tumors. Thus, chemically refined tobacco in combination with a diet high in fat, sugar, oil, and other sticky foods will combine synergistically and increase the risk of lung cancer.

Similarly, a healthy pair of lungs can withstand and neutralize a great deal of air pollution, metallic dust, or chemical irritants in the environment. This is why nonsmokers who eat a balanced diet are usually not bothered physically by cigarette smoke in their vicinity. Their lungs are working properly and naturally filter airborne particulates with no perceived discomfort. However, nonsmokers whose lungs are coated with fat, mucus, and acid from eating a meat and sugar diet or a vegetarian diet high in dairy foods and sweets will often feel irritated as these particles from the smoke enter and are trapped in their lungs. Of course, cigarette pollution should be avoided, and insofar as possible, it is not advisable to work in or live near chemical industries or hazardous waste sites. However, some people are relatively more immune than others to toxic substances owing to their daily diet and physical constitution or inherited characteristics formed primarily by their mother's diet during pregnancy.

In Far Eastern medicine, tobacco is classified as a yang substance due to its contracting and drying effects. Smokers are generally thinner (more yang) than nonsmokers, and most smokers put on weight (become more yin) when they stop. Thus, smoking contracts the body and has an alkalizing effect on the blood. As the Indians found, pure tobacco used in moderation can have a soothing effect and can increase immunity to colds, infections, and chronic ailments brought about by an overly acidic condition.

The principles of contraction (yang) and expansion (yin) can also be used to understand why many people in modern society are attracted to smoking and why they abuse tobacco by consuming it in far greater quantities than the Indians. Nicotine, the major ingredient in tobacco, is very yang. Farmers in the South have often sprayed tobacco juice on crops to ward off parasites and prevent blights. In the body, a similar process occurs. Disease-promoting bacteria cannot thrive in an alkaline environment. The human blood is normally slightly alkaline in pH. A daily diet of whole grains, cooked vegetables, and seasonal fruit produces this slightly yang condition. However, the modern diet containing a large percentage of meat and sugar has a net effect of making the blood acid. Acid-forming foods also include eggs, poultry, dairy products, refined flour and flour products, and stimulants. In order to restore proper pH and balance acidic (yin) blood, the body is physiologically attracted to nicotine (yang). Biochemically, nicotine raises sugar levels in the blood. Chain smokers are often hypoglycemic and suffer from low blood sugar and their daily diet also lacks complex carbohydrate. This condition is brought about by intake of excessive fat, protein, sugar, or alcohol and can result in pancreatic and liver malfunction, weak adrenals, and erratic emotional behavior. The weaker the blood, the greater the desire to smoke. The more one smokes, the more carbon monoxide is produced in the blood and the harder the heart has to work.

The Indians smoked at most only a handful of cigarettes a day and often went for long periods without smoking at all. Throughout history, almost all traditional societies around the world existed happily without tobacco, and there is no biological necessity to smoke. Perhaps the North American Indians alone were attracted to this extreme yang pastime because their own staple food, corn, is the most expanded, yin form of grain and this was the way they had found to achieve a balance with their natural environment.

The unifying principle of yin and yang helps us to understand the physiology of smoking and the synergistic role chemicalized tobacco plays in overworking the circulatory and respiratory systems and promoting lung cancer. Though aggravated by tobacco, the epidemic of lung cancer in the West is primarily a disease of overnutrition and corresponds with the rise of chemical agriculture and changing patterns of food consumption, especially following World War II. Return to a daily way of eating centered on whole grains, vegetables, locally grown fruit, and a minimum of animal products will make lung cancer as rare an occurrence as it was in the early part of the century. The vitamin A and beta-carotene contained in certain foods are protective, though they are some examples of several nutritional elements beneficial to the lungs. Establishment of a regionally based natural system of agriculture will result in a substantial reduction of pollution in the environment as well as improved health. Less chemicals will be needed for crops, less petroleum for transcontinental shipment of produce and livestock, and less mining of metals for heavy farm equipment.

In exploring the roots of lung cancer, we find that many social problems are also related to the way we eat, and these problems cannot be resolved apart from changing our daily way of eating.

MEDICAL EVIDENCE

• In 1773 Bernard Payrilhe, professor of chemistry at École Santé and professor-royal of the College of Surgery in Paris, urged that cancer be treated by drinking carrot juice. His proposal won first prize from the Academy of Lyon on the subject of "What Is Cancer?" In a treatise on cancer four years later, he wrote that "with respect to medicinal ailments, barley, rice, etc. will be of great use." Sources: B. Peyrilhe, M.D., *A Dissertation on Cancerous Diseases* (London, 1777) and Michael Shimkin, *Contrary to Nature* (Washington, D.C.: National Institutes of Health, p. 183, 1977).

• In the early twentieth century, cancer began to appear among North American Indians as they began to adopt the diet of modern society. In the 1920's, J.L. Bulkley, M.D., a physician who lived among native Alaskans for twelve years, reported that he did not see a trace of cancer and attributed their lack of degenerative disease to a balanced diet. "The common cereals, which they raised, were ground and baked in the ashes of their fires, unleavened, and with little if any seasoning other than salt." A U.S. government official who helped compile health statistics among tribes in the continental United States noted, "Originally the Indians lived mostly on wild game and fish, with corn and dried berries, but, of course, as their conditions have changed, their diet has changed with them. . . . Like the white man, they now live very largely from tin cans and paper bags. . . . During the first years of my service, the scarcity of cancer among the Indians was a subject of comment. Now cases frequently come to my notice." Source: J.L. Bulkley, M.D., "Cancer among Primitive Tribes," *Cancer* 4:289–95, 1927.

• In 1958 Hugh Sinclair, a researcher at Oxford University in England, reported that rats will not develop lung cancer by smoking alone, controlling for other factors. "Just let someone feed a rat a high-meat diet, rich in peroxide fat, and see how quickly it gets lung cancer when it smokes cigarettes." Source: Wayne Martin, *Medical Heroes and Heretics* (Old Greenwich, Conn.: Devin-Adair, p. 94, 1977).

• A 1967 study indicated that vitamin A protected against cancer in laboratory animals. Of 113 hamsters dosed with a tumor-inducing chemical, one of sixty animals treated with vitamin A developed lung cancer, while sixteen of fifty-three controls got cancer. Source: U. Saffiotti et al., "Experimental Cancer of the Lung," *Cancer* 20: 857–64.

• After twenty years of tobacco research, Dr. Richard Passey of London's Chester Beatty Research Institute reported an association between flue-dried tobacco, especially that to which sugar had been added, and lung cancer. However, he found no significant link between traditional sugar-free, air-dried tobacco and cancer. In one experiment, he gave twenty flue-cured high-sugar cigarettes a day to a group of twelve rats and twenty air-dried low-sugar cigarettes to another dozen rats. On the sixty-second day, three rats in the flue-cured group had died. The other high-sugar rats were too weak to continue the experiment and four more died shortly thereafter. The dead rats had lung lesions and cancerous changes. At this point, the daily quota of the air-dried low-sugar group was increased to forty cigarettes a day. After 251 days, six healthy survivors remained. Three died of heatstroke, two died of undetermined causes, and one had an abcess near the kidney but not the lungs. Epidemiological studies show that England and Wales, which have the highest male lung cancer rate in the world, also have the highest sugar content in cigarettes, about 17 percent. France, where tobacco is air-dried and contains only 2 percent sugar, has one third less lung cancer. The United States, where sugar in tobacco averages 10 percent, has one half the male lung cancer mortality rate as Great Britain. Still, the U.S. tobacco industry reportedly is the nation's second largest consumer of sugar, after the canning industry. "Investigators from some other countries where cigarettes are made of air-dried tobacco—the Soviet Union, China, and Taiwan, among them—are unable to find any correlation between smoking and cancer." Source: "Tobacco: Is There a 'Cure' for Cancer?" *Medical World News*, March 16, 1973, pp. 17–19.

• In 1977 a case-control study in Singapore among Chinese women found that those who consumed green, leafy vegetables rich in vitamin A were about one half as likely to contract lung cancer than other women. Source: R. MacLennan et al., "Risk Factors for Lung Cancer in Singapore Chinese, a Population with High Female Incidence Rates," *International Journal of Cancer* 20:854–60.

• In 1978 epidemiologists reported that cancer of the lung, breast, and colon increased two to three times among Japanese women between 1950 and 1975. During that period, milk consumption increased 15 times; meat, eggs, and poultry climbed 7.5 times; and rice consumption dropped 70 percent. In Okinawa, with the highest proportion of centenarians, longevity was associated with lowered sugar and salt intake and higher intake of protein and green-yellow vegetables. Source: Y. Kagawa, "Impact of Westernization on the Nutrition of Japan," *Preventive Medicine* 7:205–17.

• In 1979 an epidemiologist visiting Shanghai reported that "Chinese scientists are not convinced that cigarette smoking is the major cause of lung cancer." According to medical statistics, smokers in China are only slightly more susceptible to lung cancer than non-smokers and "the effect of cigarette smoking disappeared after controlling for chronic bronchitis." Source: B. Henderson, "Observations in Cancer Etiology in China," *National Cancer Institute Monograph* 53:59–65.

• In 1981 a case-control study of 375 women in Hawaii indicated that "cigarette smoking is clearly not the only cause, nor even the major cause, of lung cancer in all populations of women." The researchers found that native Hawaiians who smoked had a 10.5 relative risk of lung cancer, women of Japanese origin 4.9, and those of Chinese origin 1.8. The researchers speculated that dietary factors were possibly the primary cause of lung cancer and that smoking was a contributing factor. Source: M.W. Hinds et al., "Differences in Lung Cancer Risk from Smoking among Japanese, Chinese, and Hawaiian Women in Hawaii," *International Journal of Cancer* 27:297–302.

• A 1981 Chicago study found that regular consumption of foods containing carotene, a precursor to vitamin A, protected against lung cancer. Over a period of nineteen years, a group of 1,954 men at a Western Electric plant were monitored, and those who regularly consumed carrots, dark green lettuce, spinach, broccoli, kale, Chinese cabbage, peaches, apricots, and other carotene-rich foods had significantly lower lung cancer rates than controls. Source: R.B. Shekelle et al., "Dietary Vitamin A and Risk of Cancer in the Western Electric Study," *Lancet* 2:1185–90.

• In 1982 a British medical researcher reviewed epidemiological studies in Wales, England, the United States, Sweden, Japan, Singapore, and Thailand and concluded that tobacco was not the major cause of lung cancer. "Recorded increases in lung cancer in both sexes during this century are enormously larger than those expected from the changes in tobacco consumption . . . factors other than smoking must have been the dominant causes. . . ." Source: P.R.J. Burch, "Cigarette Smoking and Lung Cancer: A Continuing Controversy," *Medical Hypotheses* 9:293–306.

DIAGNOSIS

Doctors employ a variety of means to test for lung cancer, including chest x-rays, chest tomogram, bone, liver, and gallium scans, fluoroscopy, bronchoscopy, and sputum examination. If tumors are indicated, their location will be sought by various types of biopsies as well as a thoracoscopy, a surgical procedure in which the lung is deflated and examined, or a mediastinoscopy, a small incision in the front of the neck in which lymph nodes are removed for examination.

Oriental medicine diagnoses the condition of the lungs by observing their corresponding region of the face, the cheeks. Weak and underactive lungs, including tuberculosis, are indicated by a sallow, pale, or slightly puffy appearance on the cheeks. The person often experiences poor circulation, labored breathing, weak chest muscles accompanied by rounding and tensing of the shoulders, a drooping posture, and an inclination toward anemia or overweight. Over time, this condition of the lungs can lead to pleurisy, emphysema, asthma, and possible lung or breast cancer. This form of lung condition results from excessive consumption of hard fats, particularly eggs and cheese, as well as dry, baked, and salty foods, which lead to excessive fluid consumption, the lack of fresh or lightly cooked crisp green vegetables, excessive smoking, and a lack of exercise.

An excessive and hyperactive functioning of the lungs is reflected by a variety of other signs. These include pimples on the cheeks, showing excessive storage of fatty acid and mucus as a result primarily of dairy food and sugar. White cheeks indicate excessive animal fats from dairy foods. Red cheeks show overactive blood capillaries in the lungs caused by too much fruit and juices, spices, sugar, coffee or tea. A drawn, overly tight appearance on the cheeks is produced by overconsumption of salt, fish, or poultry as well as dry or baked goods.

This drawn appearance sometimes includes vertical lines on the cheeks indicating restricted blood flow, contracted alveoli, and tightened chest muscles and may lead to pneumonia. Brown blotches on the cheeks represent acidosis resulting from sugar consumption and is a serious precancerous condition. Green colorations on the cheeks or a light-green shadow on the outer vertical edges of the cheeks are a cancerous sign of breast or lung cancer. Beauty marks show a past fever in the lungs and moles on the cheeks indicate excess protein and sugar intake. The various signs of excess mucus and fat storage in the lungs can indicate developing allergies, nasal congestion, bronchitis, whooping cough, tuberculosis, or cancer. Overactive lungs are often accompanied by constipation or other difficulties in the large intestine, the lung's complementary opposite organ.

A skilled Oriental diagnostician will also examine the person's lung meridian, which runs along the arms and the seam between the thumb and first finger for colors and blemishes. One common sign of lung problems is a weakness or tension in the thumb, the ending of the lung meridian. The practitioner of Far Eastern medicine will also take pulses on the wrist and press the abdominal, chest, and back regions to substantiate the visual diagnosis and diagnose the exact type of lung ailment.

DIETARY RECOMMENDATIONS

Lung cancer shares similar dietary causes with cancer of the large intestine and liver cancer. Lung tumors are one of the deeper forms of cancer and usually the lungs are filled in part or in whole with mucus and fatty substances. To prevent and heal lung cancer, first, all extreme foods from the yang category are to be avoided or minimized including meat, poultry, eggs, dairy products, and seafood as well as baked flour products. It is also necessary to avoid extreme foods and beverages from the yin category, including sugar and all other sweets, fruits and juices, spices and stimulants, alcohol and drugs, as well as all artificial, chemicalized, and refined food.

Dietary recommendations for daily consumption, by volume, should be as follows:

• Fifty to sixty percent whole-cereal grains, pressure-cooked, principally medium- and short-grain brown rice. Other cereal grains such as millet, barley, whole wheat, rye, oats, buckwheat, and corn may be supplemented occasionally. Flour products such as bread, pancakes, and cookies are to be avoided to prevent mucus formation, with the exception of occasional consumption of nonyeasted whole-wheat or rye bread.

• Five to ten percent miso soup or tamari soy sauce broth. One to two bowls, prepared with sea vegetables such as kombu or wakame and with hard, leafy, and root vegetables, should be eaten daily.

• Twenty to thirty percent cooked vegetables, prepared in various forms and dishes. Cooking oil should be only unrefined sesame, corn, or other vegetable oil, used in very moderate amounts. Among vegetables, broccoli and leafy green tops of carrots, turnips, and daikon, and watercress are especially recommended. Root vegetables such as carrots, daikon, and burdock are also very beneficial, and cabbages, onions, pumpkins, and acorn and butternut squashes may also be eaten regularly. Lotus root is especially good for all sorts of lung disorders, and helps to ease breathing. Lotus root can be used frequently as a part of other vegetable dishes. Macrobiotic pickles should be of a quality that has aged for a long time.

• Five to ten percent beans and bean products, especially azuki, lentils, and smaller beans in preference to larger beans. They can be cooked with a small portion of sea vegetables such as kombu, hijiki, or arame or with sweet winter squashes or onions and carrots. Fermented soybean products such as tempeh, miso, natto, and tamari soy sauce are also recommended for supplemental use and as seasonings in moderate amount, especially miso or tamari soy sauce that has fermented for one-and-a-half years or longer.

• Five percent or less sea vegetables prepared in various ways, especially hijiki, arame, and kombu. They can be cooked in any vegetable dish or consumed as an additional small dish. Sea vegetables should be eaten frequently and are very important in detoxifying the body.

In the event that animal food is desired, a small portion of dried fish such as iriko or carp soup prepared with carp, burdock, and miso may be consumed occasionally. However, it is wiser to avoid regular consumption of animal food altogether for a few months.

Fruits may be consumed if desired, in the form of dried or cooked fruit, but only infrequently and in very small volume.

Avoid nuts and nut butters, though roasted seeds such as sesame, sunflower, and pumpkin may be consumed occasionally.

All other dietary guidelines should follow the standard cancer prevention suggestions.

As explained in the introduction to Part II, cancer patients who have received or who are currently undergoing medical treatment may need to make further dietary modifications.

HOME CARES

• Smoking should be strictly avoided by people with lung disorders, especially cancer. Nicotine, tars, and other carbon compounds in tobacco become lodged in the air sacs of the lungs. This causes further accumulation of fat, mucus, and other dietary substances that cause the tumor to form.

• In the event of coughing, drink one half cup of liquid squeezed from grated fresh lotus root. Warmed up and taken like a tea, this is particularly effective in easing throat or chest congestion. The remaining lotus root may also be cooked in soup or eaten with a little tamari soy sauce. Lotus root prepared in various forms with other vegetables is helpful in general for lung cancer and other lung and breathing disorders, including asthma and bronchitis. Raw slices of lotus root, seasoned with umeboshi juice or rice vinegar, may also be taken frequently as a side dish.

• A mustard plaster applied on the chest, preferably both front and back, can also help alleviate severe coughing.

• A lotus-root plaster, consisting of grated lotus root, mixed with white flour to hold consistency, and well mixed with 5 to 10 percent grated ginger, may be applied to loosen up the congested lung. This plaster may be kept on for a few hours.

• Lotus seeds cooked with kombu or wakame sea vegetable seasoned with a moderate amount of tamari soy sauce or miso are also helpful for the lungs. One cup of this mixture may be eaten daily.

• With a towel dipped and squeezed tightly in hot ginger water, scrub the whole body, including the chest and abdominal area, until the skin surface becomes pinkish in color. This helps improve circulation, energy, and breathing and should be done daily.

• Lung conditions are closely related to the proper functioning of the large intestine. Smooth, regular bowel movements daily can help the smooth functioning of the lungs and improve breathing. If the intestines are constipated or stagnated, it is especially necessary to chew all food very, very well, up to one hundred times, and not to overeat. This will help restore proper elimination.

OTHER CONSIDERATIONS

• In Far Eastern medicine, the lungs are viewed as the seat of the emotions, feelings, and ability to experience sadness. Lung problems are usually accompanied by a tendency toward depression, self-doubt, reclusiveness, and a sense that life is a heavy burden. As the lungs are healed, it is important to cultivate a cheerful and bright disposition. Strive to overcome feelings of self-pity by meditating on the marvelous order of the universe, nature's wonderful recuperative powers, and your opportunity to be of service and inspiration to others by overcoming your illness. Read comedies, avoid tragedies.

• Meditative exercises that focus on the breathing will help strengthen the lungs. Yoga, Do-in, tai-chi, or other exercises that stimulate the cardiovascular region and energy pathways are to be preferred over jogging, weight lifting, and more active sports.

• Avoid smoggy and dusty air as well as atmospheres contaminated with industrial gases or chemical fumes. Visit the countryside or seashore or take long walks in the woods. At home, maintain a clean orderly environment. Carbon dioxide in the house may accelerate tumor growth so place green plants in the living room and other spaces to ensure a fresh supply of oxygen.

• Avoid watching television from the front since radiation affects the chest region. Similarly, stay away from x-rays, video terminals, high-voltage lines, and other artificial sources of electromagnetic energy that can weaken your lungs and respiratory system.

• Avoid synthetic clothing; wear and sleep on cotton fibers. In addition, lung cancer patients should be careful to avoid inhaling asbestos fibers. Many household products contain asbestos, including some types of aprons, potholders, and other cooking fabrics, floor tiles, and other building and construction materials. Use natural materials and furnishings whenever possible.

PERSONAL EXPERIENCE

Lung Cancer

In December, 1981, Lucille Ré, a sixty-three-year-old widow from Manhasset, New York, first noticed that she was having trouble breathing in cold weather. It was December 9 and she was going to the Metropolitan Opera in New York City with a friend. She was rushing to the performance when she had a "horrible breathing attack" and could not catch her breath for several minutes.

The next day she made a doctor's appointment. Upon examination, he diagnosed emphysema and prescribed medicated breathalizers to clear the passage. Mrs. Ré continued using these until April 30, 1982 when the physician called with the results of a recent echocardiogram. The doctor said it appeared as though the heart was either enlarged or surrounded by water and he wanted her to be hospitalized. She left work immediately and went to a nearby hospital.

After further examinations and tests, it was discovered that her heart was surrounded by liquid and beating only 40 beats per minute. In the months that followed, Mrs. Ré had a pacemaker inserted and received further treatments for emphysema. In July her two children, Tom, a lawyer, and Elaine, a consultant, were told that she had lung cancer. The tumor was diagnosed as undifferentiated adenocarcinoma, a fatal form of lung cancer, and the doctor gave her under six months to live.

In the weeks that followed, she was given radiation therapy. On July 17 she was permitted to go home but continued with radiation in an effort to reduce the size of the lung tumor. However, by August 18, she was again gasping for breath and entered the hospital to have liquid removed from around the heart. During this period her son happened to read an article in *Life* magazine about a medical doctor whose own case of terminal cancer had been relieved on the macrobiotic diet. The Rés decided to see me and arranged for a consultation on August 31, the day after Mrs. Ré was to be released from the hospital.

"Do you know where lung cancer comes from?" I asked her.

"Smoking," she replied. Until the development of her emphysema about a year before, Mrs. Ré had smoked a pack of cigarettes a day, at which time she stopped "cold turkey."

"Smoking number two. Number one dairy," I explained.

Looking back on the rest of our conversation, Mrs. Ré later recalled:

> Patiently, Mr. Kushi specifically reviewed every facet of the diet which was soon to become my way of life and my hope for life. Toward the end of the one-hour conference, my ears perked up when I heard him say I could have ice cream.

He noticed my delight and I proudly told him, "I eat ice cream every day."

With this, a frown came over his face and he repeated, "Rice cream, rice cream, not ice cream. No more ice cream."

With that sobering remark, our conference ended and I was given specific dietary recommendations. I remember feeling exhausted, confused, and hungry. A nice tomato sandwich with mayonnaise on toasted bread would have hit the spot. Instead, we went to a restaurant called Open Sesame, where I had my first macrobiotic meal.

On the plane returning to New York, I kept wondering, How am I ever going to begin this diet, learn how to cook this food, and, most of all, how would I remember what food was what?

If you have never cooked macrobiotically, you won't know the metamorphosis a kitchen must undergo. Except for some of the pots and pans (the stainless steel ones) and the paper goods, very little was left in the kitchen to remind me of years gone by. All electrical appliances were removed, and brown bags filled with grains and beans quickly pushed out my canned goods.

In these beginning days I was unable to absorb 95 percent of what was said and shown to me because I felt so disoriented, light-headed, and unable to cope. I learned later that these symptoms are common when your body is detoxifying itself in the initial stages.

Prior to this time, a typical week's menu for Mrs. Ré consisted of meats, chicken, fish, refined flour products, cakes, dairy (including ice cream), coffee, and—one of her favorites—chocolate cream candies.

As she started to regain her strength, over about three weeks, Mrs. Ré began participating in life again. At her daughter's suggestion, she decided to go to a local fishing pier for sun, fresh sea air, and snappers. Since she had been able to walk only short distances in August, she decided to bring the wheelchair. "On this day, however, I decided to push the wheelchair and let it carry the fishing gear."

In October Mrs. Ré began feeling weak and heavy and realized that her body was retaining liquid. To reduce this excess and lessen the pain, her children, who attended her twenty-four hours a day, increased the amount of daikon in the diet and lowered the amount of salt and tamari. However, she remained bed-ridden and would fade in and out of consciousness, dreaming of cows sitting on her chest.

During this time, I was delivering seminars in Europe and Asia and, unable to contact me, the family called in a medical doctor. He told Tom and Elaine that their mother was in the last stage of lung cancer and probably would not last more than a week. If she survived longer, he said there would be no way of ridding the lymph system of the liquid and that she could count on spending the remainder of her life paralyzed.

Tom and Elaine finally got in touch with Bill Spear, head of the macrobiotic center in Middletown, Connecticut. Bill went to New York and recommended that Mrs. Ré change to fresh well water, add more seitan to her diet, and eat a bit more squash. These modifications improved her condition, and when I returned home I further recommended that she could strengthen herself by eating carp soup, squash soup, and white fish, as well as occasionally cooked tangerines. I explained that she had about a 50 percent chance of recovery.

Within a week, the swelling in her fingers and toes began to decrease visibly. By Christmas, although needing help to walk up the stairs, Mrs. Ré was feeling better and opening gifts on her own. On January 29, 1983, I saw her in New York and, observing the improvement, told her that she should be fine.

"Michio attributed my miracle to the energy and work of my family in following the dietary recommendations," she noted in February. "I personally give credit to God's power and blessing which is manifested through the talents of Mr. Kushi, the chemistry of macrobiotics, and the love and dedication of my family. Today I have the strength of mind and body to begin learning about the diet. One might ask if giving up the American diet we have come to know and enjoy is worth the effort. My answer: I was given six months by one doctor and a week by another. Thanks to God and macrobiotics, I have lived to see my sixty-fourth birthday last week. Yes, it is well worth it." Source: Elaine Ré and Associates. © 1983 by Elaine F. Ré, Ph.D., used with permission.

19.

Lymphoma and Hodgkin's Disease

FREQUENCY

Cancer of the lymphatic system will kill 13,900 Americans in 1983, while 30,700 new cases will develop. Lymphoma affects men and women about evenly and is usually divided into two types: *Hodgkin's disease*, which particularly affects people aged fifteen to twenty-four and over fifty, usually involves enlarged lymph nodes in the neck, armpit, or groin. It often spreads to the brain and adjacent lymph nodes. Depending on the case, it is treated with radiation and chemotherapy. A battery of four drugs is commonly given to control Hodgkin's disease known as MOPP (nitrogen mustard, Oncovin, procarbazine, and prednisone). Between 53 to 57 percent of those with Hodgkin's disease survive five years or longer. *Non-Hodgkin's lymphomas* are divided into eight major types depending on the type of cells affected and their state of differentiation. This form of lymphoma may appear throughout the body and in sites other than the lymph nodes such as the digestive tract. Non-Hodgkin's lymphomas metastasize in erratic manners. Radiation and chemotherapy are major methods of treatment. Depending on the type, the remission rate for these eight lymphomas is between 18 and 37 percent. There are also several rarer forms of lymphoma such as mycosis fungoides and Burkitt's lymphoma.

STRUCTURE

The lymphatic system consists of lymph capillaries, vessels, ducts, and nodes, as well as such organs as the spleen and tonsils. The lymphatic system is closely related to the blood system. When blood circulates, some of the fluid and other elements in the blood leak out due to the enormous pressure the blood is under. This clear liquid or lymph accumulates between the cells and blood capillaries. The lymph system transports this substance through a network of small, clear tubes and rejoins with the bloodstream near the collarbone. In structure, the bloodstream is generally more yang since its main function is to transport red-blood cells. The lymph stream, consisting primarily of white-blood cells, is more yin. Both comprise the circulatory system as a whole and circulate in opposite yet complementary directions. Blood circulation begins in the heart, radiates outward to the more peripheral regions, and then returns. Conversely, the flow of lymph begins in the peripheral body tissues and then enters the central bloodstream.

Unlike the bloodstream, the lymphatic system has no central organ to pump the lymph fluid. The flow of lymph is maintained by several factors such as the activity and contraction of the lungs and diaphragm during breathing and the movements of the villi and the contractions of the small intestine. The spleen is the major organ of the lymphatic system. Located opposite the liver on the left side of the body, the spleen filters substances like bacteria and worn-out red-blood cells from the lymph and body fluid. The spleen contributes to the formation of white-blood cells, especially lymphocytes; stores blood and minerals, particularly iron; produces antibodies; and contributes to the production of bile. The liver and spleen are complementary. The liver is yang (compact) in comparison and functions in coordination with the bloodstream. The more yin (expanded) spleen serves as the major focus of the lymphatic system.

Also associated with the lymph are the tonsils. The main function of the tonsils is to localize various types of toxic excess for discharging from the body. For example, after consumption of an extreme food, such as an excessive volume of sugar, oil, fats, soft drinks, fruits, juices, refined flour, or chemicals, additional white-blood cells are created in the tonsils to neutralize any harmful bacteria that may form in the lymph, while minerals start to gather in this region as a buffer for the discharge of acids. In the meantime the tonsils may become inflamed and the body temperature may rise. If, at this time, the person has the tonsils removed, the fever and inflammation may disappear, but the toxic bodily fluids will continue to circulate throughout the system, and the remaining lymphatic organs will have to work much harder to perform the cleaning and discharge function of the tonsils. The net result is a reduction in the ability of the lymphatic system to efficiently rid the body of toxic excess.

The lymphatic system also contains another major organ, which is located above the heart. Known as the thymus, this organ reaches its largest size at the age of two and then gradually declines until it disappears entirely. The thymus produces white-blood cells along with certain types of antibodies.

CAUSE OF CANCER

If the bloodstream is filled with fat and mucus, which are strong in acid, excess will begin to accumulate in the organs. Since the lungs and kidneys are usually affected first, their functions of filtering and cleansing the blood become less efficient. This situation leads to further deterioration of the blood quality and also affects the lymphatic system. General lymphatic troubles can be summarized into two types. The first involves expansion or inflammation of the lymphatic nodes and organs. In extreme cases, this overly yin condition leads to a rupture of the lymphatic vessels. These problems result when the lymph fluid contains too much fatty acid. The other, more yang condition is hardening of the lymph nodes, organs, ducts, and capillaries.

As we have seen, operations such as tonsillectomies contribute to the deterioration of the lymphatic system since they reduce the ability of this system to cleanse itself. Swollen tonsils and lymph glands result from overconsumption of refined and artificial foods, sugar, soft drinks, tropical fruits and vegetables, milk and dairy products, spices, and other extreme foods from the yin category usually higher in acid. These swellings represent a healthy reaction of the body to localize, neutralize, and discharge this excess. Continued consumption of these foods may produce a chronic deterioration of the quality of the blood and lymph. When the red blood cells begin to lose their capacity to change into normal body cells, the body starts to create a degenerate type of cell that is known as cancerous.

In Hodgkin's disease, the lymph nodes and spleen become inflamed, while in lymphomas a malignant tumor develops within the lymphoid tissue and the lymphatic organs become swollen. Both diseases involve an increase in the number of white-blood cells. Excessive intake of yin type foods and beverages is the main cause of lymphatic cancers. At the same time a decrease in the number of red-blood cells reflects a lack of minerals and other balanced foods centered around natural complex carbohydrate in the diet. Compared to other forms of cancer, especially tumors in the deep, inner organs, lymphatic cancer and leukemia are relatively easy to relieve.

MEDICAL EVIDENCE

• In a 1975 study, French researchers reported that children with chronic radiation enteritis markedly improved on a low-fat diet free of gluten, cow's milk, and milk products. The eleven-year study followed forty-four children, twenty-nine of whom had advanced lymphoma and eleven who had Wilms' tumor. The mean age of the subjects was three years, ten months. Forty-two of the children had received cobalt treatments for cancer resulting in intestinal injury prior to starting the diet. Source: S.S. Donaldson et al., "Radiation Enteritis in Children," *Cancer* 35:1167–78.

• Persons who regularly eat cereal grains, pulses, vegetables, seeds, and nuts are less likely to get lymphoma or Hodgkin's disease than persons who do not usually eat these foods, according to a 1976 epidemiological survey. The sixteen-nation study, based on World Health Organization statistics, found a high correlation between consumption of animal protein, particularly from beef and dairy products, and lymphoma mortality. "Ingestion of cow's milk can produce generalised lymphadenopathy, hepatoslenomegaly, and profound adenoid hypertrophy," the researcher commented on the mechanism of carcinogenesis. "It has been conservatively estimated that more than 100 distinct antigens are released by the normal digestion of cow's milk, which may evoke production of all antibody classes." The studies indicated that beef and dairy food increased the risk of lymphosarcoma and Hodgkin's disease by 70 and 61 percent respectively, while cereal grains lowered the risk by 46 and 38 percent. Source: A.S. Cunningham, "Lymphomas and Animal-Protein Consumption," *Lancet* 2:1184–86.

• The average American eats nine pounds of chemical additives a year including preservatives, flavoring agents, stabilizers, and artificial colors. Red Dye No. 40, found in imitation fruit drinks, soda pop, hot dogs, jellies, candy, ice cream, and some cosmetics, has been linked to lymphomas in laboratory experiments. Source: Samuel S. Epstein, M.D., *The Politics of Cancer* (New York: Doubleday, pp. 186–87, 1979).

• A California physician reported to a scientific panel on cancer and diet that a high-protein diet reduces the immune mechanism of the body by its action on the T-lymphocyte cell. A diet high in animal products also increases the blood lipids and cholesterol. This, in turn, produces an increased susceptibility to viral infections, a decrease in antibody response, and a decrease in T-cell response, which helps protect against lymphoma. Source: J.A. Scharffenberg, M.D., "Health Consequences of a Good Lifestyle," American Association for the Advancement of Science, 1981.

• Mice on a low-calorie diet live longer and have a reduced risk of cancer, including lymphoma, than mice on a high-calorie diet. Two UCLA medical researchers reported in 1982 that laboratory animals fed 28 to 43 percent less calories than a control group lived 10 to 20 percent longer and registered fewer tumors of the lymphatic system. Source: R. Weindruch and R.L. Wolford, "Dietary Restriction in Mice Beginning at One Year of Age," *Science* 215:1415–18.

DIAGNOSIS

Hodgkin's disease is diagnosed medically by laboratory tests and usually involves surgical removal of a lymph node to be examined under a microscope for malignancy. If the nodes are not involved, a variety of other methods will be used including a bone-marrow biopsy, lymphangiogram, intravenous pyelogram, liver, spleen, and bone scans, and abdominal or chest CAT scan. In some cases the abdominal wall may be opened surgically for inspection and the spleen will be removed in an operation known as a splenectomy. For non-Hodgkin's lymphomas, an upper and lower GI series is taken, and a spinal tap will be performed to check for metastases to the brain.

Oriental diagnosis focuses primarily on visual features, especially colors, to ascertain the condition of the lymphatic system. A pinkish-white color on the lips indicates weakening lymphatic functions and other disorders, including a tendency toward Hodgkin's disease. This color is caused by excessive consumption of dairy products, fats, sugar, and fruits. A reddish-yellow color inside the lower eyelids shows disorder in the circulatory system, including the spleen function. This color is caused by excessive intake of foods from the extreme yang category, such as poultry, eggs, and dairy products as well as excess yin type foods including sugar, fruits, and chemicals.

A white tone to the skin generally indicates contraction of blood capillaries and tissues and inner-organ problems, especially spleen and lymph disorders. This color is caused by excessive yang intake, especially animal food rich in fat, all dairy products, or the overconsumption of salts and minerals. A pale color on the face often arises with a light-green shade or tone in the case of lymphoma and Hodgkin's disease due to a lack of balanced minerals and an overall anemic condition.

The temples on the head correspond to the functions of the spleen and other inner organs. Green vessels appearing in this region show abnormal lymph circulation due to an overactive spleen or underactive gallbladder and are caused by excess fluid and sugar, fats and oils, alcohol and stimulants, and other extreme foods and beverages from the yin category.

The outer layer of the ear shows circulatory and excretory systems. If this area has an abnormally red color, except during vigorous exercise or after being outside in cold weather, it indicates lymphatic and spleen disorders. If the whole nose, not only the tip area, is reddish in color from expansion of the blood capillaries, disorders are indicated also in the spleen and lymph system.

By observing a combination of these and other signs, potential lymph diseases, including cancer, can be detected long before they reach the chronic or degenerative stages and appropriate dietary adjustments be made.

DIETARY RECOMMENDATIONS

The primary cause of lymph disorders, including lymphoma and Hodgkin's disease, is consumption of extreme foods from the yin category of foods and beverages. These include sugar, chocolate, honey, carob, candies, confections, other foods treated with sugar, soft drinks, ice-cold drinks, alcohol, tropical fruits and fruit juices, spices, stimulants, and refined foods. Together with these foods, all foods and beverages containing chemicals and artificially processed ingredients must not be consumed. In addition, all dairy foods including milk, cheese, creams, yogurt, ice cream, and all greasy, oily, and fatty foods must be avoided. Meat too must be eliminated from the diet, especially beef and pork, as well as chicken, other poultry, and eggs, which are all high in fat and cholesterol.

Among vegetables, potatoes, sweet potatoes, eggplant, tomatoes, asparagus, spinach, and other plants that originated in the tropics are to be avoided. In preparing food, beware of using an excessive volume of oil. However, a reasonable amount of unrefined, vegetable oil may frequently be used in sautéing vegetables. No raw uncooked foods should be eaten.

The following are general dietary recommendations for lymphoma and Hodgkin's disease (see "Baby Food Suggestions" in Part III for the nutritional advice for infants and small children with cancer):

• Fifty to sixty percent whole grains. All cereal grains, including brown rice, millet, whole wheat, rye, oats, barley, corn, and buckwheat are consumable, though brown rice and millet are preferable to other grains for daily consumption. Occasionally, for example, twice a week, these grains can be prepared in the form of fried grains with vegetables. Unrefined, nonyeasted bread may be consumed several times per week with a small portion of sesame butter as a spread if desired. Whole-wheat and buckwheat pasta or noodles may also be occasionally eaten for variety.

• Five to ten percent miso soup, prepared with barley miso or hatcho miso, using sea vegetables such as kombu or wakame and hard, root and leafy vegetables. Consume one or two bowls daily. Frequently these vegetables can be sautéed with a little sesame oil before cooking in the soup. Among vegetables, more round vegetables are preferred such as onions, pumpkins, and winter squashes, though other root and green leafy vegetables may also occasionally be used in soup.

• Twenty to thirty percent cooked vegetables. Dishes can be prepared in various ways using the above-mentioned round vegetables, together with root vegetables such as carrots, burdock, daikon, and turnip. Unlike most other cancers, some dishes for lymphatic patients may be sautéed with a moderate volume of sesame or corn oil, though vegetables should also be cooked frequently using other methods. A small volume of pressed salad or macrobiotic pickles may be consumed. However, except for this form of food, raw vegetables are to be limited. In the case of salad, a boiled salad may be eaten by dipping ingredients in a pot of boiling water for a minute or two.

• Five to ten percent beans and bean products. Smaller beans such as azukis, lentils, and chickpeas are preferable to larger beans, and they should be cooked with vegetables such as kombu, hijiki, or wakame. They can also be cooked with onions and carrots or occasionally with acorn or butternut squash. Bean products such as tempeh, natto, and tofu can be consumed occasionally in moderate volume.

• Five percent or less sea vegetables. All cooked sea vegetables are strengthening to the lymph, especially hijiki and arame.

While all animal food should be avoided, if cravings arise a small portion of white-meat fish or dried small fish cooked in soup or with vegetables may be consumed occasionally.

Fruits and fruit juices are also to be avoided, though a small portion of dried or cooked fruits may be eaten if craved.

Roasted nuts and seeds, slightly salted, can be used as a snack in moderate volume.

Use of sea salt and tamari soy sauce as a seasoning should be moderate. Sweeteners are limited only to grain-based sweeteners such as rice syrup or barley malt. For a sour taste, a grain-based product such as rice vinegar or a vegetable food such as sauerkraut is recommended. All hot spices are to be strictly avoided.

Other dietary practices should follow the standard cancer-prevention suggestions, including the use of beverages and condiments. For lymphoma and Hodgkin's disease, it is especially important to chew very well until food becomes liquid in form. Overeating must also be watched for. Eating less than three hours before sleeping also produces detrimental effects on the blood, lymph, and other bodily fluids.

As explained in the introduction to Part II, cancer patients who have received or who are currently undergoing medical treatment may need to make further dietary modifications.

HOME CARES

• A plaster of mashed tofu mixed with the same volume of mashed green leafy vegetables is recommended for swollen glands and inflammation of the spleen.

• A plaster of buckwheat flour kneaded with warm water or green clay may also be applied to inflamed lymph nodes or glands to help reduce the swelling.

• If sweating occurs at night, relief can be provided by eating a small volume of sliced burdock roots and carrot roots, sautéed with sesame oil and seasoned with tamari soy sauce.

• A cup of kuzu tea with a piece of umeboshi and a little tamari soy sauce is recommended to improve lymphatic functions. This drink should be taken once every two to three days for a period of several weeks to be effective.

• Once a day scrub the whole body with a very hot towel soaked in grated gingerroot water. This will accelerate the flow of energy, blood, and lymph fluid through the circulatory system.

• Hot baths and showers should be taken quickly. Soaking the body for a long time in the tub causes the body to lose important minerals.

OTHER CONSIDERATIONS

• Avoid synthetic clothing and wear and sleep on cotton as much as possible.

• Avoid frequent exposure to artificial radiation, including medical and dental x-rays, smoke detectors, television, and video terminals, which are weakening to the lymph and blood.

• Good exercise is strengthening to the lymph and circulatory systems, but do not exercise to the point of exhaustion. Yoga, massage, and tai chi type movements are generally preferable to strenuous activities. Walking is excellent.

• Try to be happy, positive, and outgoing. Singing, dancing, or playing are particularly beneficial to improving overall health and mentality and harmonizing with the rhythms of nature.

PERSONAL EXPERIENCE

In January 1973, nineteen-year-old Maureen Duney of Belle Mead, New Jersey, discovered a lump in the right side of her throat. In April, a biopsy of the lymph node gland proved malignant, and doctors at Memorial Hospital in New York diagnosed her condition as Hodgkin's disease, stage III B.

In June, Maureen began radiation therapy, and by August the tumors were dispersed. However, in March 1975, she noticed a thickening in the intestinal area to the left of the navel, and tests showed that the cancer had come back. There was also a tumor on the last rib on her left side.

In September 1975, she began experimental chemotherapy, but after one month friends persuaded her to try macrobiotics. At the end of the month, Maureen came to see me, and I recommended the

Cancer-Prevention Diet and an application of a ginger compress to the spleen and rib areas.

"Mr. Kushi projected that I would be cured in four to six months," she recorded. "I took the information back to my parents, family, and doctors. I began cooking and eating macrobiotically immediately. From September following my first treatment of MOPP [chemotherapy], my sediment rate was 42; in November, after eating macrobiotically for two months, it had dropped to a normal count of 14. I felt alive again, was active daily, my strength increased, and my hair stopped falling out."

Prior to this time, Maureen had always been a poor eater. She did not eat much meat but in her words "devoured sweets, ice cream, fruits, liquids, hoagies, and pizza." By early 1976, the Hodgkin's disease was gone, and she no longer suffered from itching or night sweating. "I consume none of the foods that caused my illness at the first," she concluded. "I continue to eat macrobiotically gratefully every day." Source: *Case History Reports*, Vol. 1, No. 3 (Boston: East West Foundation, 1976, pp. 5–7).

20.

Male Cancers: Prostate and Testes

FREQUENCY

Prostate cancer will cause 24,100 deaths among American men in 1983, and 75,000 new cases will arise. Cancer of the testes and other male reproductive organs will claim 950 lives, and doctors will detect 5,400 new instances of the disease. Prostate cancer is the second most common cancer in men over sixty and the incidence is higher among blacks than whites. Americans have one of the highest prostate cancer rates in the world, about ten times higher, for instance, than the Japanese.

A variety of disorders can affect the prostate gland, including both benign and malignant tumors. Depending on the particular case, the illness is treated with surgery, radiation, and hormone therapy. Techniques include a *transurethral resection* (TUR), in which a resectoscope is inserted through the penis to kill tumor cells with an electric wire loop; a *suprapubic prostectomy*, in which the bladder is opened and the prostate removed by the surgeon through the urethra; a *retropubic prostectomy*, in which the prostate and seminal vesicles are removed without going through the bladder; and a *perineal prostectomy*, in which the surgeon enters between the legs in front of the rectum. Radioactive seeds may be implanted in the prostate to reduce the tumor or external megavoltage radiation administered. Finally, to control hormone levels and retard tumor growth, estrogens in the form of DES or cortisone may be given orally. In some instances the testicles, adrenal glands, and pituitary gland may be removed to limit the spread of malignancy. Hormone therapy can result in impotence, enlarged breasts, and heart problems. Surgery may result in impotence and sterility. The current survival rate for these forms of treatment is 57 percent.

Testicular cancer is on the rise in younger American men and is the leading cause of cancer deaths among those aged twenty-nine to thirty-five. It usually affects the right testicle more than the left, seldom both, and tends to spread to the lungs. A radical orchiectomy, involving removal of one or both testicles, is the standard form of treatment. If both testicles are removed, the operation will render the patient sterile, but not impotent. If cancer has spread to the lymph nodes, radiation or chemotherapy will also be administered. If the malignancy is spreading through the blood, a lymphadenectomy may be performed, in which all the lymph nodes on one or both sides of the abdomen up to the kidneys will be removed. The survival rate for testicular cancer is between 50 and 60 percent.

STRUCTURE

The testes, located in a sac called the scrotum, are the primary organs of the male reproductive system. They produce sperm and male sex hormones. The peripheral layer of the testes contains about 250 lobules or chambers. Each chamber holds from one to three minute seminiferous tubules in which spermatozoa are formed. Sperm are discharged from each tubule, floating upward to the first portion of the duct system, called the epididymis, where they are stored for weeks, months, or even years. The seminal fluid, or semen, is a mixture of sperm from the testes and fluid from several accessory reproductive organs. The main accessory organ is the prostate gland. The prostate is situated below the bladder and surrounds the urethra, connecting the bladder and penis. The prostate secretes enzymes, lipids, and other substances, which enter the seminal fluid and are deposited in the female reproductive tract by the penis during intercourse.

CAUSE OF CANCER

In structure, the prostate is classified as yang because of its relative compactness, location deep inside the body, and the alkaline fluid it secretes, which serves to neutralize the extremely yin acids of the vagina. About 30 percent of men over fifty in the United States have enlarged prostates. As this organ presses against the upper portion of the bladder and urethra, urination becomes difficult and painful. Of these cases, about one in five develops into prostate cancer; however, any enlargement of the prostate should be suspected as a precancerous condition.

Prostate enlargement and blockage of the other semen ducts arise in the same way as hardening of the arteries. They are caused principally by the overconsumption of foods rich in fat and protein in the yang category including eggs, meat, and dairy products, all of which contain saturated fats, as well as by excessive intake of foods in the extreme yin category such as sugar, fruits, and refined flour products, which produce fat and mucus. Over time, these deposits accumulate and can turn into cysts or tumors. The blockages resulting from a high-fat diet can also contribute to impotence. However, the inability to achieve an erection is often caused by intake of too much expansive food, which causes the muscles of the reproductive system to become loose and expanded. Infertility is also caused largely from excessive intake of yin type foods, which weaken the quality of the blood, lymph, and other bodily fluids and secretions that determine the quality of the sperm. Prostate problems can be relieved by adopting a Cancer-Prevention Diet that emphasizes slightly more yin foods and style of cooking and avoids animal foods.

The testes too are extremely yang (compact) in structure. Tumors here also arise primarily from excessive animal foods, especially eggs, heavily salted meats, condensed dairy foods such as cheese, and high-fat and high-protein fish and seafood. A more centered way of eating will help relieve this condition.

MEDICAL EVIDENCE

• An international study completed in 1970 linked prostate cancer mortality directly with per capita coffee consumption. Source: P. Stocks, "Cancer Mortality in Relation to National Consumption of Cigarettes, Solid Fuel, Tea, and Coffee," *British Journal of Cancer* 24:215–25.

• In 1974 an epidemiologist found a high direct correlation between mortality from prostate cancer in forty-one countries and per capita intake of fats, milk, and meats, especially beef. Research also disclosed that people who regularly consumed rice had less incidence of the disease. Source: M.A. Howell, "Factor Analysis of International Cancer Mortality Data and *Per Capita* Food Consumption," *British Journal of Cancer* 29:328–36.

• Seventh-Day Adventist men in California have 55 percent less prostate cancer than other males, according to a 1975 study. The church members tend to avoid meat, poultry, fish, refined foods, alcohol, stimulants, and spices and consume whole grains, vegetables, and fresh fruits. Source: R.L. Phillips, "Role of Life-Styles and Dietary Habits in Risk of Cancer among Seventh-Day Adventists," *Cancer Research* 35:3513–22.

• A 1977 study based on 111 cases with prostate cancer and 111 hospital controls showed that the cancer patients consumed more high-fat foods, including beef, pork, eggs, cheeses, milk, creams, butter, and margarine. Source: I.D. Rotkin, "Studies in the Epidemiology of Prostatic Cancer: Expanded Sampling," *Cancer Treatment Reports* 61:173–80.

• A 1978 report found that U.S. counties with the highest death rates from prostate cancer also had the highest per capita intake of high-fat foods, including beef, milk and dairy products, fats and oils, pork, and eggs. Source: A. Blair and J.F. Fraumeni, Jr., "Geographic Patterns of Prostate Cancer in the U.S.," *Journal of the National Cancer Institute* 61:1379–84.

• A ten-year study of 122,261 Japanese men over forty found less prostate cancer deaths among those who regularly consumed green or yellow vegetables. The 1979 study also reported that vegetarian men had a lower incidence of prostate cancer than nonvegetarians. Source: T. Hirayama, "Epidemiology of Prostate Cancer with Special Reference to the Role of Diet," *National Cancer Institute Monograph* 53:149–54.

• In 1981 researchers found that the incidence of prostate cancer in four ethnic groups in Hawaii was highly correlated with consumption of animal fat and saturated fat and with total protein, especially animal protein. Source: L.N. Kolonel et al., "Nutrient Intakes in Relation to Cancer Incidence in Hawaii," *British Journal of Cancer* 44:332–39.

• A 1981 study suggested that lactose (milk sugar) fed laboratory animals tended to promote tumor growth, especially stones in the male reproductive glands and bladder. Source: S.N. Gershoff and R.B. McGandy, "The Effects of Vitamin A-Deficient Diets Containing Lactose in Producing Bladder Calculi and Tumors in Rats," *American Journal of Clinical Nutrition* 34:483–89.

• A 1982 case-control study reported that prostate cancer patients consumed less foods high in vitamin A and beta-carotene, such as carrots. Source: L.M. Schuman et al., "Some Selected Features of the Epidemiology of Prostatic Cancer," in K. Magnus (ed.), *Trends in Cancer Incidence* (New York: Hemisphere Publishing Corp., pp. 345–54).

• After reviewing current medical evidence, the National Academy of Sciences concluded in its 1982 report on cancer and diet: "In summary, the incidence of prostate cancer is correlated with other cancers associated with diet, e.g., breast cancer. There is good evidence that an increased risk of prostate cancer is associated with certain dietary factors, especially the intake of high fat and high protein foods, which usually occur together in the diet. There is some evidence that foods rich in Vitamin A or its precursors and vegetarian diets are associated with a lower risk." *Diet, Nutrition, and Cancer* (Washington, D.C.: National Academy of Sciences 17:21).

DIAGNOSIS

Prostate cancer is usually diagnosed by a rectal examination as well as a battery of laboratory tests, enzyme and hormone assays, and a needle biopsy if a malignancy is suspected. Skeletal and chest x-rays, bone scans, and intravenous pyelogram (IVP) will be used to check for metastases. About 60 percent of prostate tumors are currently detected before spreading to other sites. In the case of testicular cancer, many of these same diagnostic methods are used as well as an angiogram, lymphangiogram, CAT scan of chest or abdomen, and ultrasound examination of the abdomen.

Oriental medicine diagnoses potential male reproductive cancers with a variety of simple visual observations. According to physiognomy, the mouth and lower face correspond with the sex organs, and discolorations, swellings, or other abnormalities in this region may indicate improper functioning of the reproductive system. For instance, vertical wrinkles appearing on the lips show a recession of hormonal function, especially of the gonad hormones, indicating a decline in sexual function. These wrinkles may also appear in case of dehydration from lack of liquid or overconsumption of dry foods and salt, so other signs must also be observed. Generally, fatty wrinkles or sagging in the chin and upper neck indicate prostate problems in men or uterine and ovarian problems in women. Pimples that appear in the center of the cheeks and have a fatty apperance also show the formation of cysts in and around the reproductive organs.

Fat or mucus buildup in the prostate is further indicated by a yellow and white coating of mucus on the lower part of the whites of the eyes. Along the bladder meridian, cancer of the prostate shows up as a light-green coloration on the fifth toe and its extended area at the outside of the foot, below the anklebone and behind the Achilles' tendon with fatty swelling along the Achilles' tendon.

On the hands, split or uneven nails show disorders in the circulatory, nervous, and reproductive systems caused by chaotic eating habits. If one thumbnail shows this condition and the other thumbnail is normal, the testicle (or ovary in women) corresponding to the abnormal side is malfunctioning. Red, purple, and other abnormal colors appearing on the tips of the fingers also indicate disorders in the gonad region, including possible cancer or precancerous conditions.

From a combination of these and other factors, the condition of the reproductive system can be determined and appropriate corrective nutritional action taken.

DIETARY RECOMMENDATIONS

Because of the evidence that prostate and testicular cancer develops in association with dietary habits, especially food high in protein and fat, all kinds of meat, poultry, eggs, cheese, milk, and other dairy foods should be avoided. Less fatty animal food such as fish and seafood are ideally to be avoided or at least limited to small amounts. Not only animal food, but also sugar, honey, chocolate, carob, and all sugar-treated food and beverages are to be discontinued. Flour products, which have the potential to create mucus, such as refined white bread, pancakes, and cookies, are to be avoided also. All stimulants including mustard, pepper, curry, mint, peppermint and other aromatic herbs and spices, all alcoholic beverages, and coffee are to be avoided because they enhance tumor growth, though they are not the direct cause of the cancer. All chemicals artificially added or treated during food production and processing should also be avoided. Excessive consumption of oil, even of vegetable, unsaturated quality, is to be refrained from, as is excessive consumption of salts and salty food and beverages. Fruit and fruit juices, if consumed frequently, can increase the swelling of the tumor, though they can neutralize animal protein and fat. Accordingly, they should be limited. All vegetables of historically tropical origin, such as potato, tomato, and eggplant, and tropical and subtropical fruits should be avoided.

General dietary guidelines by volume of food consumption are as follows:

• Fifty to sixty percent whole-cereal grains, pressure-cooked, but comparatively softer. Brown rice and barley are recommended as daily staples, though all other grains can be used occasionally, including millet, oats, rye, whole wheat, and corn. For the first few months, it is preferable to avoid buckwheat and buckwheat products. Unleavened, unyeasted whole-wheat, rye, or other whole-grain bread may be consumed, though it is also best to limit all baked food for the initial period. For variety, whole-wheat pasta or noodles can be used occasionally.

• Five to ten percent soup. Miso soup with wakame or kombu sea vegetables and leafy vegetables, or tamari broth soup prepared with the same ingredients, can be used—one or two bowls per day. However, the volume of miso or tamari soy sauce is to be moderate so that the taste is light. Occasionally, grain and vegetable soup and bean soup can be used.

• Twenty to thirty percent vegetables. Various types of leafy vegetables—green, yellow, and white—can be cooked in different styles, as can various root vegetables such as carrots, turnips, daikon, radish, lotus root, and burdock roots, though burdock should be used much less frequently than other root vegetables. Round vegetables such as acorn and butternut squash, cabbages, and onions can also be frequently used. Seasonings such as sea salt, tamari soy sauce, and other salty condiments are to be used sparingly. A few times per week, raw fresh salad may be eaten in moderate volume, though boiled salad can be prepared frequently. The use of oil such as in sautéing or frying should be limited. Ideally, oil should be totally avoided for a period of a few weeks, though a few times a week sesame or corn oil may be harmlessly used for light sautéing.

• Five to ten percent beans and bean products. As a substitute for animal protein, smaller beans such as azuki beans, lentils, and chickpeas are recommended for frequent use. Bean products such as tempeh, natto, and cooked or dried tofu occasionally can be used also, in moderate volume.

• Five percent or less sea vegetables. As a source of various minerals, sea vegetables can be used daily or frequently in small volume. Arame, wakame, nori, and kombu are especially recommended, though other sea vegetables also may be used. They may be cooked together with vegetables or beans or cooked separately as a small side dish.

Fish and seafood are to be limited to white-meat, nonfatty, low-cholesterol fish, consumed in small volume. It is preferable to avoid fish totally for a few months, but seafood can be served once or twice a week, if craved, together with lightly cooked vegetables or with grated daikon or radish as a garnish.

Fruit, fruit juices, and fruit desserts are to be limited initially, though a small volume of cooked fruits or dried fruits may be consumed occasionally, if craved.

Nuts and nut butters are to be avoided. In the event that fat is desired, sesame butter or sesame seeds can be taken frequently as a supplement or condiment. Seeds, such as pumpkin or sunflower seeds, also can be used if lightly roasted, as a snack.

Seasoning of food should be very moderate, especially salt, though unrefined sea salt, tamari soy sauce, and miso can be used daily in cooking in moderate volume.

For sweets, barley malt, rice syrup, or other cereal-grain-based sweetener may be used in small volume, if craved.

Sauerkraut or rice vinegar can be used occasionally to satisfy the desire for a sour taste.

A small dish of grated carrots cooked with one-half teaspoon of grated ginger or a few slices of garlic is sometimes helpful for this type of cancer, if taken daily for a period of several days. Dried shiitake mushrooms cooked with carrots or daikon can be consumed frequently as a small supplemental dish, especially for prostate conditions. One or two tablespoons of grated daikon or grated carrots also can be used several times per week as a condiment at meals.

Nonstimulant teas such as bancha twig or bancha stem tea, as well as other nonfragrant traditional teas and cereal grain coffee, may be used regularly as beverages, though all liquids should not be overconsumed. Roasted grain tea or sea vegetable tea, made by boiling sea vegetables in water, also can be used as regular beverages.

An important part of dietary practice is to avoid overconsumption of food in general and not to eat for three hours before sleep. Chewing until food becomes liquid, mixing thoroughly with saliva, is very helpful for digestion and restoring the overall condition.

All other dietary practices may follow the standard recommendations for cancer patients.

As explained in the introduction to Part II, cancer patients who have received or who are currently undergoing medical treatment may need to make further dietary modifications.

HOME CARES

• For prostate cancer and enlarged prostate, a taro potato plaster may be applied for three to four hours on the lower abdomen immediately following a ginger compress for five to seven minutes. This application can be repeated daily for two to three weeks.

• For swelling of the abdominal region due to prostate cancer, it is helpful to apply a buckwheat plaster for about one hour. The plaster should be kept warm by placing roasted hot sea salt wrapped in cotton towels above it. (For ease in handling, the hot salt may be placed in a pouch made from a cotton towel, then wrapped with another towel.) This application may be repeated daily for several days.

• Pain and aches in the prostate or testicular region usually disappear after a few weeks of proper dietary practice. However, in the meantime, it is sometimes helpful to relieve pain by drinking one or two cups of hot bancha tea cooked with one umeboshi plum, two teaspoons grated daikon, one-third teaspoon grated ginger, and one-half to one teaspoon of tamari soy sauce. A kuzu drink may be served instead, using the same ingredients but substituting kuzu for bancha twigs. Also it is helpful to drink one cup of liquid in which a shiitake mushroom has been boiled for 10 to 15 minutes, seasoned with one-half to one teaspoon of tamari soy sauce.

• Scrubbing the body with a hot ginger towel or wet, hot, squeezed-out towel, once or twice a day, is very helpful for promoting better circulation of energy and blood, releasing stagnation, and improving overall conditions.

OTHER CONSIDERATIONS

• Though cancer is naturally accompanied by a decline in energy and vitality, normal sexual practice is not harmful if it does not lead to exhaustion.

• Vasectomy and other artificial birth-control methods, as well as the use of drugs or medications to control sexual performance, are to be avoided in order to prevent stagnation, interruption of energy flow, or other abnormal functions.

• Avoid the use of synthetic fibers in underwear. Use cotton clothing for direct contact with the skin.

• Exercise of any kind, especially general exercise, is helpful as long as it can be practiced comfortably without producing exhaustion.

PERSONAL EXPERIENCE

Prostate Cancer

On September 24, 1980, Irving Malow arrived at the office of Keith Block, M.D., a macrobiotic physician practicing in Evanston, Illinois. For six years, the sixty-year-old Malow had suffered from prostate cancer and now the disease had spread to his spine, pelvis, and shoulder. Prior treatments included a partial orchiectomy, radiation therapy, and chemotherapy. After being given cis-platinum, an experimental drug, Malow threw up for six hours at a stretch and decided he could no longer go on with "these debilitating and torturous treatments."

Meanwhile, some friends of his came across an article about a medical doctor who had relieved his own terminal cancer with the help of diet* in the September 1980 *Saturday Evening Post*. Malow decided to try the macrobiotic approach for himself.

Under Dr. Block's supervision, Malow began the Cancer-Prevention Diet, and his appetite quickly returned, his pain ceased, and his energy level increased. In the spring of 1981 radiologists at Weiss Memorial Hospital in Chicago found Malow's bone scans to be markedly improved. A specialist at St. Francis Hospital in Evanston found the x-rays to be "grossly normal."

Malow later stated:

I am totally convinced that we are what we eat, and that we literally destroy our bodies with the poor quality of foods, confections, etc. which we consume. When we analyze the intricate and amazing functions of our body and organs, I further decided we truly should consider the body to be a shrine, which must be given proper nourishment and care.

At age sixty, despite radiation treatment, some chemotherapy, and other minor problems associated with cancer, I continue to

---

*For a complete account of this case (primary prostate cancer with metastases to the skull, right shoulder, rib, sternum, and spine), see *Recalled by Life: The Story of My Recovery from Cancer* by Anthony Sattilaro, M.D., with Tom Monte (Houghton-Mifflin, 1982).

work full time, and also often spend some evening hours doing work. I endeavor to maintain a reasonable amount of exercise and continue to look upon cancer as something that we can overcome with diet and determination. Our amazing bodies apparently can heal themselves if we furnish the body with the proper nourishment and eliminate that which is harmful." Source: "Metastastic Prostate Cancer," *The Cancer Prevention Diet* (Brookline, Mass.: East West Foundation, 1981, pp. 81–82).

Testicular Cancer

In 1977 John Jodziewicz, a twenty-year-old college student from Henningsville, Pennsylvania, noted a pea-size hardness in his left testicle. During the winter of 1979 to 1980, it increased in size and a lump appeared in his neck. On March 20, 1980, doctors at Sacred Heart Hospital discovered that he had advanced (fourth stage) choriocarcinoma and surgically removed his left testicle. Two oncologists and a resident physician told him that this particularly malignant form of testicular cancer had spread to his left kidney, both lungs, and neck and that he had "a one percent chance to live out the year, even with chemotherapy."

The findings came as a shock to John and his fiancé, Ingrid Koch. John had observed a vegetarian diet for a few years, kept active physically, and felt that he was in good health. "I was sure that my 'anything goes but meat' diet, megadoses of vitamins and supplements, and rugged outdoor activities protected me from disease," he later recalled. "But here Ingrid and I sat, being told that I would most probably die before my twenty-fourth birthday."

During the next four months, John underwent chemical therapy, including receiving intravenous injections for seven days at a stretch at two-week intervals. During the period that he received drugs he suffered fevers, nosebleeds, constipation, difficulty breathing, a persistent cough, total hair loss, chills, lack of appetite, headaches, fatigue, severe mouth ulcers, nausea, vomiting, bone-marrow depression, total body arthritis pain, dizziness, hypersensitivity of the scalp, ringing in the ears, and loosening teeth. "This was the most horrible time in my life; and these symptoms were not as a result of the cancer, but of the treatment."

After two cycles of chemotherapy, the tumors remained, and doctors began administering cis-platinum, an experimental drug, in high dosages. John's prognosis was reduced to two months, and after a series of wretchings and convulsions he was given last rites by a priest.

Two events, however, coincided to change the course of John's life and forestall imminent death. First, just before the last round with drugs, a friend introduced Ingrid's mother to macrobiotics and later encouraged John and Ingrid to visit the East West Foundation in Philadelphia. There John met director Denny Waxman, who explained the yin/yang approach to cancer and gave him several books to read. The second turning point came in the hospital. One night John had a dream in which his mother, who had died seven years earlier, told him to go to St. Joseph's Cathedral in Montreal and pray. As a child, John and his family had often visited the shrine where Brother André reportedly performed many healing miracles until his death in 1937. (He was proposed for sainthood by the Vatican in 1982.) At St. Joseph's, pilgrims from around the world came to crawl up the long flight of steps to the top on their knees in hope that God would reward their humility and relieve their illness.

On June 16, 1980, Ingrid and John arrived in Montreal. There were throngs of tourists, but for some reason no pilgrims that time of day. Nevertheless, John determined to climb the steps alone. As he placed his knees on the first step, he experienced what he described as a transcendent moment of illumination and felt that he had become united with the mountain on which the cathedral rested. As he ascended each step, John prayed for others whom he knew also to be in need of help and he felt his mother's spirit close by. At the top, he got up and walked into the cathedral. A priest was holding up a wafer at the altar as if in anticipation of his arrival, and John took communion. He knew that if he changed his way of life and began eating macrobiotically he would live.

Returning to Pennsylvania, John and Ingrid attended the East West Foundation's summer camp. I met them there for the first time and assured John that he would recover completely if he followed the Cancer-Prevention Diet faithfully. Back home, John and Ingrid drove three times a week to Philadelphia, seventy miles away, for macrobiotic cooking classes and other instruction in Oriental medicine and philosophy. In two weeks, John's pain had entirely disappeared, and in two months the tumor in his neck had shrunk to half its previous size. In August, John went on a strenuous thirty-eight-mile hike in the woods, alone except for his dog.

In May 1981, blood tests confirmed that his body no longer had any signs of cancer. John had been off medication, including chemotherapy, for a year. Reviewing his case, John listed five reasons why he survived:

1. Total support from his family and friends.
2. Correct macrobiotic practice, including cooking classes and discipline in avoiding extreme foods.
3. A strong natural immune system.
4. The will to get better.
5. Faith in God and willingness to accept life's difficulties as opportunities for personal growth and understanding.

"I'm not only physically healthy, but I feel spiritually healthy as well," John explained in 1982, two years after his remission. "The clean, macrobiotic diet and way of life has enhanced and broadened my perspective of the Catholic tradition in which I was raised. Ingrid and I plan to study and teach macrobiotics for the rest of our lives and have a large family."

John and Ingrid were married in the summer of 1982 and are implementing their dream. Sources: Tom Monte, "Triumph Over Cancer: A Young Man's Journey Back to Life," *East West Journal*, April 1982, pp. 32–40; "Choriocarcinoma," *Cancer and Heart Disease: The Macrobiotic Approach to Degenerative Disorders* (New York: Japan Publications, pp. 157–59, 1982).

21.

Pancreatic Cancer

FREQUENCY

Nearly 22,600 Americans will die from pancreatic cancer in 1983, and 25,000 new cases will arise. The illness is about evenly divided among men and women and accounts for between 2 and 3 percent of all cancers in the United States. About 90 percent of pancreatic cancers are *adenocarcinomas*, affecting the tissue of the organs, and most of these are accompanied by pancreatitis and obstruction of the ducts. The other 10 percent are *tumors of the islet cells*. Pancreatic cancer may spread to the liver or small intestine.

Modern medical treatment calls for surgery, but because the disease is difficult to diagnose in early stages, many tumors have already metastasized and are considered inoperable. If operable, a partial or total pancreatectomy is performed. The first procedure calls for removal of part of the organ, adjacent lymph nodes, the duodenum, part of the stomach, and the common bile duct. A total pancreatomy involves removing the whole pancreas. Radiation and chemotherapy may be given after surgery to control pain. The survival rate for pancreatic cancer is 1 percent. Many patients die within a few months of diagnosis.

STRUCTURE

The pancreas is six to eight inches in length and weighs about three ounces. It is situated behind the stomach and is connected to the duodenum through a common bile duct with the liver and gallbladder. The sections of the pancreas are known as the head, body, and tail. The head secretes pancreatic juice into the duodenum, and this juice aids in the digestion of carbohydrates, fats, and protein. The body of the pancreas produces enzymes and hormones, including insulin, which regulate sugar levels in the blood. These hormones are secreted by the islets of Langerhans, a network of cells scattered throughout the pancreas, which vary in number from 200,000 to 1,800,000. They are most numerous in the tail portion of the pancreas, which touches the spleen.

CAUSE OF CANCER

Diabetes and hyperinsulinism are the two major degenerative diseases associated with the pancreas and are related to the rise of tumors in this organ. To understand the progressive development of pancreatic disorders, it is necessary to consider the effects of the three different forms of sugar on the body. Simple sugars or *monosaccharides* are found in fruits and honey and include glucose and fructose. Double sugars or *disaccharides* are found in cane sugar and milk and include sucrose and lactose. Complex sugars or *polysaccharides* are found in grains, beans, and vegetables and include cellulose.

In the normal digestive process, complex sugars are decomposed gradually and at a nearly even rate by various enzymes in the mouth, stomach, pancreas, and intestines. Complex sugars enter the bloodstream slowly after being broken down into smaller saccharide units. During the process, the pH of the blood remains slightly alkaline.

In contrast, simple and double sugars are metabolized quickly, causing the blood to become overacidic. To compensate for this extreme yin condition, the pancreas secretes a yang hormone, insulin, which allows excess sugar in the blood to be removed and enter the cells of the body. This produces a burst of energy as the glucose (the end product of all sugar metabolism) is oxidized and carbon dioxide and water are given off as wastes. Diabetes is a disease characterized by the failure of the pancreas to produce enough insulin to neutralize excess blood sugar. After years of excessive consumption of refined sugar, fruit, dairy products, chemicals, and other highly yin substances, the islet cells in the pancreas become expanded and lose their ability to secret insulin. Sugar begins to appear in the urine, the body loses water, and reserve minerals are depleted. To offset these symptoms, modern medicine treats diabetes with artificial injections of insulin.

Much of the sugar that enters the bloodstream is originally stored in the liver in the form of glycogen until needed, when it is again changed into glucose. When the amount of glycogen exceeds the liver's storage capacity of about fifty grams, it is released into the bloodstream in the form of fatty acid. This fatty acid is stored first in the more inactive places of the body, such as the buttocks, thighs, and midsection. Then, if refined sugars continue to be eaten, fatty acid becomes attracted to more yang organs such as the heart and kidney, which gradually become encased in a layer of fat and mucus.

This accumulation can also penetrate the inner tissues, weakening the normal functioning of the organs and causing their eventual stoppage such as in atherosclerosis. The buildup of fat can also lead to various forms of cancer, including tumors of the breast, colon, and reproductive organs. Still another form of degeneration may occur when the body's internal supply of minerals is mobilized to offset the debilitating effects of simple sugar consumption. For example, calcium from the bones and teeth may be depleted to balance the effects of excessive intake of candy and soft drinks.

As a small, compact organ, the pancreas is yang in structure. Pancreatic cancer results primarily from long-time consumption of eggs, meat, seafood, poultry, refined salt, and other strong yang animal foods high in protein and saturated fat in combination with refined sugars and other strong yin foods and beverages, chemicals, and drugs. Tumors in the pancreas may follow the development of pancreatitis (the acute or chronic inflammation of the organ) and hyperinsulinism (an overly contractive condition in which blood sugar levels are abnormally low from secretion of too much insulin). The overproduction of insulin attracts fatty acids and coagulates into tumors in the bile duct or the islets of Langerhans. Diabetes may be treated and relieved by adopting a slightly more yang macrobiotic diet consisting of whole grains and vegetables, prepared with a slightly longer cooking time and heavier taste, while cancer of the pancreas can be reversed by a slightly more yin diet consisting primarily of whole grains and vegetables prepared with a little bit less cooking and a lighter taste.

MEDICAL EVIDENCE

• A 1968 Japanese study of mortality in men found a direct association between high meat consumption and pancreatic cancer. High vegetable intake was found to be inversely associated with the disease. Source: K. Ishii et al., "Epidemiological Problems of Pancreas Cancer," *Japan Journal of Clinical Medicine* 26:1839–42.

• A 1975 epidemiological study found a direct correlation between sugar intake and pancreatic cancer mortality among women in thirty-two countries. Source: B. Armstrong and R. Doll, "Environmental Factors and Cancer Incidence and Mortality in Different Countries, with Special Reference to Dietary Practices," *International Journal of Cancer* 15:617–31.

• A 1977 Japanese study reported that men who ate meat daily risked pancreatic cancer 2.5 times more than those who did not. Source: T. Hirayama, "Changing Patterns of Cancer in Japan with Special Reference to the Decrease in Stomach Cancer Mortality," in H.H. Hiatt et al. (ed.), *Origins of Human Cancer, Book A* (Cold Spring Harbor, N.Y.: Cold Spring Harbor Laboratory, pp. 55–75).

• In 1979 the American Diabetes Association revised its dietary recommendations, stating that "carbohydrate intake should usually account for 50-60 percent of total energy intake," with "glucose and glucose containing disaccharides (sucrose, lactose) . . . restricted." In addition, the guidelines recommended that "whenever acceptable to the patient, natural foods containing unrefined carbohydrate with fiber should be substituted for highly refined carbohydrates, which are low in fiber" and "dietary sources of fat that are high in saturated fatty acids and foods containing cholesterol should be restricted." Source: "Principles of Nutrition and Dietary Recommendations for Individuals with Diabetes Mellitus: 1979," *Journal of The American Dietetic Association* 75:527–30.

• Mormons, whose diet is high in whole grains, vegetables, and fruits, moderate in meat, and low in stimulants, alcohol, and tobacco, have substantially less pancreatic cancer than the general population, according to a 1980 epidemiological survey. Male Mormons have 36 percent less and females 19 percent less. High church officials, who adhere more faithfully to the group's dietary recommendations, have 53 percent less pancreatic cancer. Source: J.E. Engstrom, "Health and Dietary Practices and Cancer Mortality among California Mormons," in J. Cairns et al. (ed.), *Cancer Incidence in Defined Populations, Banbury Report 4* (Cold Spring Harbor, N.Y.: Cold Spring Harbor Laboratory, pp. 69–90).

• People who drink a cup of coffee a day are nearly twice as likely to develop cancer of the pancreas as non-coffee drinkers, according to a 1981 study by the Harvard School of Public Health. Source: B.

MacMahon et al., "Coffee and Cancer of the Pancreas," *New England Journal of Medicine* 304:630–33.

• The per capita intake of several foods has been associated with pancreatic cancer in a number of international studies. Analyses of mortality data have produced direct associations with intake of fats and oils, sugar, animal products, eggs, milk, and coffee. Source: *Diet, Nutrition, and Cancer* (Washington, D.C.: National Academy of Sciences pp. 17:12–13, 1982).

DIAGNOSIS

In the hospital, pancreatic cancer is diagnosed by a variety of means, including lab tests, a fasting blood sugar test, liver scans, upper and lower GI series, CAT scan, ultrasound, and an ERCP (endoscopic retrograde cholangiopancreatography). The ERCP is a kind of endoscope or tube, which is swallowed and woven into the duodenum. It contains a tiny catheter, which is inserted into the duct of the pancreas. X-rays may then be taken of a dye injected into the pancreas. If a tumor is indicated, cell and tissue samples will be taken in a biopsy or a major surgical procedure called a laparotomy in which the abdominal wall is opened and the inner organs palpated by the surgeon.

Oriental medicine relies on simpler, visual cues to ascertain the condition of the pancreas. In facial diagnosis, two major areas correspond with the pancreas: 1) the upper bridge of the nose, and 2) the outside of the temples. Swellings, discolorations, or other abnormal markings in these locations indicate pancreatic and sometimes also spleen disorders. For instance, a dark color shows overburdening of the pancreas and elimination of excessive sugars including cane sugar, honey, syrups, chocolate, fruit, and milk. Red pimples and patches in these regions are caused by excess sugar, sweets, juice, and fruits. Whitish-yellow pimples are caused by fats and oils from both animal and vegetable sources including dairy foods. Dark patches and pimples are caused by excessive sweets or by salt and flour products. Moles here are caused by excess animal-quality protein and fat and show an overactive spleen and pancreas. A light-green color appearing together with whitish, reddish, or dark fatty, oily skin textures in either of these areas indicates possible pancreatic cancer.

Blisters on the eyes may also reflect tumor development in the pancreas. A reddish-yellow color in the pink area inside the lower eyelid is caused by consumption of excess yang animal food together with excess yin. A blue-gray color in the middle regions of the white of the eye further suggests cancer in the pancreas.

Above the bridge of the nose, hair growing between the eyebrows shows that the person's mother ate a high amount of dairy food and fatty animal food during the third and fourth months of pregnancy. A person with this type of eyebrows is particularly susceptible to pancreatic, spleen, and liver disorders and should be careful to avoid meat, poultry, eggs, dairy foods, and oil and fatty foods.

Oily skin in general shows disorders in fat metabolism, including pancreatic troubles. A yellowish color to the skin from excess yang foods also shows bile troubles and probable pancreatic malfunctioning.

Finally, cancer of the pancreas, spleen, or lymph is indicated by the presence of a light-green color along the spleen meridian. Observe especially the area of the foot below the anklebone extending to the outside of the big toe.

Oriental diagnosis allows us to quickly scan these and other areas and accurately determine the condition of the pancreas and other internal organs. A propensity to cancer can be identified long before it develops and corrective dietary adjustments taken.

DIETARY RECOMMENDATIONS

The primary cause of pancreatic cancer is the long-time overconsumption of animal food, including eggs, beef, pork, poultry, and cheese and other salted dairy food. All animal food should be avoided, except, occasionally, nonfatty white-meat fish in small volume, if it is desired. Pancreatic cancer is also accelerated by the overconsumption of salty food and hard, baked food, as well as sugar and sugar-treated food, soft drinks, spices, stimulants, tropical fruits and fruit juices, and chemicals used in various ways for food production and processing. All these foods and beverages are to be avoided. Though not the cause of pancreatic cancer, refined flour and flour products easily tend to produce mucus and should therefore also be avoided. Commercial seasonings, sauces, and dressings, in which artificial chemical processing is involved, should also be discontinued.

The following are general guidelines for dietary practice, by volume of daily food consumption:

• Fifty to sixty percent whole-cereal grains. Brown rice and barley are most recommended, together with oats, though all other grains can be used occasionally. However, it is recommended not to consume buckwheat and buckwheat products for an initial few months. Grains are to be pressure-cooked with water and a pinch of sea salt. They should not be consumed in the form of flour or flour products such as bread, pancakes, or cookies. However, if craved, unleavened whole-wheat or rye bread may be consumed infrequently with a small volume of sesame butter, especially after steaming. Whole-wheat pasta or noodles can also be used occasionally for variety, but buckwheat pasta and noodles are to be avoided for several months until the condition improves.

• Five to ten percent soup. One or two cups of miso soup cooked with wakame or kombu sea vegetables and green or white leafy vegetables can be eaten daily. Occasionally, grains may be added to the soup. If more strength is needed, pumpkin or fall-season squash soup can be consumed several times per week. Miso can be replaced with tamari soy sauce or sea salt, though all seasonings should be used moderately so that the taste of the soup is light.

• Twenty to thirty percent vegetables, cooked in a variety of styles, including boiling, steaming, and sautéing. Sautéed dishes can be made with a moderate volume of sesame oil or corn oil, and a small dish may be consumed several times a week. Green and white leafy vegetables as well as round vegetables, including hard autumn squash, cabbages, and onions may be used proportionately more than root vegetables, though leafy, round, and root types should all regularly be consumed. Overcooking should be avoided, and lighter cooking is more recommended. Vegetable dishes may be seasoned with sea salt, tamari soy sauce, or miso. However, any salty taste should be moderate, and the natural taste of cooked vegetables is more to be emphasized. If desired, boiled salad and occasionally a raw fresh salad with many hard, leafy greens may be served in small volume. Heavy, oily salad dressings are to be avoided.

• Five to ten percent beans and bean products. Small beans such as azuki beans, lentils, and chickpeas can be used daily or every other day as one of the regular dishes. They can be cooked with a small portion of sea vegetable such as kombu, fall-season squash, or vegetables like onions and carrots. Bean products such as cooked tofu, tempeh, and natto may be used a few times per week as an alternative to whole beans. Beans and bean products may be seasoned with a very small volume of sea salt, tamari soy sauce, or miso.

• Five percent or less sea vegetables. All edible sea vegetables are recommended. However, nori and arame are especially beneficial. A small volume of roasted nori may be used daily, and a side dish of cooked arame may be consumed a few times a week.

Except for grains and beans, it is important that all side dishes, especially vegetables, not be overcooked or have a strong salty taste. Lighter cooking, which leaves some freshness anad crispness, is recommended. Prepare at least one dish every day in this way.

In the event that animal food is desired, nonfatty white-meat fish may be prepared in small volume with one to two tablespoons of grated daikon or radish with one-half to one teaspoon grated ginger if desired, together with a small volume of tamari soy sauce for taste. This dish may be eaten once or twice a week.

Fruits and fruit juices are primarily to be avoided, though, if craved, cooked apples, peaches, grapes, strawberries, and other berries may be used two to three times a week in small volume. In the event that fresh fruit is desired, strawberries and other berries, melons, or apples may be used occasionally in small volume.

Nuts and nut butters are generally to be avoided, though if craved, a small volume of roasted peanuts or peanut butter may be used on rare occasions. Roasted seeds such as sesame seeds, pumpkin seeds, and sunflower seeds may be consumed occasionally as a snack in moderate volume.

If a sweet taste is craved, naturally sweet vegetables should be prepared more often including fall-season squash, carrots, cabbages, and onions. If a sweet taste is further craved, barley malt, rice syrup, or other cereal-grain-based natural sweetener can be consumed in moderate volume.

For pancreatic disorders, dried shiitake mushroom can frequently be used together with sliced daikon in miso soup along with other leafy vegetables. Shiitake can also be used often as a part of regular vegetable dishes. Daikon radish can be used often as well, in various forms and in small volume, for example, raw and grated, dried and cooked, boiled or steamed.

Daily beverages may include bancha twig tea or bancha stem tea, cereal-grain coffee or tea, and other nonaromatic, nonstimulant herb teas, as well as natural spring water and well water.

Chewing food well is essential to restoring health, and the volume of eating should be moderate. Also, eating later than three hours before sleeping should be avoided. All other dietary practices, including use of pickles and condiments, may follow the standard guidelines for cancer prevention described in the recipe section.

As explained in the introduction to Part II, cancer patients who have received or who are currently undergoing medical treatment may need to make further dietary modifications.

HOME CARES

• For pancreatic growths and tumors, a taro potato plaster can be applied on the area every day for three to four hours, immediately following a hot ginger compress applied for five to ten minutes. This application may be continued for the initial two- to three-week period and thereafter occasionally two to three times per week.

• In the event that pain arises, a cup or two of boiled dried shiitake mushrooms and nori or wakame kombu may be consumed for several days. The taro potato plaster and ginger compress, as mentioned above, are also helpful to reduce pains.

• In the event of swelling from fluid retention in the pancreatic and abdominal regions, a buckwheat plaster can be applied for one to two hours daily for several days. Full-body shiatsu massage or palm healing to the abdominal region, one-half to one hour daily, can also be helpful.

• Scrubbing the whole body daily with a very hot towel that has been immersed in water containing grated gingerroot and squeezed out will help improve circulation of blood, body fluids, and energy as well as promote general metabolism.

OTHER CONSIDERATIONS

• Physical exercises are always beneficial to health, but should not lead to exhaustion. Mental relaxation is also helpful, as well as meditation, prayer, visualization, chanting, and similar practices.

• It is important to keep air quality clean and fresh and avoid a heavy, stuffy environment. For this purpose, green leafy plants can be placed in the home and windows opened often to circulate air.

• For undergarments, pillowcases, and bedsheets, cotton is recommended instead of synthetic fabrics. Avoid exposure to artificial electromagnetic radiation, including that from prolonged television viewing.

PERSONAL EXPERIENCE

Pancreatic Cancer

On August 21, 1973, Jean Kohler, a professor of music at Ball State University in Muncie, Indiana, underwent exploratory surgery at Indiana University Medical Center. The fifty-six-year-old pianist had always been healthy and kept fit by gardening and lifting weights. During the summer he had experienced an itching spreading from his leg and thought he had contracted poison oak. Initial medical tests turned up nothing. However, chief surgeon John Jesseph, M.D. discovered a tumor the size of a fist on the head of Kohler's pancreas. Moreover, the cancer had spread to the duodenum. Like most other pancreatic cancer patients, Kohler's condition was discovered too late to operate. Dr. Phillip Christiansen, the other doctor in the case, concluded pessimistically, "I know nothing coming out in research in the next ten years that could possibly help him." Kohler was told he would live anywhere from one month to three years and was advised to take chemotherapy to control the pain.

After five days of drug treatment, Kohler suffered badly swollen hands and arms as well as a cough, chills, and general stress. With the help of his wife Mary Alice, he decided to search for an alternative treatment. An Indiana nutritionist referred him to me, and the Kohlers arrived in Boston for a consultation on September 25. Visual diagnosis, especially the presence of a small blister on Jean's right eye, confirmed the presence of pancreatic cancer.

Kohler expressed a sincere desire to follow the Cancer-Prevention Diet for pancreatic tumors outlined above, and I told him that he would be out of danger within three to six months. Prior to this time, Jean had consumed meat twice a day, eaten much canned and packaged food, and had a well-developed sweet tooth. He especially enjoyed milk, cocoa, soft drinks, milkshakes, and desserts topped with whipped cream. A threat of diabetes several years earlier made him switch to diet sodas and saccharin and sucaryl instead of sugar.

In Boston the Kohlers spent a few days learning to cook according to yin and yang. "One of the most amazing, and totally unexpected, benefits for us personally was that after only five days of macrobiotic food, Jean's hands were suddenly much more flexible," Mary Alice later recalled. "He could reach farther on the keyboard than ever before! This condition has remained to the present time."

On April 7, 1974, after following the diet faithfully for about six months, Kohler returned to Boston. Visual diagnosis indicated that all signs of cancer activity had disappeared. There was a small tumor, the size of a walnut, but it was no longer malignant. Back home Jean continued the Cancer-Prevention Diet for another three months and in July was healthy enough to add a little maple syrup to his way of eating. He continued to improve steadily over the next two years, and his medical tests, including the CEA, which tests for cancer cells in the bloodstream, returned to normal.

For seven years from initial discovery of the tumor, Kohler led a completely normal, active life. In addition to continuing his academic duties and performing musical concerts, he tirelessly wrote letters to scientists around the country about his medical case, delivered hundreds of speeches, and published a book on his recovery. Many thousands of people were helped by his example. As he often said, "The best thing ever to happen to me was having so-called terminal cancer."

The medical world, however, tended to discount his case even though he had compelling scientific documentation. He was often told that only an autopsy would show whether his surgeon's original diagnosis of cancer was accurate and whether it had truly disappeared. In September 1980, Kohler became suddenly ill and checked into Boston's Beth Israel Hospital. Doctors, looking at his medical records, suspected that the pancreatic cancer had come back and asked permission to perform exploratory surgery. Kohler's friends and relatives strongly opposed it, but Jean consented, saying, "I'm too weak to explain, but I have to do this."

On September 14, Kohler died in the hospital. According to Dr. Michael Sobel, the surgeon who performed two operations on him and examined the autopsy, Jean's death had "nothing to do with cancer." Microscopic signs of previous cancer were discovered showing that the diagnosis of his original doctors in Indiana was correct. However, no current cancer activity was found. "For someone to survive seven years with cancer of the pancreas without being treated is extremely rare, if not unheard of," Dr. Sobel commented. Kohler's death was attributed to a liver infection and complications resulting from hemorrhaging following surgery.

In death, as in life, Jean Kohler showed that cancer is not incurable and can be reversed by a balanced diet centered around whole grains and vegetables, accompanied by faith in nature and a strong will to live. Sources: Jean and Mary Alice Kohler, *Healing Miracles from Macrobiotics* (West Nyack, N.Y.: Parker, 1979); Tom Monte, "The Legacy of Jean Kohler," *East West Journal*, March 1981, pp. 14–18.

Pancreatic Cancer

In May, 1982 sixty-four-year-old Bob Williams from Dousman, Wisconsin, learned that he had pancreatic cancer. A former nuclear scientist, advertising executive, and businessman, Williams was told by his doctors that he would be dead within sixty days. While awaiting diagnostic results in the hospital, his wife came across two copies of *Healing Miracles from Macrobiotics* by Jean and Alice Kohler at a local health foods store. She bought both copies, one for her husband and one for herself.

"I devoured the book in ten days," Williams recalled, "I made up my mind this was the route I would go. I turned down medical treatment cold, no chemotherapy, no radiation. My doctors got mad at me and said I was stupid, a layman, and had no background or training."

Prior to this time, Williams had eaten a fairly typical modern diet, high in meat, cheese, yogurt, juices, and sweets. "I used to drink a gallon of milk a day," he recalled.

On June 12, Williams came to Chicago. When my wife Aveline and I first saw him, he was in a wheelchair and could barely speak. He looked near death, and we thought because of the advanced state of the malignancy he might not survive, even with the diet. However, we underestimated his will and reservoirs of inner strength. We learned that during World War II, Bob participated in the Manhattan Project and contributed to the development of the atomic bomb. As the time neared for its employment, he and a small group of other top scientists suggested that the weapon should first be demonstrated over an uninhabited site rather than dropped on hundreds of thousands of civilians. He faced strong opposition because of his views but he stuck to his position. Clearly, the same spirit on behalf of life, this time his own, helped him overcome the ordeal of cancer.

"Within ten days after starting the diet," he noted, "I knew I'd made the right decision. I felt some energy in my body for the first time, not enough to go out and chop the trees down. And as I gained weight, my wife, who also went on the diet and was completely supportive, lost weight."

In addition to changing his way of eating, Bob used the buckwheat plaster to discharge water which had accumulated in his legs. Ever the scientist, he carefully measured the drained off liquid and reported that it amounted to eighteen pounds.

With the further guidance of macrobiotic physician Keith Block, M.D. in Chicago, Bob rapidly recovered, and by the end of July, after little more than a month, he was out of the wheelchair and back on his feet. By August 2 he could walk six miles, and by the autumn he had roto-tilled the garden, built a greenhouse, and reroofed part of his house.

"My surgeon couldn't believe it when I walked into see him," he said. "Fortunately I didn't have that medical attack on my body to overcome as well."

In the fall, Bob began to speak on his recovery to groups throughout the Midwest as well as counsel many individuals with cancer similar to his. When we saw him in Boston on December 6, we hardly recognized him. "It's really a miracle," Aveline exclaimed. "You have given us a very great gift and will inspire and encourage many people." Bob proudly showed us the manufacturer's design for a new airplane, which he intends to build from scratch in the months ahead. "I'll take you up for a flight on my next visit to Boston," he promised. Source: Michio Kushi and Alex Jack, "Back from Death," *East West Journal*, March, 1983.

22.

Skin Cancer and Melanoma

FREQUENCY

About 400,000 new cases of skin cancer are diagnosed each year in the United States, and about 1,900 people die annually of this disease. Because detection is comparatively easy, tumors are slow to spread, and survival is high, skin cancer is not included in many cancer statistics. However, there is a more deadly form of skin cancer, called malignant melanoma, which comprises about 1 to 2 percent of all cancers in the United States. In 1983 it will take 5,200 lives, and an estimated 17,400 new cases will arise. The incidence of melanoma is on the rise and in some countries has doubled over the past twenty years. It affects men and women about equally.

Eighty percent of common skin cancers are classified as basal-cell carcinomas and occur primarily on the face or back of the hands. They do not metastasize but spread by invasion to bone and tissue. Skin cancer is often treated by surgery in a doctor's office under local anesthesia. Methods include electrosurgery with a small electric needle and curette, surgical excision with a scalpel, or chemosurgery with zinc chloride or other chemicals to remove the tumor and a portion of normal tissue around it. Radiation is sometimes used, especially on the face where surgery would result in disfigurement. Chemotherapy and immunotherapy may also be employed.

Melanoma usually appears initially on an existing mole under the skin and spreads quickly through the lymph or blood to the lungs, brain, liver, eye, intestines, reproductive organs, or other sites. Standard treatment is surgery. Melanoma tends to recur, and patients may have many operations, supplemented with chemotherapy. Surgeons say that nearly all persons who have malignant melanomas removed in the early stages of the disease will survive five years or more. For melanoma that has spread to the lymph nodes, the remission rate is between 10 and 20 percent.

STRUCTURE

The main function of the skin, the body's largest organ, is to control adjustment between the external environment and the internal body condition. The skin protects the body's surface, helps regulate body temperature, and excretes waste material and water through sweat glands. Sweat glands come in two types. The exocrine glands, which are located over the entire surface of the body, serve to cool the body and guard against infection. They secrete a watery solution consisting of various fats, sugar, salts, proteins, and toxins. The second type of gland is called apocrine and is found only in certain areas such as under the arms, the nipples, the abdomen, and reproductive areas. The apocrine glands secrete stronger solutions and give rise to body odors.

The color of the skin is regulated by melanin, a pigment that varies from brown to black in color. The less melanin in the skin, the lighter the skin color. Such factors as climate, exposure to sunlight, and daily diet influence the production of melanin.

CAUSE OF CANCER

Normally the body is able to eliminate wastes through such normal functions as urination, bowel movements, respiration, and perspiration. Imbalanced foods or beverages will trigger a variety of abnormal discharge mechanisms in the body such as diarrhea, frequent urination, fever, coughing, or sneezing. Chronic discharges are the next step in this process, and continued poor eating will usually take the form of some kind of skin disease. These are common in cases where the kidneys have lost their ability to properly clean the bloodstream. For example, hard, dry skin arises after the bloodstream fills with fat and oil, eventually causing blockage of the pores, hair follicles, and sweat glands. The mechanism of skin cancer, including the synergistic role that sunlight plays in combination with a high-fat diet, was described in Chapter 10 (Part I).

Melanoma, while classified as a skin cancer, is actually more like a muscular disorder, falling in structure between yin skin-surface tumors, occurring on the periphery of the body, and yang bone tumors, occurring in the deep, compact region of the body. Melanoma usually begins to manifest on existing moles. These are tiny dark-brown mounds under the skin, which serve to eliminate excess protein and fat from the body. This protein and fat does not necessarily come from the consumption of protein itself, but is produced by a combination of consuming too many extreme yin foods such as sugar, fruits, and chemicals and general overconsumption of yang foods, including animal foods, especially poultry, eggs, heavy dairy foods, and other high-protein and high-fat foods. Skin cancer can be relieved by adopting a more yang Cancer-Prevention Diet, while a centrally balanced way of daily eating is recommended for malignant melanoma.

MEDICAL EVIDENCE

• In 1930 researchers reported that dietary fat could influence tumor growth in laboratory animals. Increasing the amount of butter in the diet from 12.5 to 25 percent increased induced skin cancer incidence from 34 to 57 percent. Source: A.F. Watson and E. Mellanby, "Tar Cancer in Mice; Condition of Skin When Modified by External Treatment or Diet, as Factors in Influencing Cancerous Reaction," *British Journal of Experimental Pathology* 11:311–22.

• In 1931 a cancer study with male rats suggested a direct relationship between the amount of protein in the diet and skin tumors. Source: J.R. Slonaker, "The Effect of Different Per Cents of Protein in the Diet," *American Journal of Physiology* 98:266–75.

• In 1941 and 1943 mice fed a diet supplemented with 15 percent corn oil, coconut oil, or lard experienced a rise in induced skin tumors from 12 to 83 percent. Source: P.S. Lavik and C.A. Baumann, "Dietary Fat and Tumor Formation," *Cancer Research* 1:181–87 and "Further Studies on Tumor Promoting Action of Fat," *Cancer Research* 3:749–56.

• In 1966 a medical doctor reported that a special protein-restricted diet helped regress melanoma. Dr. Harry B. Demopoulos put five of his patients with advanced malignant melanoma on a diet high in vegetables and fruits and a supplement that decreased serum levels of several amino acids thought to promote tumor growth. In addition, patients were not allowed to eat high-protein foods such as meat and dairy products, nuts and nut butters, as well as potatoes, bread, and flour products. However, they were allowed to eat oils, stimulants, sugar, and syrups. In three of five patients he reported an "abrupt cessation of tumor growth" and "in all three cases one or more tumors completely regressed." The fourth patient improved while on the diet but the cancer spread when she discontinued it. The fifth patient showed no change. Source: H.B. Demopoulos, "Effects of Reducing the Phenylalanine-Tyrosine Intake of Patients with Advanced Malignant Melanoma," *Cancer* 19:657–64.

• Methylchloromethylether, a corrosive liquid used in refining cane sugar and in gelatin production, causes skin and lung cancer in laboratory animals. Source: "Carcinogens, Job Health Hazards Series" (Washington, D.C.: Occupational Safety and Health Administration, pp. 7–8, 1975).

• PCB's (polychlorinated biphenyls), industrial chemicals used in such things as heavy-duty electrical equipment, air conditioning, microwave ovens, and fluorescent lighting, have become assimilated into the North American food chain and are associated with cancer of the skin and liver. In foods PCB's are found only in animal products, especially fish, milk, eggs, and cheese, and when eaten accumulate in the adipose tissue of humans, in breast milk, and in the blood. Studies in 1976 and 1977 reported higher incidences of melanoma in workers exposed to these chemicals. Source: *Diet, Nutrition, and Cancer* (Washington, D.C.: National Academy of Sciences pp. 14:22–23, 1982).

• In 1980 investigators reported that soybeans contain substances called protease inhibitors, which retard the growth of tumors. In laboratory experiments with mice, skin tumors were blocked when soybeans, lima beans, or other seeds and beans containing this factor were added to the diet. Source: W. Troll, "Blocking of Tumor Promotion by Protease Inhibitors," in J.H. Burchenal and H.F. Oettgen (eds.), *Cancer: Achievement, Challenges, and Prospects for the 1980s, Vol. 1* (New York: Grune and Stratton, pp. 549–55).

• In 1981 a medical doctor from Auburn, California, reported that in conjunction with a natural foods diet, sunlight could inhibit cancer as well as contribute to overall health. Dr. Zane Kime, author of *Sunlight Could Save Your Life*, asserted that when exposed to sunlight, saturated and unsaturated fats in the body turn rancid. Oxidation of these fats damages the tissues, stimulates the development of tumors, and ages the skin. However, he found that a diet high in whole grains and green leafy vegetables is rich in antioxidants and will help protect the body from cancer and other ailments. When the skin is not blocked by an underlying layer of fat and oil, sunlight increases white-blood cells, especially the lymphocytes, which protect against harmful bacteria, and lowers blood pressure. In an address before a cancer society, he cited the case history of a woman who restored her health following a mastectomy for breast cancer by eliminating refined, polyunsaturated fats and oils from her diet, switching to whole foods, and taking regular sunbaths. Source: E.K. Roosevelt, "Sunlight and Cancer," *Natural Food and Farming* 27:1–4.

DIAGNOSIS

Precancerous skin conditions include a variety of lesions and leukoplakia, the growth of white patches on the mucous membranes. Modern medicine distinguishes skin cancer from these conditions by taking a biopsy. In testing for melanoma, patients will also usually be administered a lymphangiogram, chest x-rays, brain and liver scans, and sometimes a cardiac catheterization.

Oriental medicine tends to look at all skin ailments on a spectrum and focuses on three major characteristics: condition of the skin, skin color, and skin marks. Normal, healthy skin should be clean, smooth, slightly shining, and slightly moist. Wet skin indicates an overconsumption of liquid, sugar, and other sweets and results in a thin quality to the blood, rapid metabolism, a faster pulse, and excessive perspiration and urination. Wet skin can accompany a variety of disorders ranging from diarrhea, fatigue, hair loss, and aches and pains to epilepsy and various hyperactive psychological disorders.

Normal skin is slightly oily, but excessively oily skin—showing up on peripheral parts of the body such as the forehead, nose, cheeks, hair, or palms—shows overconsumption of oil and fats or disorders in fat metabolism. Dry skin also results from overconsumption of fats and oils and is caused by a formation of fat layers under the skin, preventing the elimination of moisture toward the surface. Depending on other related symptoms, dry or oily skin accompanies a wide variety of chronic and degenerative conditions.

Rough skin reflects an overconsumption of protein and heavy fats or excess intake of sugar, fruit, and drugs. The second, more yin cause is accompanied by more open sweat glands and a slightly red color. People with hardening of the arteries and accumulations of fat and cholesterol around the organs often have rough skin. Doughy skin, which appears white and flabby and lacking in elasticity, indicates overconsumption of dairy products, sugar, and white flour. A variety of illnesses are connected with this condition, affecting primarily the breasts and reproductive organs.

Aside from natural skin colors, many abnormal colors may appear on the skin. In the case of cancer, a light-green color, reddish-white color, or pinkish-red color from excessive yin or yang food reflects decomposition of tissues and cells and development of cysts and tumors.

Abnormal markings on the skin may also reflect a chronic or degenerative condition. Freckles are the elimination of refined carbohydrates, especially sugar, honey, fruit sugar, and milk sugar. Moles are eliminations of excess protein and fat and appear along the corresponding meridians of the organs affected or muscle areas. Warts signify the elimination of a mixture of protein and fat and indicate developing skin diseases and possible future tumors of the breast, colon, or sex organs. White patches, the result of excess milk, ice cream, and other dairy products, indicate accumulation of fat and mucus throughout the respiratory and reproductive systems. Eczema, dry, hard, raised areas of skin, show a massive elimination of excess fats, especially from dairy foods, more particularly from cheese and eggs cooked with butter.

According to traditional iridology, clogged skin is indicated by a dark circle on the periphery of the iris of the eye. The color, intensity, and width of the ring varies in each case.

DIETARY RECOMMENDATIONS

For skin cancer, avoid all extremes in the yin category of food including refined sugar and foods and beverages treated with sugar such as soft drinks; artificial and chemicalized food; oily and greasy food; all dairy foods including cheese, milk, butter, cream, and yogurt; all foods having stimulant and aromatic qualities including curries, mustard, peppers, and various fragrant beverages and teas; all sorts of alcohol; fruits, fruit juices; nuts; and raw vegetables. It is also necessary to avoid extreme foods in the yang category, especially all sorts of fatty, greasy animal food including meat, poultry, eggs, and oily fishes. In cooking, all foods are to be cooked, and the use of oil should be either avoided or minimized. Frying and oily salad dressings are to be avoided. In addition, it is necessary to avoid all flour products including breads, pancakes, cookies, and cream-of-wheat type cereals, except for the occasional use of whole-grain flours baked without yeast. Avoid vegetables that originally came from tropical climates and are too expansive (yin) for regular use. These include potato, sweet potato, tomato, eggplant, beets, green peppers, and avocado.

In the case of melanoma, in addition to avoiding the above foods, take special caution to avoid poultry such as chicken and eggs completely as well as any use of oils in cooking.

For both skin cancer and melanoma, all foods are to be cooked and not eaten raw. The use of sea salt, tamari soy sauce, miso, and various condiments should be moderate. Recommended daily food for these forms of cancer, by volume of daily intake, should consist of:

• Fifty to sixty percent brown rice and other whole grains, by volume of total intake. Other grains may include millet, barley, rye, whole wheat, oats, buckwheat, and corn. Bread made of whole flour without yeast may be consumed occasionally, without butter. A little bit of sesame butter may be used if desired.

• Five to ten percent miso soup or tamari broth cooked with vegetables and sea vegetables such as wakame or kombu. Occasionally a grain soup or a bean soup may also be eaten.

• Twenty to thirty percent cooked vegetables, prepared in a variety of styles. Among vegetables, round vegetables such as cabbages, onions, pumpkins, acorn and butternut squash are especially recommended as well as root vegetables such as burdock, carrots, and daikon. Many other hard, green, leafy vegetables are also to be used.

• Five to ten percent beans, prepared in various forms. Smaller beans such as azuki, lentils, and chickpeas are preferred to larger beans. Soybean products such as tempeh, tofu (dried or cooked), and natto can be used occasionally but only in moderate volume.

• Five percent or less daily cooked sea vegetables, especially kombu, arame, or hijiki, with a little tamari soy sauce added for taste. Other kinds of sea vegetables may also be consumed frequently.

As supplemental food, a small portion of white-meat fish, which is less fat than red-meat fish, may be cooked without oil and consumed with garnishes of grated fresh daikon or radish, possibly one or two times per week in the event animal food is desired. Fruits are to be minimized, and only cooked seasonal fruits can be consumed in a small volume from time to time if craved. Avoid nuts and nut butters of all kinds, though roasted seeds may be used occasionally as a snack. These include sesame, sunflower, and pumpkin seeds.

All other dietary practice, including condiments and beverages, can follow the standard cancer-prevention suggestions.

As explained in the introduction to Part II, cancer patients who have received or who are currently undergoing medical treatment may need to make further dietary modifications.

HOME CARES

• A compress made from dried daikon leaves and grated ginger can help speed up the process of discharge. Boil daikon leaves; grate fresh gingerroot, and wrap in cheesecloth. Turn down the flame, and place this "ginger sack" (which should contain a lump of grated ginger about the size of a golf ball) in the water. Then, dip a towel into the water, squeeze, and apply to the affected area.

• A rice bran (nuka) skin wash is also beneficial. Wrap nuka in cheesecloth. Place in hot water and shake. The nuka will melt and the water will begin to turn yellow. Then, wash the affected area with a towel or cloth that has been dipped in this water.

• The skin may also be washed with wood ash. Place ashes that are left over after burning wood in a fireplace into hot water and stir very well. Let sit until the ashes settle to the bottom, and then use the water to wash the skin. Pat dry with a towel.

• In cases where a person with a skin disease suffers itching, rub a piece of cut fresh daikon directly onto the affected area. If you don't have a daikon, use a scallion or onion.

• Sesame oil can be applied directly to the affected area in cases where the skin becomes ruptured. Afterward, cover the area with cotton cloth to protect from external contact.

OTHER CONSIDERATIONS

• Wool and synthetic fabrics are particularly irritating to the skin. Wear cotton and sleep on all-cotton fabrics to allow your skin to breathe naturally.

• Avoid cosmetics or antiperspirants made with synthetic or toxic ingredients. Most commercial deodorants contain aluminum salts that temporarily close the openings of the sweat glands and stop "wetness." They also contain chemical antibacterial agents that are harmful to the body. Body odor is largely caused by consumption of animal food, including all kinds of dairy foods, and naturally lessens as the diet becomes more centered on grain-and-vegetable foods. Even natural deodorants should be minimized since they may contain ingredients such as beeswax, which can also stop up pores. Among natural cosmetics, one of the safest is clay. A pure clay powder sprinkled on the body can have an antiperspirant effect. Clay also naturally draws wastes and toxins from the skin and can be used as a basis for a facial mask or a compress.

• A sauna, steam bath, or Japanese hot tub can help open clogged skin pores. However, cancer patients should steam or bathe only occasionally, such as a few times a week, and for a short period of time, ten minutes. Prepare a thermos of tamari-bancha tea or miso soup to drink when you come out in order to replace lost fluids and to thicken the blood quality. Unless proper foods have been consumed, this form of inducing sweat is preferable to running, working out in a gym, or other strenuous activity, which may generate more waste products—chiefly urea and lactic acid—than are lost through sweating.

• Vigorous daily brushing of the skin with a squeezed wet towel or loofa vegetable sponge will help unblock pores and release excess fat and protein through the skin. When washing, avoid the use of soaps. Skin and scalp normally have a slightly acid pH and this is upset by most commercial soaps, which are alkaline. Soaps do not really cleanse the skin and can actually prevent excess cholesterol from coming out of pores. Rice bran wrapped in cheesecloth or natural vegetable-quality soaps should be used instead of chemicalized or animal-quality soaps and shampoos.

• Do-in or shiatsu massage is beneficial to restoring proper respiration and elimination through the skin. Yoga, martial arts, and other exercises that are grounded in an understanding of the energy meridians can also be used to complement dietary adjustments.

• The sun has an overall healthy effect on the body, mind, and spirit as long as you are eating a balanced diet. Try to spend some time each day outside walking, gardening, or relaxing. You do not have to be in the direct glare of the sun. Reading a book in normal daylight under a tree is very peaceful and centering.

• Avoid x-rays, television sets, and other artificial sources of electromagnetic radiation, which are extremely weakening (yin) to the body and accelerate the spread of tumors. Similarly, avoid the sunscreen creams recommended for skin-cancer patients.

PERSONAL EXPERIENCE

Skin Cancer

In early 1975, Roger Randolph, a sixty-one-year-old lawyer from Tulsa, Oklahoma, observed three red spots on his chest and one on his back which did not go away over the course of several weeks. A skin specialist diagnosed his condition as skin cancer and prescribed two types of medicine: one to be applied to these spots twice daily for three weeks, followed by the other medicine for another three weeks. The doctor said the spots on his chest would probably clear up but recommended surgery or radiation therapy to excise the malignancy on his back before it spread.

Randolph discussed his case with his wife and children, and they recommended that he try the macrobiotic approach. Randolph agreed and told his doctor that he would experiment with the Cancer Prevention-Diet and report back in three months.

On April 28, Randolph came to see me and I examined him carefully. The spots on his chest had cleared up, but the one on his back was definitely malignant. I recommended the diet described above for three months with particular emphasis on chewing each mouthful fifty to seventy times. "Mr. Kushi said the cancer would probably continue to grow for a month or two," Randolph recorded, "but that soon thereafter it would definitely disappear. On May 1, I commenced the strict diet and followed it faithfully for three months."

On August 18, Randolph returned for a medical examination, and his doctor was astonished to find that the tumor on his back had disappeared. "He was flabbergasted and suggested that the cure must have been produced by a delayed reaction to the medicine which I had ceased to apply four-and-a-half months earlier," Randolph wrote. "He urged me to return in three weeks to verify the cancer was gone."

On September 9, Randolph went back and received a clean bill of health. Two months later, in November, he had a final medical check and received a discharge as cured. "In my opinion the macrobiotic diet was the sole cause of the cure," Randolph concluded, "permitting my body to cure itself by providing it with proper nutrition and insulating it from the dreadful food most of us eat." Source: *Case History Report*, Vol. 1 No. 3 (Boston: East West Foundation, 1976, pp. 1–2).

Malignant Melanoma

In August 1978, Virginia Brown, a fifty-six-year-old mother and registered nurse from Tunbridge, Vermont, noticed a black mole on her arm that kept getting bigger and blacker. She had lost a lot of weight and felt very dull mentally. Doctors at Vermont Medical Center in Burlington performed a biopsy and discovered that she had an advanced case of malignant melanoma (Stage IV). The physicians told her that without surgery she could expect to live only six months. "Even though I had been trained and practiced in the medical profession for years," she later recalled, "I could not go along with surgery. I had professed alternatives for years, but did not really practice them."

At home, her son and daughter-in-law encouraged her to try macrobiotics, and shortly thereafter she attended the East West Foundation's annual cancer conference, meeting that year in Amherst, Massachusetts. At the conference she listened to fifteen cancer patients discuss their experiences on the diet and was impressed with their accounts.

Prior to that time she had followed the standard American way of eating, high in refined foods and fat, especially animal fat from dairy foods, beef, poultry, and fish. At the time she started the diet, she was so sick that she could hardly make it upstairs and slept most of the day. After three weeks eating the new food, which her children prepared for her, she experienced a change in her energy level, attitude, and mental clarity. "I was a new person, I could get up and walk around."

In September she came to Boston to see me, and I made more specific dietary recommendations and advised her to study proper cooking. With the support of her family, she adhered faithfully to the diet, supplemented by Korean yoga exercises, prayer and meditation, and a two-mile walk each morning after breakfast.

She noted afterward:

I amazed myself at my perseverance, not one of my better qualities. There have been all kind of days—angry, crying, pain, weakness, tension, sadness, and hopelessness, but also thankful times. . . . The most difficult thing has been to see other loved ones go the chemotherapy and radiation route and suffer so.

The most impressive thing was when I first saw Michio. He

looked at me and said, "You're doing it. You can get rid of it." He had faith. This was such a contrast to the doctors. The way they look at you is unbelievable.

In October 1979, I met with her again and found that she no longer had any cancer in her body. Medical exams subsequently confirmed this diagnosis. After restoring her health, Virginia went on to study at the Kushi Institute and is now working in the macrobiotic health program at the Lemuel Shattuck Hospital in Boston, promoting a more natural way of living among other medical professionals and patients. Sources: "Malignant Melanoma, Stage IV," *Cancer and Diet* (Brookline, Mass.: East West Foundation, 1980, pp. 69–70); interview with Alex Jack, September 30, 1982.

23.

Stomach Cancer

FREQUENCY

In the United States, an estimated 13,900 persons will die from stomach cancer in 1983, and 24,500 new cases will develop. Men suffer the illness about one-and-a-half times as often as women, blacks slightly more than whites. It is more prevalent in older than in middle-aged or younger persons. Stomach or gastric cancer, as it is also known, accounts for about five percent of all cancers in the United States. In Japan, however, it is the leading type of cancer, with an incidence six times higher than in the United States.

Surgery is the standard medical treatment, though many cases are considered inoperable because stomach cancer is usually detected only in the late stages of development. The operation is called a gastrectomy, and the stomach may be partly or totally removed. In total gastrectomies, regional lymph nodes, the spleen, and part of the small intestine are also removed. Chemotherapy or radiation may follow. From 12 to 14 percent of patients who undergo this treatment survive five years or more. In his book, *When Cancer Strikes* (Prentice-Hall, 1979), John A. MacDonald, M.D., a cancer surgeon for twenty years, describes the surgical approach to stomach cancer as "discouraging" and "ineffective." "We are uncertain as to what causes gastric cancer," he writes, "but it is quite likely that it has to do with what we eat and how we prepare our food."

STRUCTURE

The stomach is a relatively hollow gourd-shaped organ located in the upper left of the abdominal cavity between the esophagus and the small intestine. The layers of the stomach include 1) the mucosa, or interior lining of the stomach, which secretes digestive enzymes; 2) the connective tissue between the submucosa and the muscles of the stomach; 3) the muscular coat, which enables the stomach to contract and expand and move decomposing food toward the intestines; and 4) the serosa, or outer coating.

The mucosa contains millions of tubular glands, which secrete hydrochloric acid or pepsin as well as small amounts of mucin, anti-anemia materials, and inorganic salts. The upper, expanded region of the stomach, known as the fundus and the body, secretes hydrochloric acid, the stronger of the two acids. The lower, more compact section of the stomach, called the pylorus, secretes pepsin. These acids decompose protein into its various amino acids. Together with muscular peristalsis, enzymatic actions convert solid food into semi-liquid chyme, an acid substance that relaxes the lower pyloric valve allowing the chyme to pass from the stomach into the duodenal section of the small intestine.

CAUSE OF CANCER

In order for the digestive juices in the stomach to be secreted properly, food must first be alkalized by saliva in the mouth. Hence the necessity for thorough chewing of each mouthful of food. Whole grains, especially those cooked with a pinch of sea salt, pass through the stomach to the small intestine, where they are absorbed in the villi and converted into red-blood cells and other healthy circulatory fluids. In contrast, morsels of food from refined grains such as white flour and white rice, as well as refined sugar, start to be absorbed directly in the stomach and enter the body fluids prematurely, producing a thinner quality of blood and lymph. Stomach cancer results from long-term consumption of extreme yin foods and beverages such as refined grain, flour, sugar and other sweets, soda and ice-cold drinks, alcohol, aromatic and stimulant beverages, chemicals and drugs. Strong yang foods, which overtax the stomach, can also cause cancer, including foods high in animal protein and salts, as well as high-fat, oily, and greasy foods. Repeated oversecretion of stomach acids to neutralize and process an excess of these foods results in irritating the stomach lining, ulcerations, and eventually the formation of tumors. Depending on the location and type, stomach cancer can metastasize to nearby lymph nodes, the pancreas, liver, or ovaries (Krukenberg tumor). It can also spread to the lungs, bones, and occasionally the skin through the lymphatic system.

The yin form of stomach cancer, affecting the upper expanded region of the stomach, is caused by overconsumption of extremely expansive substances, especially refined grains, sugar, foods containing chemical additives or preservatives such as MSG, food grown with chemical fertilizers, or pesticides. Cancer in the more compact pylorus in the lower stomach results from overconsumption of meat, eggs, fish, or other overly yang products. Over the last twenty years, the rate of stomach cancer in the United States has fallen about 75 percent. In a recent issue of *Life* magazine, in an article "The Endless Quest for a Cure," medical writer Jeff Wheelwright concludes, "The trend towards more vegetables, fruit, and fiber in the American diet . . . may be the main reason for the decline."

MEDICAL EVIDENCE

• In 1558 Venetian-born architect and counselor Louis Cornaro wrote an essay on health and diet describing how he suffered from a terminal stomach disorder (though not necessarily cancer) in middle-age which he overcame by adopting a grain-based diet and avoiding certain kinds of animal food, raw salads, fruit, pastries, and sweets. "O Happy Life!" he recorded in another essay in his eighty-sixth year, "Thou, besides all the aforesaid manifold blessings thou grantest to thy old disciple, hast brought his stomach to so good and perfect a condition that he now relishes plain bread more than he ever did the most delicate viands in the years of his youth. All this thou dost because thou art reasonable, knowing that bread is the proper food of man when accompanied by a healthful appetite . . . we cannot partake of a more natural food." Cornaro lived to age 102, and his book became one of the most influential books on health and diet during the Renaissance. Source: Louis Cornaro, *The Art of Living Long* (Milwaukee: William F. Butler, pp. 44–46, 86, 1935 edition).

• In 1713 Japanese physician Ekiken Kaibara wrote a book on health and longevity in which he recommended balanced diet to protect against chronic diseases. "A person should prefer light, simple meals. One must not eat a lot of heavy, greasy, rich food. One should also avoid uncooked, chilled, or hard food. . . . Of everything one eats and drinks, the most important thing is rice, which must be eaten in ample amounts to ensure proper nutrition. . . . Bean paste has a soft quality and is good for the stomach and intestines." Source: Ekiken Kaibara, *Yojokun: Japanese Secret of Good Health* (Tokyo: Tokuma Shoten, 1974 edition).

• In 1887 Ephraim Cutter, M.D., a physician from Albany, New York, wrote a book in which he postulated that "cancer is a disease of nutrition." Cutter presented nine case histories of cancer relieved by putting the patient on a balanced diet and concluded that the question was not vegetable versus animal food, but the "proper proportion of animal to vegetable food." He listed mental depression and stress as contributing factors and reported one case of stomach cancer "evidently caused by living in the suburbs and having business in the city, taking a light lunch there, and returning late in the day, all tired out, and having a hearty supper with much condiments." Cutter speculated that "cancer may be cured in times to come by food." Source: Ephraim Cutter, M.D., *Diet in Cancer* (New York: Kellogg, pp. 19–26, 1887).

• From 1904 to 1911 British surgeon Robert McCarrison traveled in the Hunza, a remote Himalayan kingdom in the then Northwest Territory of India. There he was astonished to discover a completely healthy culture in which the infectious and degenerative diseases of modern civilization, including colonial India, were unknown. "I never saw a case of asthenic dyspepsia, of gastric or duodenal ulcer, of appendicitis, of mucous colitis, or of cancer," he informed his medical colleagues. McCarrison hypothesized that the unusual health and longevity of the Hunza people was due primarily to their daily diet consisting of whole-wheat chapatis, barley, and maize, supplemented by leafy green vegetables, beans and legumes, apricots, and a small amount of dairy products and goat's milk only on feast days. The Hunzas did not eat refined white rice, sugar, black tea, or spices as did most of the Indian population. In 1927 Sir Robert McCarrison assumed the post of Director of Nutritional Research in India and to test his theory began a series of laboratory experiments. Feeding the Hunza diet and the regular Indian diet to rats over a period of four years, he discovered that animals fed the modern, refined diet of Bengal and Madras contracted cysts, abscesses, heart disease, and cancer of the stomach. Rats fed the Hunza whole-grain diet remained healthy and free of all disease. Sources: Robert McCarrison, M.D., "Faulty Food in Relation to Gastro-Intestinal Disorder," *Journal of the American Medical Association* 78:1–8, 1922 and G.T. Wrench, M.D., *The Wheel of Health* (London: O.W. Daniel, 1938).

• A 1966 case-control study found that stomach cancer cases had consumed fried foods more frequently than controls, especially bacon drippings and animal fats used for cooking. Source: J. Higginson, "Etiological Factors in Gastrointestinal Cancer in Man," *Journal of the National Cancer Institute* 37:527–45.

• In 1971 a Japanese cancer researcher reported a significant negative association between per capita tofu intake and stomach cancer. Source: T. Hirayama, "Epidemiology of Stomach Cancer," in T. Murakami (ed.), *Early Gastric Cancer. Gann Monograph on Cancer Research, 11* (Tokyo: University of Tokyo Press, pp. 3–19).

• A 1974 case-control study observed that high-starch foods such as refined white bread and sugar were consumed more frequently by gastric cancer cases than controls. Source: B. Modan et al., "The Role of Starches in the Etiology of Gastric Cancer," *Cancer* 34:2087–92.

• In 1978 medical researchers reported that brussel sprouts, cabbage, turnips, cauliflower, broccoli, and other vegetables high in a substance identified as indoles lessened the incidence of stomach and breast cancer in laboratory animals by 77 percent. Source: L.W. Wattenberg and W.D. Loub, "Inhibition of Polycyclic Hydrocarbon-Induced Neoplasia by Naturally Occurring Indoles," *Cancer Research* 38:1410–13.

• In 1981 Japan's National Cancer Center reported that people who eat miso soup daily are 33 percent less likely to contract stomach cancer than those who never eat miso soup. The thirteen-year study, involving about 265,000 men and women over forty, also found that miso soup is effective in reducing the risk of "hypertensive diseases, ischemic heart disease and all other causes of death." Source: T. Hirayama, "Relationship of Soybean Paste Soup Intake to Gastric Cancer Risk," *Nutrition and Cancer* 3:223–33.

• A 1981 case-control study of 100 gastric cancer patients and controls in Shanghai showed significantly lower cancer risk among those who regularly consumed soy milk. Source: S.K. Xing, "Personal Communication," *Chinese Journal of Preventive Medicine* 15:2.

• In 1979 researchers at Tokyo Medical and Dental University reported that traditional Oriental diagnostic techniques for stomach cancer compared favorably with Western detection methods. Using a Meridian Imbalance Diagram based on twenty-three different ratios of measurements along the yin and yang meridians of the upper and lower limbs, the scientists compared Oriental and Western diagnosis in twenty-two patients complaining of stomach problems and nineteen healthy controls. These findings were then evaluated against postoperative reports. For example, ten of the patients were later confirmed to have stomach cancer. "This shows the existence of a pattern of Oriental diagnosis corresponding to a specific Western diagnosis," the researchers concluded. Source: Jean Pierre Garnery, M.D. et al., "Oriental Diagnosis in Stomach Cancer Patients," *American Journal of Chinese Medicine* 7(1):91–99.

DIAGNOSIS

Stomach cancer is difficult to diagnose by modern medical methods. Only 18 percent of current stomach cancers are detected in the local stage before spreading to other organs of the body. Cancer of the stomach is commonly confused with other abdominal disorders, especially gastric ulcers, and the patient may feel no unusual symptoms. The normal hospital procedure is called a gastroscopy and allows direct x-ray viewing of the entire stomach. A biopsy is performed if cancer is suspected, and the lining of the stomach may be brushed and washed to obtain cell samples. Follow-up chest and skeletal x-rays and a liver scan are taken to determine possible metastases.

The condition of the stomach is relatively easy to diagnose by traditional Oriental medicine, and the tendency toward acidosis, ulcerations, or tumors can be monitored long before they actually develop so that preventive dietary action can be taken. To diagnose stomach problems, corresponding areas in the face can be observed: the upper lip and the bridge of the nose. The entire digestive system is reflected in the mouth as a whole, and the upper lip mirrors the upper digestive tract, especially the stomach. More specifically, the left side of the upper lip corresponds with the upper, more yin part of the stomach, while the right side shows the lower, more yang region. Swelling in the upper lip shows an expanded stomach condition caused by consumption of refined grains, sugar and other sweeteners, alcohol, tropical fruit and juices, or overeating. A contracted upper lip reflects a tightening in the stomach due to excessive intake of meat, eggs, salt, or dry baked goods. Both of these conditions reflect overacidity in the stomach, and the tendency or presence of ulcerations may be indicated by inflammation, a blister, or discoloring on the upper lip.

Brown blotches or freckles on the upper part or bridge of the nose indicate chronic stomach acidosis, ulcerations, hypoglycemic and diabetic tendencies, or possible stomach cancer. In the case of stomach cancer, a slight green tinge may show up in this area. The skin as a whole also shows the condition of the stomach. A splotchy brown or dirty skin color suggests chronic acidity in the stomach as a result of excess sugar or fruit consumption. Discolorations along the stomach meridian, especially in the area below the knee or on top of the foot in the extended region of the second and third toes, are a good indicator of stomach imbalances. Again, a green shading in either of these locations indicates possible stomach cancer.

The near back of the tongue also may be examined to observe developing stomach problems. A dark-red color indicates inflammation, ulcerations, and a potential development of stomach cancer. A white or yellow color or white patches indicates accumulations of fat and mucus in the stomach. Blue or purple signifies overconsumption of sugar, soft drinks, alcohol, drugs, medications, and other extreme yin substances. Small mushroomlike eruptions are signs of acidity, ulcerations, and possible nausea and regurgitation.

DIETARY RECOMMENDATIONS

The cause of stomach cancer is chiefly the overconsumption of strong foods and beverages in either/or both the yin and yang categories. Accordingly, it is necessary to avoid all overly expansive foods including all refined food such as white rice, white bread, and other refined flour products; sugar, honey, chocolate, carob, and similar sweeteners; sugar-treated food and beverages; artificial soda and soft drinks; coffee, black tea, and alcohol; cold, icy beverages; all stimulants and spices including curry, mustard, and pepper; all aromatic foods and beverages; butter, milk, and cream; chemicalized food, seasonings, and beverages; oily, greasy food; tropical fruits, juices, and vegetables of tropical origin including potato, sweet potato, yam, tomato, and eggplant. In the yang category, beef, pork, poultry, and eggs; all types of dairy food including cheese; very salty food; hard, baked flour products such as hard bread and cookies; all baked animal food; and high-protein and high-fat food are to be avoided.

Following are the general guidelines for daily dietary practice:

• Fifty to sixty percent whole-cereal grains, by volume of total food consumed each day. All whole grains including brown rice, barley, whole-wheat berries, rye, millet, oats, corn, and buckwheat can be prepared as main dishes. However, for regular daily usage, brown rice is the first choice and barley and millet the second choices. Grains are to be pressure-cooked with water and a pinch of sea salt. In the event flour products are desired, steamed unleavened, non-yeasted whole-wheat or rye bread may be served. Whole-wheat and buckwheat pasta and noodles can be used occasionally for variety.

• Five to ten percent soup. One or two cups of miso or tamari soy sauce soup in which wakame or kombu sea vegetables are cooked together with vegetables can be used daily. Occasionally, cooked whole grain can be added to soup to make grain and vegetable soup. Occasionally hard autumn squash can be used to make a sweet soup.

• Twenty to thirty percent vegetables. A variety of leafy, round, and root vegetables may be prepared in different cooking styles. Among vegetables, daikon and its greens are particularly recommended for frequent use. The taste of vegetables should be mild, using a small volume of sea salt, tamari soy sauce, or miso in cooking. If a sour taste is desired, a small quantity of rice vinegar or umeboshi vinegar may be used for boiled salad or a small portion of sauerkraut can be served. Besides boiling and steaming, vegetables can be sautéed with sesame or corn oil applied in small volume two to three times a week. Avoid deep frying, which uses a large volume of oil. Fresh salad is to be refrained from, though boiled salad may be used regularly. Pickled vegetables—long time rather than light, quick pickles—should be used in small volumes as a garnish, if desired.

• Five to ten percent beans and bean products. Smaller beans such as azukis, lentils, and chickpeas are preferred to large beans and can be cooked with sea vegetables such as kombu, fall-season squash, onions and carrots, or other vegetables. Bean products such as tempeh, natto, and tofu are also recommended for occasional use, cooked in soup or with other vegetables. However, beans and bean products are to be used in moderate volume. They can be lightly seasoned with sea salt, tamari soy sauce, miso or, if sweetness is craved, with cereal-grain-based sweeteners such as barley malt or rice syrup.

• Five percent or less sea vegetables. All sea vegetables are recommended, but arame, nori, and hijiki may be used more frequently than others. They are to be consumed in small volume and cooked and seasoned with a small amount of tamari soy sauce. Occasionally one or two drops of sesame oil can be added during cooking.

Fish and seafood are generally to be avoided. However, if desired, a small portion of nonfatty white-meat fish can be cooked in miso or tamari soy sauce soup with sea vegetables and vegetables to make a fish soup. This soup can be served with one to two tablespoons of grated fresh daikon or radish as a garnish. It can also be cooked with dried shiitake mushrooms.

Fruits and fruit juices should generally be avoided. However, if desired, a small volume of either dried or cooked fruits such as apples, peaches, grapes, cherries, strawberries and other berries, and melons can be used infrequently.

If a sweet taste is desired, naturally sweet vegetables such as fall-season squash, carrots, onions, cabbages, and parsnips can be prepared more often. If still more sweetness is craved, cereal-based natural sweeteners such as barley malt and rice syrup may be used in moderate volume.

Nuts and nut butters are primarily to be avoided, though roasted seeds such as sesame, pumpkin, or sunflower may be used occasionally in small volume as a snack.

Scallion-miso condiment can be used frequently in small volume as one of the regular condiments. This is made by cooking chopped scallions and an equal volume of miso with a small amount of sesame oil. However, condiments should not be used in excess and a salty or strong taste should be avoided.

Daily beverages are to be nonaromatic, nonstimulant drinks such as bancha twig or stem tea, roasted barley or roasted rice tea, and cereal-grain coffee. Clean, natural well or spring water is also recommended.

Chewing food well until it becomes liquid in the mouth is absolutely essential to improving stomach cancer and other serious illnesses. It is also important to avoid overconsumption of food and beverages and not to eat within three hours before sleeping. All other dietary practice may follow the standard guidelines for cancer prevention.

As explained in the introduction to Part II, cancer patients who have received or who are currently undergoing medical treatment may need to make further dietary modifications.

HOME CARES

• A taro potato plaster may be applied for three to four hours or overnight on the stomach region, immediately after a hot ginger compress applied for ten to fifteen minutes. They can be used daily for two to three weeks or whenever necessary to help reduce tumor development and to provide relief in the case of pains and aches.

• Application of warmth on the stomach region as well as palm healing for one-half to one hour also can help ease pain or ache in the stomach region.

• In the event the stomach has been removed in part or whole by surgery, genuine brown-rice cream can be used. Two to three bowls may be consumed per day with a small volume of condiments such as scallion-miso, gomashio (sesame salt), tekka, or umeboshi plum for the initial several days. After that period, regular brown rice and other cereal grains can be served, gradually shifting toward more complete meals, including various side dishes. During both times, it is very important to chew the food thoroughly until it assumes a liquid form, up to 100 or more times per mouthful. The removed portion of the stomach will often restore itself as time passes. Even if the amputated section is not restorable, chewing well can sufficiently serve for digestion.

• Scrubbing the whole body daily with a tightly squeezed towel that has been immersed in water containing grated gingerroot is very helpful to improve circulation, activate energies, improve overall conditions, and stimulate the appetite.

OTHER CONSIDERATIONS

• Light exercises, including breathing fresh air outdoors and ten to fifteen minutes a day practicing long exhalations through the nostrils, will promote harmonious mental and physical metabolism and contribute to overall relaxation.

• Underwear, clothing, pillowcases, and bedsheets should be made of cotton material rather than synthetic fabrics or wool.

• Exposure to contaminated air including smoky, heavy air and artificial radiation should be avoided. Neither watching television for long periods nor staying under white fluorescent light is advisable.

PERSONAL EXPERIENCE

Stomach Cancer with Metastases to the Esophagus

In October 1982 (Charles) Duane Moyer, a forty-three-year-old well-drilling contractor from Lehighton, Pennsylvania, experienced difficulty swallowing. Medical tests showed a stricture of the esophagus, and a biopsy indicated cancer of the stomach with metastases to the esophagus. Moyer's doctors wanted to operate and remove three-quarters of his stomach, but Duane's brother, a physician, recommended that he seek a second opinion. Doctors at the Mayo Clinic in Minneapolis confirmed the diagnosis. Exploratory surgery further showed that the malignancy had spread to the lymph nodes, and there was a large tumor on the outside of the gullet, strangulating the heart and windpipe. The surgeons told Moyer that his condition was terminal and that he could expect to live six months. They recommended chemotherapy to reduce the pain and told him that possibly a tube could be inserted into his throat so that he could die in peace.

Shortly after this unhappy prognosis, a neighbor gave Moyer a copy of a book describing the macrobiotic approach to cancer. On October 31, after a consultation with Murray Snyder at the East West Foundation in Philadelphia, Duane decided to begin the Cancer-Prevention Diet. Up until this time, he had consumed lots of meat, cheese, pizza, milk, ice cream, fruit, coffee, and tea. For example, a big eater and robust outdoors worker, Duane customarily devoured three sandwiches at a time consisting of white bread and luncheon meat.

After practicing the diet for about a month, Duane and his wife Connie came to see me, and I suggested further modifications in the new way of eating as well as special home cares. In addition to regular ginger compresses and a ginger bath for his abdomen and chest, I recommended that he eat daily a side dish of grated daikon or grated lotus root for two months in order to help keep his esophagus open.

Mrs. Moyer was very supportive of her husband's dietary approach and took macrobiotic cooking classes in Doylestown. The family switched from an electric to gas range and replaced their color TV with black and white. "Duane was able to make the transition smoothly," Connie reported several months later. "He even enjoys the seaweed. We have five children. Three are living at home, and we are eating macrobiotically and adjusting just fine, though it is harder on the teenager."

In addition to the diet, Duane continued to take chemotherapy upon the recommendation of his doctor, consisting of 5FU and Adreomycin four times a month. The Moyers also had a strong faith in God, and in the face of this challenge, the family grew closer spiritually.

On December 13, 1982, an oncologist in Bethlehem examined Moyer. "I had the pleasure of seeing Duane, again today," the cancer specialist wrote. "He looks absolutely great and is feeling very well. He has been hunting and leading a perfectly normal life and working full time. He stays rather faithfully on his macrobiotic diet, in fact he swears by it and I have no qualms about it. He has no further dysphagia, as he did in the past; he can eat at the same pace as his family." The doctor went on to say that his lymph, lung, and liver functions were clearing up and that his blood counts, including both red-blood and white-blood cell levels, were "within normal limits." About six weeks later, chest x-rays confirmed that Moyer no longer had a tumor in the esophagus. Similar medical tests to check his stomach are scheduled for later in the spring.

While it would be premature at this writing to say that Duane is healed, it is fair to say that his progress has been steady and the future is optimistic. "Unlike last fall when his cancer was diagnosed," his wife observed, "today Duane is full of energy. He jogs five miles a day, he is active, gets up early, cuts firewood. There has been a dramatic change. Now he makes me tired." Mrs. Moyer went on to say that over the winter she and her husband met about ten other cancer patients and felt grateful for the opportunity to share with them the benefits of their experience. She also noted that in view of her husband's renewed vitality, the cancer specialist was "reading up on macrobiotics" and Duane's brother, the doctor, had become convinced of its value.

The Moyers' story is an inspiring example of how a modern family can maintain their faith and hold together in the most difficult of times, and how macrobiotic counselors and medical professionals can cooperate to ensure a smooth recovery. Source: Telephone interview with Connie Moyer by Alex Jack, February 5, 1983, and report from Duane Moyer's oncologist.

24.

Upper Digestive Cancers: Esophagus, Larynx, Mouth, and Pharynx

FREQUENCY

Cancers of the upper digestive system, including the mouth, throat, and esophagus, will account for 21,350 estimated deaths in the United States in 1983 and some 47,100 new cases. Men are about twice as likely to contract these forms of cancer as women. The incidence of upper digestive cancer is particularly high in the Far East.

Cancers in the head and neck do not usually metastasize, but spread by local invasion. About 90 percent of these tumors are classified as squamous-cell carcinomas. They grow slowly and tend to recur within several years of treatment. Cancer of the esophagus often spreads to the liver, lungs, or the membrane surrounding the lungs.

Surgery and radiation are widely used by modern medicine to treat these forms of cancer. In the case of esophageal cancer, partial removal of the diseased section will be rectified by taking a portion of the large intestine and surgically linking it with the remaining part of the esophagus and the stomach. This procedure is called an esophagogastric anastomosis. If the whole esophagus is taken out, the spleen and end of the pancreas are usually removed as well. Again, part of the intestinal wall or plastic tubing will be inserted to connect the severed ends of the digestive tract.

For head and neck tumors, surgery is usually employed to remove the tumor and part of the healthy tissue surrounding it. Plastic surgery will follow if this results in the disfiguration of the face. The voice is often lost as a consequence of surgery to the throat area. Radiation therapy may also be used as a primary treatment, depending on the type and size of the tumor. Chemotherapy may be used in conjunction with radiation if the tumor is advanced or has spread to the bone. The survival rate for esophageal cancer is 3 percent. The five-year cure rate is higher for head and neck cancers: lips, 84 percent; tongue, 32 percent; mouth, 45 percent; larynx, 63 percent; and pharynx, 21 percent.

STRUCTURE

The upper digestive tract extends from the lips to the stomach and consists of the mouth, the larynx, the pharynx, and the esophagus. The larynx is also known as the voice box, the pharynx as the throat, and the esophagus as the gullet. Food enters the body through the mouth and moves spirally up and down in the process of chewing. Digestion alternates between alkaline (yang) and acidic (yin) secretions at various stages along the alimentary canal. From the mouth, where alkaline substances are released, food travels to the stomach, where acids are secreted. From there it moves to the duodenum, where alkaline enzymes from the small intestine and pancreas are activated. Finally, remaining foodstuffs are absorbed by the acidic substances in the villi of the small intestine.

In the mouth the digestive process begins with the secretion of saliva, a clear, watery fluid that has a pH of 7.2, making it slightly salty or alkaline. The main function of saliva is to begin gradually breaking down carbohydrates for further absorption in the stomach and complete digestion in the small intestine. Ptyalin, an enzyme in saliva, is released during chewing and initiates this process.

The pharynx is a mucus-lined tube situated at the back of the mouth, nasal cavity, and larynx. Its muscles push food to the esophagus, a flat canal about ten to twelve inches long extending from the lower neck through the chest to the stomach.

CAUSE OF CANCER

Tumors of the upper digestive system, except for the tongue, are a more yin form of cancer. They are caused primarily by long-term consumption of expansive yin substances including milk and dairy products, oily and greasy foods, sugar and other sweeteners, tropical fruits and vegetables, coffee and black tea, spices, vitamin pills and protein supplements, alcohol, drugs, and medications. In the Far East, a diet centered around refined white rice, the use of sugar and refined oil, the increasing use of chemical seasonings and flavors, and the popular practice of chewing betel-nut leaves, a gumlike wad of spices, are the main factors contributing to the high rise of mouth, throat, and esophageal cancers in that part of the world.

As we have seen, digestion begins in the mouth, and the primary function of saliva is to alkalinize (make more yang) entering foodstuffs. A meal consisting primarily of whole grains and other balanced foods will begin to be broken down in the mouth as the enzyme in saliva slowly metabolizes starch into maltose, a disaccharide. Thorough chewing is essential for this process, and it is especially necessary to balance the acidity of extreme yin foods, drinks, and medications. If chewing is minimal or light, not enough saliva will be secreted to neutralize the excess volume or strong quality of incoming yin. As a result, these expansive substances will be prematurely absorbed into the blood system in the mouth, throat, esophagus, or stomach. This makes for a thinner condition of the blood and other bodily fluids, ultimately giving rise to illness, loss of vitality, and degeneration of the organism.

The progressive development of disease in the upper digestive system, as in other systems of the body, takes the form of localized inflammations, ulcers, cysts, and, finally, tumors. Mouth cancer is often preceded by leukoplakia, a disease characterized by the growth of thick white patches on the inside of the cheeks, gums, or tongue. Cancer of the esophagus is commonly accompanied by difficulty in swallowing as the gullet moves to restrict the passage of harmful and irritating substances by creating a natural obstruction.

Cancer of the tongue, a small compact organ, is a more yang form of mouth cancer and is caused by the excessive intake of yin accompanied by overly yang food. Cancer of the tongue could result from long-term consumption of sardines and cream cheese, smoked white fish cooked with spices, overconsumption of salt and fatty, greasy, and oily foods, or other extreme combinations.

Cancer of the throat is caused by consumption of both extreme yin and yang foods and beverages, including overconsumption of greasy and oily foods, dairy food, flour products, sugar and sweeteners.

MEDICAL EVIDENCE

• The Yellow Emperor's Classic of Internal Medicine, dating in written form to about the third century B.C., discusses the application of yin and yang to treating sickness. Although it does not mention cancer, it recommends a balanced diet to prevent and relieve other degenerative diseases. "The Yellow Emperor asked the heavenly teacher: I have heard that people of ancient times had lived as long as 120 years with no signs of weakening in movements, but people nowadays become weakened in their movements at the age of less than sixty years old. Is this due to a change in natural environments or due to man's faults? Chi-Po replied: The ancient people who knew the proper way to live had followed the pattern of Yin and Yang which is the regular pattern of heaven and earth, remained in harmony with numerical symbols which are the great principles of human life, eaten and drunken with moderation, lived their daily lives in a regular pattern with neither excess nor abuse." The text goes on to record that in former days people treated disease "by cereal soups to be drunk for ten days" but that medicine had degenerated and now people treated illness with herbs, acupuncture, and moxibustion. Source: *A Complete Translation of Nei Ching and Nan Ching*, translated by Dr. Henry C. Lu (Vancouver: The Academy of Oriental Heritage, pp. 1–2, 84–87, 1978).

• A 1961 study found that consumption of green and yellow vegetables was lower for esophageal cancer patients than controls. Source: E.L. Wynder and I.J. Bross, "A Study of Etiological Factors in Cancer of the Esophagus," *Cancer* 14:389–413.

• A 1975 study in the Caspian littoral region of Iran, an area of high esophageal cancer, indicated lower intake of lentils and other pulses, cooked geen vegetables, and other whole foods. Source: H. Hormozdiari et al., "Dietary Factors and Esophageal Cancer in the Caspian Littoral of Iran," *Cancer Research* 35:3493–98.

• Heavy consumption of alcohol increases the risk of cancer of the mouth, throat, larynx, esophagus, and liver. These forms of cancer appear about fifteen times more frequently in heavy drinkers and smokers than in those who neither smoke nor drink. Source: Samuel S. Epstein, M.D., *The Politics of Cancer* (New York: Doubleday, pp. 474–75, 1979).

• Mormon males in California have 55 percent less esophageal cancer and females 39 percent less than other Californians. A 1980 epidemiological study associated lowered cancer risk with the Mormons' diet high in whole grains, vegetables, and fruit, moderate in meat, and low in stimulants, alcohol, tobacco, and drugs. Source: J.E. Engstrom, "Health and Dietary Practice and Cancer Mortality among California Mormons," in J. Cairns et al. (ed.), *Cancer Inci-*

dence in Defined Populations, Banbury Report 4 (Cold Spring Harbor, N.Y.: Cold Spring Harbor Laboratory), pp. 69–90.

• A 1981 epidemiological study found that populations with a low risk of esophageal cancer in Africa and Asia consume more millet, cassava, yams, and peanuts than high-risk groups. Source: S.J. van Rensburg, "Epidemiologic and Dietary Evidence for a Specific Nutritional Predisposition to Esophageal Cancer," *Journal of the National Cancer Institute* 67:243–51.

• Research studies in Colombia, Chile, Japan, Iran, China, England, and the United States have indicated an association between increased cancer of the esophagus and stomach and exposure to high levels of nitrate or nitrite in the diet and drinking water. Foods generally containing or producing these substances include hams, sausages, bacon, and other cured meats, baked goods and breakfast cereals, and fruit juices. Source: *Diet, Nutrition, and Cancer* (Washington, D.C.: National Academy of Sciences, pp. 12:19–21, 1982).

DIAGNOSIS

Cancers of the mouth and throat are commonly detected by x-rays to the chest, skull, and jaw; an upper GI series; various endoscopies; and a biopsy. Esophageal tumors will be diagnosed with these methods as well as liver and bone scans to check for metastases and a bronchoscopy to see whether the tumor has spread to the bronchial tubes.

Cancers of the upper digestive organs can be pinpointed, however, without the intervention of high technology, including potentially harmful x-ray radiation. In visual diagnosis, the upper lip corresponds with the condition of the upper digestive system. Specifically, the top part of the upper lip reflects the condition of the esophagus, the lower part of the upper lip reveals the state of the stomach. Swellings, discolorations, or patches in this region indicate corresponding troubles in the respective digestive organs. For example, a pinkish-white hue on the lips shows overconsumption of sugar, fruits, fats, and dairy products. White patches show excessive intake of dairy foods and fat.

The condition of the gums and mouth cavity offers other clues to general health. Swollen gums, often accompanied by pain and inflammation, are caused by overconsumption of liquid, oil, sugar, fruits, and juices. Receding gums are caused by either the overconsumption of yang foods—including animal food, salts, and dried food—or overconsumption of yin foods, including sugar, honey, chocolate, soft drinks, and fruit juices. Abnormally red or purple gums that are not swollen are caused by a combination of yang animal food or salts and yin sugar, fruits, juices, soft drinks, and chemicals. Similar colors accompanied by swelling are caused by the overconsumption of yin foods and drinks. Pale, whitish gums indicate poor circulation as well as a lack of hemoglobin in the bloodstream, due to anemia caused by nutritional imbalance.

Pimples appearing on the inner wall of the mouth cavity are eliminations of excessive protein, fat, oil (from either animal or plant sources), sugar or sugar products. Bleeding gums, in most cases, are caused by broken blood capillaries, which have been weakened by a lack of salt and other minerals in the bloodstream. In rare cases, they can also be caused by an overconsumption of animal food, dry flour products, salts and minerals, and a lack of fresh fruits and vegetables, as in the case of scurvy. Inflammation deep in the throat, with or without swollen tonsils, is caused by the overconsumption of such yin foods as fruits, juices, sugar, soda, ice-cold drinks, and milk.

The back region of the tongue, the root area below the uvula, also corresponds to the esophagus. Discolorations, inflammation, pimples, or patches here indicate disorders in the gullet.

DIETARY RECOMMENDATIONS

For all cancers in the upper digestive tract, including the mouth, gums, lips, tongue, larynx, pharynx, and esophagus, it is of primary importance that fatty and oily foods, including animal foods such as meat, poultry, eggs, dairy food of any kind, as well as vegetable oil, be avoided. Sugar, chocolate, fruits, juices, soda, and all food and beverages treated by sweeteners, as well as heavily chemicalized and artificialized food and beverages, are to be avoided. All stimulants including alcohol, coffee, black tea, aromatic herb drinks, curry, mustard, and peppers should be discontinued. Avoid refined flour products and limit even unrefined flour products.

Following are the dietary guidelines, by daily volume, to be practiced:

• Fifty to sixty percent whole-cereal grains, especially brown rice as the staple. All other grains can occasionally be substituted or added, including barley, millet, buckwheat groats, oats, whole-wheat berries, and rye, though corn should be minimized. These grains have to be pressure-cooked or boiled a long time with a pinch of unrefined sea salt added before cooking. Whole-grain flour products such as unyeasted bread and pastas can be used for change, but the amount should be limited.

• Five to ten percent miso soup, occasionally alternated with tamari broth soup. These soups should be cooked with sea vegetables such as kombu or wakame and hard, leafy vegetables. Occasionally, grains or beans can be cooked with either soup. One or two cups of soup should be consumed daily.

• Twenty to thirty percent vegetables. Hard, leafy vegetables are to be emphasized, supplemented with root vegetables and round vegetables such as onions, pumpkin, autumn squash, and cabbages. These vegetables may be cooked in various styles and seasoned with either sea salt, tamari soy sauce, or miso, in moderate volume. It is best not to use any oil in cooking for the initial period. Very occasionally, sautéed vegetables may be eaten if they are cooked with high quality natural unrefined sesame oil in small volume.

• Five percent beans and bean products. They are to be limited to smaller beans such as azuki, lentils, and chickpeas during the initial two to three months. Larger beans can be consumed later as the condition improves. These beans can be cooked with sea vegetables such as kombu, kelp, hijiki, or arame. They also can be cooked with land vegetables such as onions and carrots and moderately seasoned with unrefined sea salt, tamari soy sauce, or miso.

• Five percent or less well-cooked sea vegetables of any kind, especially hijiki, arame, or kombu that have been cooked for a long time. They may be seasoned moderately with tamari soy sauce.

People with cancer of the upper digestive system need to avoid all fruits, fruit dessert, and juices, regardless of whether the fruit is dried, cooked, or fresh, until the condition improves.

All animal food is to be avoided, including fish and seafood. However, in the event that cravings arise for animal food, dried small fish such as iriko or a small portion of nonfatty white-meat fish, served together with grated daikon and/or grated ginger, may be consumed occasionally. The fish may be moderately seasoned with sea salt, tamari soy sauce, or miso. It may also be cooked together with two to three times more vegetables.

All nuts and nut butters are to be avoided, though roasted sesame, sunflower, and pumpkin seeds may be consumed as a snack.

In the event cravings arise for sweets, autumn squash or other sweet vegetables can be served more frequently. If the desire for sweets persists, a small amount of a grain-based natural sweetener such as barley malt or rice syrup may be used on occasion.

A small volume of condiments such as umeboshi plum and gomashio can be consumed daily. The gomashio can be made with one part roasted sea salt to twelve to sixteen parts roasted unhulled sesame seeds that are mixed together in a suribachi until half crushed. Other regular condiments may also be used in small volume.

Buckwheat noodles or buckwheat paté, made with buckwheat flour cooked with chopped scallions, is helpful for upper digestive cancers if consumed two to three times per week.

A cup of kuzu drink can be helpful if drunk daily for a one- to two-week period and occasionally thereafter. This is made by dissolving a teaspoon of kuzu (kudzu) powder in two teaspoons of water, adding one cup of spring water, and bringing to a boil with one umeboshi plum, slices of garlic and/or grated ginger, and tamari soy sauce to taste.

One teaspoon of miso sautéed with sesame oil together with the same volume of scallions and a small volume of grated ginger or garlic added while cooking may be used as a condiment for the meal.

Chewing thoroughly is essential for all types of cancer, but especially for cancers in the mouth and upper alimentary tract. Liquefying and mixing food well with saliva contributes to the prevention and improvement of this condition. Also it is important to avoid overconsumption of liquid, though bancha tea or water should be consumed if thirst arises.

As explained in the introduction to Part II, cancer patients who have received or who are currently undergoing medical treatment may need to make further dietary modifications.

HOME CARES

• For throat and esophageal cancers, a taro potato plaster can be applied to the area daily for three to four hours, immediately following a ginger compress for about ten minutes. In some cases, a taro plaster causes mucus and fat to gather too rapidly for comfort, in which event a lotus root plaster can be applied to slow the discharge. This is made by mixing an equal volume of grated fresh lotus root and grated taro potato with a small amount of white flour to hold them together, and mixing with 5 to 10 percent grated fresh ginger. The lotus plaster may be applied for a few hours daily over a few weeks period.

• Scrubbing the whole body with a hot ginger towel is very helpful for promoting circulation of blood and energy. This includes the front chest, throat, neck, and lower jaws.

• In the event that the esophagus is blocked by a tumorous obstruction and the person is unable to eat, or if the tumor has been removed and a tube has been inserted from the nose, the diet should be liquefied by cooking with more water and by mashing food substances. Rice cream is also helpful and may be consumed with miso soup as well as other mashed and liquefied vegetables, beans, and sea vegetables.

OTHER CONSIDERATIONS

• Avoid synthetic clothing, especially around the area of the throat, neck, head, and chest and use cotton underwear, clothing, and sleepwear if possible.

• Avoid exposure to artificial electromagnetic radiation in the upper body from such sources as television, video terminals, electric shavers and hair dryers, and other hand-held electrical devices.

PERSONAL EXPERIENCE

Granular Myoblastoma on the Vocal Cord

In the spring of 1979, Laura Anne Fitzpatrick discovered that her voice had become raspy when she tried out for cheerleader at her high school in Sherborn, Massachusetts. Doctors told her that she had a benign tumor on the vocal cords known as a granular myoblastoma, and in August she had it surgically removed. By January 1980, however, the tumor had reappeared, and Laura underwent a second operation, this time with advanced laser-beam surgery, at University Hospital in Boston. A month later the swelling returned, and doctors feared yet another recurrence of the obstruction.

During this period, Laura and her family saw a television program on macrobiotics. After attending a seminar on cancer and diet at the East West Foundation, Laura came to see me for a consultation, and I recommended the Cancer-Prevention Diet. I warned her to completely avoid oil in cooking and advised her to go to bed with a taro plaster wrapped around her neck. Laura's family, including her parents and two sisters and three brothers still living at home, were very supportive and started the macrobiotic way of eating as well. "John and I both wanted to support Laura, and we also began to eat in this new way as much as we could," her mother later noted. "We changed our stove from electric to gas, and the adventures continued as we truly tried to understand the principles behind the diet."

Laura experienced many changes in her body as the toxins from many previous years of imbalanced eating were rapidly released. She began to feel more energy and her voice started improving. In the spring of 1980, she returned for a medical checkup, and her doctor was surprised to find that the operation was unnecessary. Laura continued to improve through the fall. However, in November, she began to deviate from the diet and use oil in cooking. On Thanksgiving she had turkey. By Christmas, her symptoms started to return and her voice grew weak. The doctors told her the tumor had returned and would have to be removed.

Laura and her family asked the hospital for a two-month reprieve from surgery and returned to see me. "[Michio] scolded me humorously," Laura recalled of that visit, "and I decided I was ready to get back to basics and resume the diet he had recommended. . . . I again began to discharge a lot of mucus and felt a tremendous cleansing coming very rapidly. I resumed the taro potato compresses each night. One humorous sidelight of this was that my father's T-shirts were disappearing, and he would find them with mysterious brown spots from the remains of the taro potato. I found that whenever I missed the ginger and taro potato plaster compress for a few days, the mucus would not discharge as freely. I prepared all the compresses by myself and the routine became normal."

At the college she was now attending, Laura found it difficult to get the proper food and care she needed. But with the help of her family she succeeded. In March 1981, she returned for a medical checkup, and her doctor told her the condition had improved and stabilized and there was no need for surgery. "I learned from this experience that the diet makes sense," Laura concluded. "I feel I am well on my way to a full and complete recovery." Source: "Granular Myoblastoma on the Vocal Cord," *The Cancer Prevention Diet* (Brookline, Mass.: East West Foundation, 1981, pp. 87–89).

25.

Urinary Cancer: Bladder and Kidney

FREQUENCY

Cancers of the kidney, bladder, and other parts of the urinary tract will claim an estimated 19,200 American lives in 1983, and in the same year 56,700 cases will develop. About one third of all urinary cancers occur in the kidney and two thirds in the bladder, ureters, and urethra. Kidney cancer occurs about evenly in men and women and is found among both adults and children. Bladder cancer is much more prevalent in men, especially those in the fifty-five to seventy-five age group.

Standard medical treatment calls for surgical removal of the afflicted kidney along with adjacent lymph nodes and adrenal glands in an operation called a radical nephrectomy. In a rarer form of kidney cancer known as renal pelvis carcinoma, the ureter will be removed along with the kidney in a procedure called a nephroureterectomy. A person can survive with only one kidney. If both kidneys are removed, a kidney transplant may be performed or kidney dialysis instituted. A kidney dialysis machine performs the functions of the kidneys by filtering fluids through tubes imbedded in the patient's arms. The patient must undergo this treatment two or three times a week for three or four hours' duration each time. Radiation therapy is sometimes used prior to kidney surgery to shrink a tumor. The five-year survival rate for kidney cancer is a little above 40 percent.

In the case of bladder cancer, superficial tumors are generally removed by burning or cutting with the use of a cystoscope, a flexible tube inserted through the urethra, or an abdominal incision. Total removal of the bladder, in advanced cases, is called a cystectomy. In men the prostate is often malignant and is removed as well. An artificial bladder is then constructed, usually with a section of the small intestine, and connected to a disposable bag on the outside of the body for the elimination of urine. Radiation in the form of external voltage or internally implanted radioactive seeds is also sometimes employed before bladder surgery in order to destroy invasive tumors. Chemotherapy is not used as a primary treatment for urinary cancers, but may be used to control pain following surgery. Sixty-two percent of bladder-cancer patients treated by these methods live five years or more.

STRUCTURE

The two kidneys are bean-shaped organs located in the upper part of the abdominal cavity near the spinal column. The main tasks of the kidneys are to filter impurities from the blood and to discharge excess fluid from the body in the form of urine. About a quart of blood passes through the kidneys every minute, and these organs serve to regulate the amount of salt, water, and other constituents of the bloodstream. Urine is formed in the kidney by filtration of urea and other wastes from the blood vessels and the absorption and excretion of other substances from the filtrate.

In general, urine is amber in color, forms a mildly acidic reaction, has a slight odor, and a salty taste. The quantity of urine discharged varies with the amount of fluids consumed, but usually amounts to between 1,000 and 1,500 cubic centimeters a day. The quantity of solids in the urine changes with the diet and is significantly higher following consumption of foods higher in fat and protein. People eating the modern diet excrete about forty to seventy-five grams of solid waste daily in their urine, of which 25 percent is urea, 25 percent chlorides, 25 percent sulfate and phosphates, and the rest organic acids, pigments, hormones, and so on. In unhealthy urine, high levels of albumin, sugar, blood, pus, acetone, fat, chyle, cellular material, and bacteria may be present.

The adrenal glands, attached to the upper part of the kidneys, are part of the endocrine system. They secrete hormones, including adrenalin, regulating mental and emotional stress. The ureters are long, narrow tubes that convey the urine from each kidney to the bladder by muscular action. The bladder is a hollow Y-shaped organ situated in the pelvis, which serves as a reservoir for urine. It can hold about one pint. The urethra is the canal through which the urine is discharged from the body. The urethra extends from the neck of the bladder to the genital region. In men, the urethra is divided into the prostatic portion and the penile portion. In women, the urinary system is largely separated from the reproductive system.

CAUSE OF CANCER

Kidney disorders may be divided into two groups. 1) Overly contracted, tight, and inflexible (yang) kidney conditions result in the restriction of blood flow and urination; and 2) Loose or swollen (yin) kidney conditions prevent complete filtration of the blood and can lead to excessive retention or elimination of liquids. Preliminary signs of contracted and hardening kidneys are tossing and turning during sleep, insomnia, nightmares, and rising early in the morning. Tight kidneys are caused by overconsumption of extreme yang foods such as eggs, meat, other animal products, dry baked goods, commercial salt, as well as overactivity and a pressure-filled environment. Initial symptoms of overly expanded kidneys are snoring, groaning, bedwetting, lower back pain, getting up to urinate at night, and getting up late in the morning. This yin condition may be caused by a high intake of beverages (especially milk, fruit juices, and coffee) as well as foods of tropical origin, fruit, sugar, and sweets. A sedentary lifestyle contributes to weak, sluggish kidneys.

Over time, excessive consumption of a combination of extreme yin and yang foodstuffs and beverages can lead to the formation of stones, cysts, or tumors in the urinary tract. These obstructions develop when an excess of solid wastes cannot pass through the fine network of cells in the interior of the kidneys, the ureters, or the bladder. The kidneys are a frequent site of mucus and fatty-acid accumulation. In this condition, the kidneys often retain water and become chronically swollen. Since the process of elimination is impaired, excess fluid is often deposited in the legs, producing periodic swelling and weakness. At the same time, excessive perspiration will also usually develop. If someone with this swollen condition continues to consume large amounts of expansive foods, the deposited fat and mucus will crystallize into kidney stones. Stones are principally caused by long-term eating of high-fat foods combined with chilled or frozen foods, particularly ice cream, sherbet, yogurt, orange juice, soft drinks, ice water, and other beverages that make the body cold.

Over a long period of time, cysts and stones will culminate in the formation of tumors as the kidney fights back in self-defense to restrict the flow of excess waters and irritating fluids through its system. In the case of bladder cancer, excessive toxins and other irritants in the urine, especially from processed foods and chemicalized water, can ultimately give rise to cancer. Kidney cancer, affecting the more tight, compact part of the urinary system, is a relatively more yang form of cancer. Bladder cancer, affecting the expanded, hollow portion of the urinary system, is relatively more yin. To restore balance, a slightly more yin macrobiotic diet is recommended for kidney cancer, a more yang diet in the case of bladder cancer.

MEDICAL EVIDENCE

• In his essay on health and diet, poet Percy B. Shelley discussed a cure for cancer and other maladies. "There is no disease, bodily or mental, which adoption of vegetable diet and pure water has not infallibly mitigated wherever the experiment has been fairly tried." Percy B. Shelley, *A Vindication of Natural Diet* (London, 1812).

• In 1881 New York physician Thomas Low Nichols, M.D. wrote a book on relieving degenerative diseases with natural food. Describing the mechanism by which the internal organs cleansed the body of impurities, he wrote:

The effort to free the body from too great a quantity of food, or some irritating quality it contains, produces fevers. Coarse and fatty animal food disturbs the liver and kidneys. The skin cannot throw off the superfluous matter. . . . The impure blood made of unnatural and often diseased food, produces scurvy, scrofula, tubercular disease, consumption, leprosy, cancer. In a word there is not one of the diseases that afflict and destroy humanity, which may not be produced by an unnatural diet. . . . I have no doubt about the natural food of man. Fruit, and seeds, and nuts, which are but larger seeds, contain all that man requires. Millions of men live almost entirely on rice, millions live on oatmeal, or barley, or rye; millions on maize, on wheat. . . ." Source: Thomas L. Nichols, M.D., *Eating to Live: The Diet Cure* (New York: M.L. Holbrook and Co., p. 11, 1881).

• Looking back over four decades of medical work in French Equatorial Africa, Dr. Albert Schweitzer reported that he had never had any cancer cases in his hospital and that its occurrence among the African people was very rare. He attributed the rise of degenerative diseases to the importation of European foods including condensed milk, canned butter, meat and fish preserves, white bread, and especially refined salt. "It is obvious to connect the fact of increase of cancer with the increased use of salt by the natives. In former years there was only available the little salt extracted from the ocean. . . . So it is possible that the formerly very seldom and still infrequent occurrence of cancer in this country is connected with the former very little consumption of salt and the still rare use of it." Source: Albert Schweitzer, M.D., *Briefe aus dem Lambarenespital*, 1954.

• In 1948 laboratory tests first linked saccharin, an artificial sweetener used in diet colas, toothpaste, cosmetics, and animal feed, with bladder cancer and cancer of the reproductive organs. A controversial 1977 study, published in a British medical journal, observed that men who used saccharin regularly faced a 60 percent greater risk of bladder cancer. However, other studies showed no significant relationship. Sources: G.R. Howe et al., "Artificial Sweeteners and Human Bladder Cancer," *Lancet* 2:578–81 and *Diet, Nutrition, and Cancer* (Washington, D.C.: National Academy of Sciences, 14:1–5, 1982).

• A 1971 study reported that women who drank coffee regularly had about 2.5 times higher risk of developing urinary cancer than non-users. The relative risk for men was 24 percent. The test controlled for cigarette smoking and high-risk occupational exposure to chemicals known to affect the bladder and kidneys. Source: P. Cole, "Coffee-Drinking and Cancer of the Lower Urinary Tract," *Lancet* 1:1335–37.

• Bottled spring water can reduce the risk of cancer, according to an Illinois experiment. Mice on a high-protein, high-sugar diet were divided into two groups. One group received bottled spring water and the control group received Chicago tap water. The mice on spring water lived 20 percent longer. Source: Dr. Hans Kugler, *Slowing the Aging Process* (New York: Pyramid, 1973).

• A 1975 epidemiological study reported that Seventh-Day Adventists in California have 72 percent less bladder cancer than the general population. The church members avoid meat, poultry, fish, rich and refined food, coffee, tea, hot condiments, alcohol, and spices and eat proportionately more whole grains, vegetables, fresh fruit, and nuts. Source: R.L. Phillips, "Role of Life-Styles and Dietary Habits in Risk of Cancer among Seventh-Day Adventists," *Cancer Research* 35:3513–22.

• A 1975 epidemiological study found a direct association of bladder-cancer deaths with per capita intake of fats and oil, especially in women. The scientists also linked kidney cancer with higher intake of meat, milk, total animal protein, and coffee. Source: B. Armstrong and R. Doll, "Environmental Factors and Cancer Incidence and Mortality in Different Countries, with Special Reference to Dietary Practices," *International Journal of Cancer* 15:617–31.

• A New York study found that women in seven counties with chlorinated municipal drinking water ran a 44 percent greater chance of dying from cancer of the urinary or gastrointestinal tract than women whose water was unchlorinated. Source: *Washington Post*, May 3, 1977, p. A3.

• A 1979 case-control study reported an inverse association with consumption of foods high in vitamin A and bladder cancer. Source: C. Mettlin and S. Graham, "Vitamin A and Lung Cancer," *Journal of the National Cancer Institute* 62:1435–38.

DIAGNOSIS

When kidney cancer is suspected, modern medicine offers the following diagnostic methods: laboratory tests including urinalysis; x-rays; an intravenous pyelogram (IVP) to locate tumors; ultrasound examination of the abdomen; a renal angiogram to determine the location and extent of tumor growth; a tomogram of the kidney to distinguish between a cyst and a tumor; and a CAT scan of the pelvis and upper abdomen. Sometimes a needle aspiration biopsy is performed, but this procedure has been implicated in spreading cancer along the path of the needle and is increasingly avoided. Many kidneys are nearly completely damaged before being diagnosed as cancerous, and one third of patients have metastases to other locations. In the case of bladder cancer, diagnostic procedures include lab tests, IVP, cystoscopy, cystogram, bone scan, liver scan, ultrasound, lymphangiogram, and a cystourethrogram in which the bladder and urethra are observed during urination. About 82 percent of bladder cancers are diagnosed in local stages before spreading to regional areas or other organs. In men, bladder surgery can result in impotence.

Traditional visual diagnostic techniques do not rely on potentially harmful x-rays or mechanical invasions of the body. Simple visual methods allow the kidneys to be monitored long before the onset of serious illness and permit corrective dietary adjustments to be made. These nutritional measures will safeguard against the development of kidney troubles in healthy individuals and offset any tendency toward urinary cancer in those who already are sick.

In physiognomy, the area under the eyes corresponds to the kidneys. Darkness or black coloring of the skin in this region signifies kidney stagnation and toxic blood due to kidney malfunction. During adulthood, but increasingly even during youth in modern society, many people develop eyebags under the lower eyelid. Eyebags may have one of two causes, though the appearance may be similar: 1) eyebags due to a pool of liquid and 2) eyebags due to pooled mucus. The first type of eyebag appears watery and swollen. Both types of eyebags show disorders of the kidney, bladder, and excretory functions. The first type, due to excess liquid, indicates swelling of the kidney tissues and frequent urination. Excessive intake of any kind of liquid, including all kinds of beverages, fruits, and juices, may cause this condition. The second type of eyebag does not necessarily accompany frequent urination but shows mucus and fat accumulation in the kidney tissue. If small pimples or dark spots appear on these mucus-caused eyebags, accumulated mucus and fat in the kidney tissues may be forming kidney stones. If these eyebags are chronic, mucus accumulation is developing in the ureter, the wall of the bladder, and the reproductive organs (ovaries, Fallopian tubes, and uterus in women and prostate gland in men), creating bacterial activity, inflammation, itching, vaginal discharge, ovarian cysts, and eventually the growth of tumors and cancers in these areas.

Both types of eyebags also indicate the decline of physical and mental vitality as a natural result of the above conditions. Overloaded body systems, fatigue, laziness, forgetfulness, indecisiveness, and loss of clear judgment are developing. The water-caused eyebag is easily corrected by the restriction of liquid intake, while the mucus-caused eyebag can be corrected by the restriction of all mucus- and fat-forming food, including dairy products, meat, poultry, sugar, refined flour, and all sorts of oil. This type of eyebag takes longer than the watery eyebag to clear up. In visual diagnosis, the right eye and its surrounding area corresponds to the right kidney, the left eye to the left kidney. Relative darkness, swelling, tightness, or other markings indicate which kidney is more affected.

The ears, which are shaped like kidneys, also mirror the internal condition of the urinary tract and should be checked carefully. Redness around the edge of the ear indicates an overly yin condition of the kidneys caused by excessive consumption of sugar, dairy food, fruit, and juices. Overconsumption of oil, fat, and other strong yin items will also overburden the kidneys and show up in ears that are oily to the touch. Moles or warts on the ears show deposits of mucus in the kidneys caused by an accumulation of animal protein. The left ear shows the left kidney, the right ear, the right kidney, and the location of these abnormalities indicates precisely where troubles in the kidneys are occurring. Bumps or pimples on the ears show deposits of fat and developing kidney stones. Deafness is often connected with buildup of fat in the kidney. Excessive wax in the ears indicates fatty deposits in the ureter.

The kidneys can be aggravated by too much fluid consumption, and this shows up in generally wet or damp hands and feet. Kidney disorders, including cancer, are indicated by pain or hardness on the initial point of the kidney meridian at the bottom of the foot. Calluses here represent an effort on the part of the kidneys to discharge excess mucus, protein, and fat through the meridian or energy channel in the foot. Flour products, fats and oils, and sugar and sweets especially give rise to this condition.

Urine itself can be inspected for general clues to the condition of the kidneys and bladder. Urine that is healthy is light gold or yellow in color. Too much salt will turn the urine darker, and too little salt or too yin a diet will result in urine that is much lighter in color. If too much fluid is consumed, urination will become very frequent. Normally, we should urinate about three or four times a day. More than this indicates that too much fluid is being consumed, while less means that not enough is being consumed.

The upper part of the forehead corresponds with the bladder, and lines or ridges in this area indicate troubles in this organ.

Posture is a further clue to kidney condition. Leaning forward while sitting, standing, or walking indicates overly contracted kidneys. This yang condition may also be shown by a stiff back, walking brusquely, or running, or wearing shoes with elevated heels. On the other hand, leaning backward, leaning against things, or slouching as well as wearing shoes with elevated toes are all signs of overly expanded (yin) kidneys.

DIETARY RECOMMENDATIONS

Cancer of the kidney is caused mainly by overconsumption of dairy food and animal food rich in saturated fats, together with sugar, chemicals, and artificial beverages. Cancer of the bladder is largely caused by dairy foods, sugar products, chemicals, stimulants, fruits, juices, and food that produces fat and mucus. All these foods are to be avoided. Overconsumption of salt tends to solidify the mass of cancer cells and therefore moderate use of natural, unrefined sea salt is advisable. Refined table salt should be avoided. All oily and greasy food as well as all refined flour products, including bread, pancakes, and cookies, are to be avoided. Food and beverages that lower the body temperature, including fruits, icy drinks, and artificial beverages, are to be discontinued. For improvement of urinary cancer, eating baked flour products is not advisable. All spices including mustard, peppers, curry, and any fragrant, aromatic condiments and supplements are to be avoided.

Following are the general dietary guidelines, by daily volume, for urinary cancer, including cancer of the kidney and bladder:

• Fifty to sixty percent whole-cereal grains, especially pressure-cooked brown rice and barley, with occasional use of oats, millet, and other grains. It is advisable to minimize corn, though occasional use of buckwheat groats is helpful. In the event that bread is craved, unrefined whole-wheat or rye bread made without yeast may be consumed two to three times a week. Beans such as azuki beans or lentils may be cooked together with cereal grains and consumed two to three times a week. Whole-flour pasta such as whole-wheat noodles and buckwheat noodles may be used two to three times per week with tamari or miso broth in which sea vegetables and land vegetables are cooked.

• Five to ten percent soup. Miso soup cooked with sea vegetables such as wakame or kombu and with root and hard, leafy vegetables can be consumed daily, one to two bowls. Grain as well as beans may be added to soups occasionally.

• Twenty to thirty percent vegetables cooked in various styles. Fresh raw salad should be avoided, except for a small volume of homemade pickles and salad that is boiled in water one to two minutes. Among vegetables, root vegetables such as carrots, daikon, and burdock roots should be consumed daily, in moderate volume, though hard, leafy vegetables are also to be eaten. The use of oil in large volume for sautéing and frying should be avoided, though a moderate volume may be used occasionally in cooking.

• Five to ten percent beans and bean products. Azuki and other small beans such as lentils are recommended for frequent use in small volume, cooked with kombu and other sea vegetables or with onions, carrots, and hard autumn squash. Cooked tempeh, natto, and tofu may be used in moderate volume. Beans can be cooked with cereal grains also.

• Five percent or less sea vegetables. All edible cooked sea vegetables are recommended for frequent use in small volume, especially arame and hijiki for the kidneys and nori for the bladder. The sea vegetables may be used in soup, in vegetable dishes, or in bean dishes, as well as for an independent side dish.

All animal food including fish and seafood should be limited. However, carp soup (koi koku) cooked with burdock and seasoned with miso and a little ginger may be consumed, if craved.

All fruits, juices, and fruit desserts are to be avoided, though a small volume of cooked fruits such as cooked apples, peaches, strawberries, and other berries may be consumed, if craved. Natural sweeteners are to be used sparingly, if at all. Fall-season squash, cabbages, and other sweet vegetables can be used daily in various cooking styles to help satisfy the desire for a sweet taste.

All nuts and nut butters are to be avoided, though roasted seeds such as sunflower, sesame, and pumpkin may be used occasionally.

The use of regular macrobiotic seasonings and condiments is to be moderate. Be especially careful of salt consumption, which should be light on most dishes. To help relieve urinary cancer, special dishes may be necessary. For example, brown rice cooked with kombu (five percent or so by volume) can often be served as the main grain dish of the meal. Rice juice, which arises to the surface while cooking brown rice, can be used daily or frequently as a beverage.

A special dish of sliced burdock roots and carrots, sautéed together with sesame oil and seasoned with miso or tamari soy sauce, can help to improve kidney and bladder functions if consumed frequently in small volume.

Beverages are to be all warm or hot. Cold beverages are to be avoided. All liquid intake should be limited to actual thirst.

Chewing food thoroughly and even mixing beverages in the

mouth with saliva is an essential factor in restoring health. All other dietary practices can follow the general recommendations for cancer patients.

As explained in the introduction to Part II, cancer patients who have received or who are currently undergoing medical treatment may need to make further dietary modifications.

HOME CARES

• One or two cups of azuki bean juice cooked with a little sea salt or a piece of kombu may also be used often to help kidney functions and restore smooth urination.

• A plaster combining an equal volume of grated fresh lotus root and taro potato (mixed with a little white flour for consistency and 5 to 10 percent grated ginger) applied from the back on the area of the kidneys for three to four hours is helpful for kidney cancer if used daily for two to three weeks. This should be preceded by a ginger compress for five to ten minutes.

• A ginger compress applied for ten to fifteen minutes once a day on the abdomen helps reduce blockage of the urethra. This compress should be repeated for several days.

• Drinking one or two cups of hot water in which two tablespoons of grated daikon (or red radish), one roasted crushed nori sheet, and one-half teaspoon of grated ginger (seasoned with one teaspoon of tamari sauce) have boiled for three to five minutes is helpful for stimulating the bladder and proper urinary passage.

• Massage, acupuncture, or moxibustion (burning an herb on the skin) can help to relieve pain. A ginger compress on the painful area for ten to fifteen minutes can also help, together with the use of all the above home cares.

• A daily hot bath or shower should be quick and not frequent (i.e., not two to three times a day). In the event that fatigue is experienced after washing, one cup of ume-sho-kuzu can help to restore vitality. This is a drink cooked with kuzu, one umeboshi plum, and seasoned with tamari soy sauce.

• Scrubbing the whole body daily, including the areas of the kidneys, urethra, and bladder, with a hot towel soaked in gingerroot water is helpful for activating circulation of the blood and general metabolism.

OTHER CONSIDERATIONS

• Psychologically, keeping a positive mind and a strong will are important. Also, any comfortably manageable exercises, including walking outdoors, contributes to improvement. Visualization, prayer, meditation, and other spiritual practices, performed daily, will also be beneficial.
• The kidneys and bladder are particularly susceptible to cold weather and chills. Keep these organs protected and warm at all times, especially during the winter. In the Far East, a cotton band is commonly worn around the abdomen and back to keep these organs warm.
• Avoid wearing synthetic clothing next to the area affected and replace with cotton as soon as possible.

PERSONAL EXPERIENCE

Cancer with Terminal Kidney Condition

In 1968 Terry Klemens, a twenty-year-old living in Chicago, became a vegetarian. He had grown up on the standard American diet high in meat and animal products. For four years he ate a meatless diet high in milk and other dairy food. During the fifth year he became a fruitarian and lived primarily on fruit, juices, and raw foods. In March 1973, Klemens moved to a mountain retreat in southern Arizona and switched to a diet of grains and vegetables. During the cold weather in this new location, he became seriously ill, with pains in the back and on both sides of the lower abdomen. At a local clinic, a medical doctor took x-rays and told Klemens that his kidneys were pulled down, a condition similar to floating kidneys. He was also diagnosed as having stomach ulcers and cancer of the colon. "As he put it, I was 'a mess,'" Klemens later reported. "He said the kidney condition would eventually prove fatal, and he gave me one year to live."

Klemens returned home with several medications to reduce the pain. But he could not accept his fate and determined to practice macrobiotics, which he had just adopted, correctly. "I started reading *Zen Macrobiotics* again," he explained. "After reading it another four times, I started to understand what I had been doing wrong: 1) I wasn't chewing my food properly. 2) I wasn't taking enough vegetables. 3) I was taking too much liquid. 4) I was using honey. 5) I was using marijuana. 6) I was taking an excess of fruit and fruit juice."

Klemens stopped these excesses and in a few days felt much better. Within two weeks he felt on the way to recovery. Klemens continued macrobiotics over the next five years. When he wrote his case history, he asserted that he had been in good health ever since. Source: "Floating Kidneys," *Macrobiotic Case Histories*, No. 5 (Boston: East West Foundation, 1978, p. 24).

PART III

Recipes and Menus

26.

General Dietary Recommendations

The following dietary guidelines are a summary of material presented in Part I, Chapter 5. They are intended for use by reasonably healthy individuals or families. Modifications for patients with cancer are discussed in the individual chapters in Part II and summarized in the following chapter. Persons with sicknesses other than cancer may safely follow these standard guidelines for grains, soup, vegetables, beans, sea vegetables, and beverages. However, they should minimize or avoid animal food, fruit, salad, and sweets until they have consulted an experienced macrobiotic counselor or medical professional for proper evaluation of their condition and dietary recommendations suited to their unique case. Chapter 28, "Making a Smooth Tradition," should also be read carefully to help implement these guidelines. In the lists of foods that follow, *regular* use means daily or every other day, *occasional* means once or twice a week, and *avoid* means refrain completely or limit. The lists of items are for temperate climates and do not include many lesser known and regional varieties.

WHOLE-CEREAL GRAINS

The principal food of each meal is whole grain, comprising from 50 to 60 percent of the total volume of the meal. Cooked whole grains are preferable to flour products. Whole-cereal grain and whole-grain products include:

Regular Use

Short-grain brown rice	Whole oats
Medium-grain brown rice	Wheat berries
Millet	Rye
Barley	Buckwheat
Corn	Other cereal grains

Occasional Use

Sweet brown rice	Rice kayu (porridge) bread
Mochi (pounded sweet rice)	Rice cakes
Long-grain brown rice	Whole-wheat crackers
Udon (whole-wheat noodles)	Whole-wheat matzo
Soba (buckwheat noodles)	Cracked wheat, bulgur
Somen (fine whole-wheat noodles)	Steel-cut oats, rolled oats
Whole-wheat spaghetti noodles	Corn grits, corn meal
Whole-wheat pasta such as elbows, spirals, flat noodles, lasagna, etc.	Rye flakes
	Couscous
	Seitan (wheat gluten)
Unleavened whole-wheat or rye bread	Fu (puffed wheat gluten)

SOUPS

One or two bowls of miso, tamari broth, or soup seasoned with sea salt is recommended every day (approximately 5 percent of daily intake). Prepare soups with a variety of ingredients, including sea vegetables, seasonal vegetables, grains, and beans. Occasionally soups may include small pieces of white-meat fish or seafood.

VEGETABLES

About one quarter (25 to 30 percent) of each meal includes fresh vegetables prepared in a variety of ways, including steaming, boiling, baking, or sautéing (with a small amount of unrefined sesame or corn oil). In general, up to one third of vegetables may be eaten in the form of pickles or salad. In selecting vegetables, observe these guidelines:

Regular Use: Green and White Leafy Vegetables

Broccoli	Daikon greens
Bok choy	Dandelion greens
Brussels sprouts	Kale
Cabbage (green)	Leeks
Carrot tops	Mustard greens
Cauliflower	Parsley
Chinese cabbage	Scallion
Chives	Turnip greens
Collard greens	Watercress

Regular Use: Ground Vegetables

Acorn squash	Hubbard squash
Buttercup squash	Hokkaido pumpkin
Butternut squash	Pumpkin

Regular Use: Stem/Root Vegetables

Burdock	Parsnip
Carrots	Radish
Daikon	Rutabaga
Dandelion root	Salsify
Lotus root	Turnip
Onion	

Vegetables for Occasional Use

Bamboo Shoots	Mushrooms
Beets	Patty pan squash
Celery	Red cabbage
Cucumber	Romaine lettuce
Endive	Shiitake mushrooms
Escarole	Snap beans
Green peas	Snow peas
Iceberg lettuce	Sprouts
Jerusalem artichoke	String beans
Jinenjo (mountain potato)	Summer squash
Kohlrabi	Swiss chard

Vegetables to Avoid or Limit

Asparagus	Purslane
Avocado	Shepherd's purse
Curly dock	Sorrel
Eggplant	Spinach
Fennel	Sweet potato
Ferns	Taro (albi)
Green and red peppers	Tomato
Plantain	Yams
Potato	Zucchini

BEANS

A small portion (about 10 percent) of daily intake includes cooked beans or bean products. The most suitable include:

Regular Use

Azuki beans	Chickpeas	Lentils (green)

Occasional Use

Black-eyed peas	Lentils (red)
Black soy beans	Navy beans
Black turtle beans	Pinto beans
Great northern beans	Soybeans
Kidney beans	Split peas
Lima beans	Whole dried peas

Regular Use: Bean Products

Tofu (bean curd)	Tempeh (soy meat)	Natto (fermented soybeans)

SEA VEGETABLES

These important foods are served in small quantities and comprise about 5 percent of daily intake.

Regular Use

Agar-agar	Kelp
Arame	Kombu
Dulse	Nori
Hiziki	Wakame
Irish moss	

FISH

For those in good health, once or twice a week, a small amount of white-meat fish or seafood may be eaten.

Occasional Use

Carp	Iriko (small dried fish)
Cod	Little necks
Chirimen iriko (tiny dried fish)	Oysters
Clams	Red snapper
Eel	Scallops
Flounder	Shrimp
Haddock	Smelt
Halibut	Sole
Herring	Trout

Avoid

Red meat or blueskinned fish such as salmon, sword fish, blue fish, etc. (raw-meat tuna may be served occasionally with tamari soy sauce and a garnish of grated daikon or mustard).

NUTS AND SEEDS

A small volume of roasted seeds or nuts, lightly salted with sea salt or seasoned with tamari soy sauce, may be enjoyed as snacks. It is preferable to minimize the use of nuts and nut butters as they are difficult to digest and high in fats.

Occasional Use

Sesame seeds	Filberts
Sunflower seeds	Peanuts
Pumpkin seeds	Pecans
Chestnuts	Spanish peanuts
Almonds	Walnuts

Avoid: Tropical Nuts

Brazil	Pistachio
Cashew	Hazel

DESSERTS AND FRUIT

Desserts may be enjoyed two or three times a week and are best when sweetened with a high-quality sweetener, especially any made from grain such as rice syrup, barley malt, amasake, and mirin. Fresh fruit and dried fruit may be eaten on occasion by those in good health. Fruit juice is not recommended as a regular beverage. Many desserts can be made with naturally sweet vegetables, including cabbage, carrots, daikon, onions, parsnips, pumpkins, and squash.

Occasional Use: Sweeteners

Rice syrup (yinnie syrup)	Chestnuts
Barley malt	Apple juice or cider
Amasake	Dried raisins
Mirin	Dried temperate-climate fruit

Avoid: Refined Sugars

Sugar (white, raw, brown, turbinado)	Fructose
	Chocolate
Molasses	Carob
Corn syrup	Honey
Saccharine and other artificial sweeteners	Maple syrup

Occasional Use: Temperate-Climate Fruit

Apples	Honeydew melon
Apricots	Peaches
Blackberries	Pears
Blueberries	Plums
Cantaloupe	Prunes
Cherries	Raspberries
Cranberries	Strawberries
Currants	Tangerines
Grapes	Watermelon

Avoid: Tropical Fruits and Juices

Bananas	Limes	Figs
Grapefruit	Mangoes	Coconut
Oranges	Papayas	Kiwi
Lemons	Dates	

BEVERAGES

Spring or well water may be used for teas and drinks.

Regular Use

Bancha twig tea (Kukicha)	Spring or well water
Bancha stem tea	Other grain-based teas or
Roasted rice tea	traditional, nonstimulant herb
Roasted barley tea	tea
Boiled water	

Occasional Use

Grain coffee	Umeboshi tea
Dandelion tea	Mu tea
Kombu tea	Other traditional, nonaromatic
	root and herb teas

Less Frequently

Nachi green tea	Beer
Green magma	Sake
Soy milk	Other grain, bean, and herb
Vegetable juice	beverages
Fruit juice (temperate climate)	

Avoid

Coffee	Soda, cola, artificial beverages
Decaffeinated coffee	Alcohol
Black tea	Chemicalized or distilled water
Stimulating aromatic teas (mint, rose hips, etc.)	

CONDIMENTS

The following condiments are recommended for daily or special use:

Tamari soy sauce	Shio kombu
Gomashio (sesame salt)	Nori condiment
Roasted sea vegetable powder	Tekka
Umeboshi plum	

PICKLES (types)

Regular Use

Bran	Sauerkraut
Brine	Takuan
Miso	Tamari
Miso-Bran	Umeboshi
Pressed	

Avoid

Dill	Spices
Garlic	Vinegar (apple, wine, etc.)
Herbs	

COOKING OIL

For cooking oil, we recommend that only naturally processed, high quality, cold-pressed, unrefined vegetable oil be used. Oil should be used in moderation for fried rice, fried noodles, and sautéing vegetables. Generally, two to three times a week is reasonable. Occasionally, oil may be used for deep frying grains, vegetables, fish, and seafood.

Regular Use

Sesame oil	Corn oil
Dark sesame oil	Mustard seed oil

Occasional Use

Safflower oil	Peanut oil
Sunflower oil	Cottonseed oil
Soybean oil	Other traditional vegetable oils
Olive oil	

Avoid

Butter or margarine
Lard, shortening, or all animal fats
Refined, chemically processed vegetable oils
Soy margarine

SEASONINGS

Naturally processed, unrefined sea salt is preferable to refined table salt. However, heavy gray crude sea salt is not suitable. Miso and tamari soy sauce (both containing sea salt) may also be used as seasonings. Use only naturally processed, nonchemicalized varieties. In general, seasonings are used moderately.

Regular Use

Miso	Rice or other grain vinegar
Tamari soy sauce (shoyu)	Umeboshi vinegar
Tamari	White or light gray
Umeboshi plum or paste	unrefined sea salt

Occasional Use

Vegetable oil	Rice syrup
Sauerkraut vinegar	Barley malt
Ginger	Green mustard
Horseradish	Other traditional, naturally
Mirin	processed seasonings

Avoid

Herbs	All unnatural, artificial, or
Spices (cayenne, cumin, etc.)	chemically processed
Iodized salt	seasonings
Wine- or apple-cider vinegar	Mayonnaise
Ginseng	Soy margarine

FOODS TO AVOID FOR BETTER HEALTH

In addition to some of the items noted above, the following foods should be reduced or avoided.

Animal Products

Red meat (beef, lamb, pork)	Poultry
Cured meat (ham, bacon,	Wild game
salami, etc.)	Eggs
Sausage (hot dogs, etc.)	

Dairy Products

Cheese	Ice cream
Butter	Cream
Milk (whole, raw, skim,	Sour cream
buttermilk, etc.)	Whipped cream
Yogurt	Margarine
Kefir	

Processed Foods

Instant foods	Foods processed with
Canned foods	Chemicals
Frozen foods	Additives
Refined (white) flour	Artificial coloring
Polished (white) rice	Artificial flavoring
Sprayed foods	Emulsifiers
Dyed foods	Preservatives
Irradiated foods	Stabilizers

Vitamins and Supplements

Vitamin pills (synthetic or natural)	Mineral supplements
B-complex	Bone meal
B_1	Calcium
B_2	Dolomite
Niacin	Iron
Niacinamide	Selenium
Folic acid	Zinc
B_6	Lecithin capsules
B_{12}	Brewers yeast
Biotin	Bran tablets
Choline	Herbal tablets
Inositol	Papaya tablets
Pantothenic acid	Desiccated liver
PABA	Ginseng tablets or pills
Vitamin C	Bee pollen
Vitamin E	Diet pills
	Other similar products

27.

Guidelines for Cancer Patients

When properly applied, the Cancer-Prevention Diet can help to restore an excessively yin or yang condition to one of more natural balance. However, slight modifications are needed in every case. Below is a summary of the common types of cancer and the general dietary adjustments for the category in which they fall. Specific nutritional advice for each cancer is given in the individual chapters in Part II under the section "Dietary Recommendations." Cancer patients should consult an experienced macrobiotic counselor or medical associate to make sure the evaluation of their condition is accurate and to help formulate a diet suited to their unique case and personal needs.

Kind of Food	More Yin Cancer	Combination of Both	More Yang Cancer
	Mouth (except tongue Esophagus Stomach (upper) Breast Skin Lymphoma and Hodgkin's Disease Brain (outer regions) Leukemia	Lung Bladder/Kidney Stomach (lower) Uterus Melanoma Spleen Liver Tongue	Colon Rectum Prostate Ovary Bone Pancreas Brain (inner regions)

Kind of Food	More Yin Cancer	Combination of Both	More Yang Cancer
Grains	Minimize use of corn	Minimize corn and buckwheat	Minimize buckwheat
Soup	Slightly stronger flavor (more miso or tamari soy sauce)	Moderate flavor	Milder flavor (less miso or tamari soy sauce)
Vegetables	Slightly greater emphasis on root varieties (burdock, carrot, turnip, etc.)	Greater emphasis on ground varieties (cauliflower, acorn and butternut squash, pumpkin)	Greater emphasis on leafy green varieties (daikon, carrot, or turnip greens, kale, watercress, etc.)
Beans	A little more strongly seasoned, use less often	Moderately seasoned and moderate volume	More lightly seasoned, may use regularly
Sea Vegetables	Longer cooking, slightly thicker taste	Moderate cooking, medium taste	Quicker cooking, lighter taste
Pickles	More long-time pickles	More medium-time pickles	More short-time pickles
Condiments	Stronger use	Moderate use	Lighter use
Animal Food	Occasional small volume of white fish or dried fish, only if craved	Avoid completely or minimize	Avoid completely
Salad	Avoid raw salad, occasional boiled salad	Limit raw salad, frequent boiled or pressed salad	Occasional raw, frequent boiled or pressed salad
Fruit Dessert	Avoid completely	Small amount of dried or cooked fruit (locally grown and seasonal), if craved	Small amount of dried or cooked fruit (locally grown and seasonal), if craved; occasional fresh fruit in small volume

Kind of Food	More Yin Cancer	Combination of Both	More Yang Canc
Seeds and Nuts	Occasional roasted seeds, avoid nuts	Occasional roasted seeds, limit nuts	Occasional roasted seeds, avoid nuts
Oil	Sesame only, as little as possible. Apply with brush to prevent burning. No raw oil.	Sesame or corn only, as little as possible. Apply with brush to prevent burning. No raw oil.	Sesame or corn for cooking, small amount occasionall for sautéing. No ra oil.
Beverage	Longer cooked, thicker tasting tea	Medium cooked, medium tasting tea	Shorter cooked, lighter tasting tea

28.

Making a Smooth Transition

During the Lebanese crisis in 1982, a Midwest hamburger chain air-lifted several thousand hamburgers to Beirut for the American marines. While this was more a publicity stunt in the ongoing burger wars at home than an exercise in peacekeeping abroad, it symbolized a widespread recognition that adjusting to a new environment is difficult and that our desire for familiar foods persists when circumstances change.

The transition to a more natural diet and way of life should present no serious conflict. However, sometimes we approach the process too ambitiously and go to great lengths to avoid the foods to which we were previously accustomed. If we rush things and try to change overnight, we are bound to make mistakes and within a short period will revert to our former lifestyle or go onto sample something else. This desire for instant satisfaction is part of the modern consumer mentality, and we can make the mistake of approaching the Cancer-Prevention Diet in this way as well as anything else.

In selecting natural foods, we begin to appreciate crops that have matured in the fields and weathered the elements in contrast to those that have been produced in a factory and artificially aged. Similarly, we must respect our own biological rhythms and personal rates of growth. In many cases, it has taken ten, twenty, or thirty years or more of poor eating for the cancerous condition to develop. Depending upon our own unique situation, it will take several months and, in some cases, a few years to recover our normal digestive, respiratory, circulatory, excretory, and nervous functions. The healing process should not be artificially hurried up.

When starting the new way of eating, it is best to begin with just a few basic preparations, such as pressure-cooked brown rice, miso soup, a few vegetable dishes, one sea vegetable, and bancha tea. Then, day by day, week by week, we can gradually widen our selection of natural foods and introduce new cooking styles. In the meantime, we can still be eating some of the same types of foods we have been eating in the past, including salads and fruit, flour products and seafood. Rather than eliminating certain categories of food from our diet, it is better to initially reduce their intake and then switch to a better quality of intermediary food until a taste and appreciation for the new foods are developed.

The important thing is to begin to change in the right direction. Ideally the rate of change should be more like walking long distances where we gradually build up our endurance rather than like sprinting or marathon running where we get off to a fast start but inevitably get worn out. If we throw away all of our old food the first day and memorize the yin and yang tables like a catechism, we will soon either leave the diet as abruptly as we adopted it, or we will become missionaries, preaching to the nutritionally unconverted. Such behavior is childish and violates the macrobiotic way of life, which respects all lifestyles and understands opposites as complementary aspects of the whole.

On the other hand, there is a danger of taxiing so slowly down the dietary runway that our plane never takes off. Sometimes we can remain in a holding pattern for years, never realizing that we are still on the ground. We are conscious of the importance of proper food and eat a little brown rice and a little miso soup, but we never really experience looking at things from a healthy perspective. If we adopt a middle way between proceeding too quickly or too slowly, we will soon find ourselves pleasantly aloft.

Of course, these reflections on making a smooth transition apply to people already in relatively healthy shape. Those with cancer or other serious conditions may need to adopt a strict form of the diet at once without the luxury of integrating it into their previous way of eating. However, in practice the reduction in pain and discomfort quickly convinces the person of the value of the new approach.

As far as obtaining natural foods, growing our own grains and vegetables, of course, is best if the situation allows. We should all try to cultivate a garden, even if it is a very small one in an urban environment. Next best is to obtain food at an organic farmers market or a natural foods coop so that we can actually experience some of the living energy of the food before it reaches the market shelf or dinner table. In most North American and European cities, there are now natural foods and health food stores, which supply most of the staple items in the Cancer-Prevention Diet as well as a regular supply of fresh, seasonal produce. It is important to shop around and learn what each store offers in terms of quality, availability, service, and price. Buying in bulk saves on packaging and is more ecological and less expensive. Ethnic markets, such as Oriental, Latin America, Afro-American, and Middle Eastern food shops, are also potential sources of basic items, such as grains and beans, and often have a wider selection of vegetables than elsewhere. Even the local supermarket often has a natural foods section and suitable locally grown produce. For those people who do not have access to any of these sources or who are confined, a list of whole foods distributors and mail order stores can be obtained from the East West Foundation.

As far as possible, we should try to make our own bread, tofu, pickles, and traditionally processed foods. Homemade dishes have a much fresher quality, are more delicious, and contribute to the peaceful energy of the home. Each week, each month, or each season of the year, we can try out a new food preparation or style of cooking and slowly build up a reservoir of experience that can become translated into well-balanced recipes and menus.

During the transition period, there will be times when we crave the taste, texture, odor, and other characteristics of previous foods and drinks, especially those we had in childhood. Often, when eating such foods, we suffer from feelings of guilt. These feelings should be put aside and a more relaxed attitude developed. Instead of feeling as if we have committed a sin, we should reflect and try to understand why such cravings arose. Usually, during the first weeks or months of the new diet, these cravings reflect a natural discharge process. As our condition improves, the toxins and mucus that have accumulated in our bloodstream and internal organs are eliminated from the body through the bowels, urination, perspiration, and other excretory functions. As they leave the body, the discharged food particles often impress themselves in our consciousness and we experience them as cravings. At other times, after our condition has stabilized, these occasional cravings signify that our diet is imbalanced in the opposite yin or yang direction from the food to which we are attracted. Thus if we are attracted to fruit juice or ice cream, our diet is probably too salty, overcooked, and generally yang. If we are attracted to fish, eggs, or other animal products, we are consuming too many sweets, liquids, and other strong yin foods. These promptings are one of the body's way of alerting us to a disequilibrium in our way of eating.

Rather than suppress these natural urges, it is better to acknowledge them and take a tiny volume of the previous type of food from time to time until such cravings lessen and finally go away, as they ultimately will. During the transition period, the following table may serve as a guide in substituting better-quality foods for the previous items that we miss.

Cravings	Replacement	Goal
Meat	Fish, seafood	Grains, beans, seitan, tempeh, tofu
Sugar, molasses, chocolate, carob, and other highly refined sweeteners	Honey, maple syrup	Rice syrup, barley malt, and ultimately natural sweeteners from whole grains and vegetables
Dairy food, cheese, milk, cream, butter	Organic dairy food, in small volume; nuts and nut butters; soy milk	Traditional soy products such as miso and tofu; tahini and other seed butters
Tropical and semi-tropical fruits and juices such as orange, grapefruit, and pineapple; artificial juices and beverages	Organic fruits and fruit juices	Organic temperate-climate fruit (fresh, dried, and cooked) and juices in small volume and in season
Coffee, black tea, soft drinks, diet drinks	Herb teas, green tea, mineral water	Bancha twig tea, grain coffee, and other traditional nonaromatic teas

In addition to cravings, the discharge process is often accompanied by some abnormal physical manifestations that may last from three to ten days and, in some cases, up to four months until the quality of the blood fully changes. If our native constitution is strong and well structured, such reactions are usually negligible. However, if our embryonic and childhood development suffered from chaotic dietary habits, if we have ingested many chemicals, drugs, or medications, or if we have had surgery or an abortion, these discharge reactions will be more pronounced.

Whatever the case may be, we should not worry if these reactions occur. They are part of the natural healing process and signify that our systems are regenerating themselves, dislodging and throwing off the excess that has accumulated over many years. These reactions may be generally classified as follows:

General Fatigue

A feeling of general fatigue may arise among people who have been eating an excessive amount of animal protein and fat. The energetic activity that they may have previously experienced was the result of the vigorous caloric discharge of these excessive foods rather than a more healthy, balanced, and peaceful way of activity. Often these people initially experience physical tiredness and slight mental depression until the new diet starts to serve as an energy supply for activity. Such a period of fatigue usually ends within a month.

Pains and Aches

Pains and aches may sometimes be experienced, especially by people who have been taking excessive liquid, sugar, fruits, or any other extremely yin quality of food and beverages. These pains and aches—such as headaches and pains in the area of the intestines, kidneys, and chest—occur because of the gradual contraction of abnormally expanded tissues and nerve cells. These aches and pains disappear—either gradually or suddenly—as soon as these abnormally expanded areas return to a normal condition. This usually takes between three and fourteen days, depending upon the previous condition.

Fever, Chills, and Coughing

As the new diet starts to form a more sound quality of blood, previous excessive substances—excessive volume of liquid, fat, and many other things—begin to be discharged. If at this time the functions of the kidneys, urinary system, and respiratory system have not yet returned to normal, this discharge sometimes takes the form of fever, chills, or coughing. These are temporary and disappear in several days without any special treatment.

Abnormal Sweating and Frequent Urination

As in the symptoms described above, unusual sweating may be experienced by some people from time to time, for a period of several months, and other people may experience unusually frequent urination. In their previous diets, these people have been taking excessive liquid in the form of water, various beverages, alcohol, fruits, fruit juices, milk or other dairy food. By reducing these excessive liquids and fats accumulated in the form of liquid, the body returns to a normal, balanced, healthy condition. When metabolic balance has been gradually restored, these discharges will cease.

Skin Discharge and Unusual Body Odors

Among the forms of elimination is the discharge of unusual odors from the entire body surface, through breathing, urination, or bowel movements and often, in the case of women, through vaginal discharges. This usually occurs among people who were previously taking excessive volumes of animal fat, dairy food, and sugar. In addition, some people experience—for only short periods—skin rashes, reddish swelling at the tips of the fingers and toes, and boils. These types of elimination arise especially among people who have taken animal fat, dairy food, sugar, spices, chemicals, drugs, and among those who have had chronic malfunctions of the intestines, kidneys, and liver. However, these eliminations naturally heal and usually disappear within a few months without any special attention.

Diarrhea or Constipation

People who have had chronically disturbed intestinal conditions, caused by previous improper dietary habits, may temporarily experience either diarrhea (usually for several days) or constipation (for a period lasting up to twenty days). In this case, diarrhea is a form of discharge of accumulated stagnated matter in the intestines, including unabsorbed food, fat, mucus, and liquid. Constipation is the result of a process of contraction of the intestinal tube, which was abnormally expanded due to the previous diet. As this contraction restores normal elasticity to the intestinal tube, the elimination of bowels resumes.

Decrease of Sexual Desire and Vitality

There are some people who may feel a weakening of sexual vitality or appetite, not necessarily accompanied by a feeling of fatigue. The reason for such a decline is that the body functions are working to eliminate imbalanced factors from all parts of the body and excessive vitality is not available to be used for sexual activity. Also, in some cases, the sexual organs are being actively healed by the new quality of blood and are not yet prepared to resume normal activity. These conditions, however, last only for a short period, usually a few weeks and, at most, a few months. As soon as this recovery period is over, healthy vitality and desire for sexual activity return.

Temporary Cessation of Menstruation

In a few women, there may be a temporary cessation of menstruation. The reason for this cessation is that in the healing of the entire body, once again the vital organs need to receive energy first. Less vital functions, including reproductive activities, are healed later. The period of cessation of menstruation varies with the individual. However, when menstruation begins anew, it is healthy and natural, and begins to adjust to the normal twenty-eight-day lunar cycle and presents no discomfort, as was previously often the case. Mental clarity and emotional calm are strengthened as well as physical flexibility.

Mental Irritability

Some people who have been taking stimulants, drugs, and medications for long periods experience emotional irritability after changing their dietary practices. This irritability reflects adjustments taking place in the blood and various body functions, following the change to the different quality of food, and generally passes within one week to several weeks, depending upon how deeply affected the body systems were by the previous habitual use of such drugs and medications. The consumption of sugar, coffee, and alcohol for long periods, as well as long-time smoking, also produces temporary emotional irritability when the new diet is initially practiced.

Other Possible Transitory Experiences

In addition to the above conditions, some people may experience other manifestations of adjustment, such as bad dreams at night or a feeling of coldness. These too will pass.

In many instances, the discharge process is so gradual that none of these more visible temporary conditions arises. However, when they do appear, the symptoms vary from person to person, depending upon their inherited constitution and physical condition, and usually require no special treatment, naturally ceasing as the whole body readjusts to normal functioning. In the possible event that the symptoms are severe or uncomfortable, the discharge process can be slowed down by modifying the new diet to include continuous consumption of some previous food in small volume—about 10 to 30 percent of the meal—until balance is restored. The important thing is to understand that the discharge mechanism is part of the normal healing process and these symptoms are not to be suppressed by taking drugs or medications, resorting to vitamin or mineral supplements, or going off the diet altogether in the mistaken belief that it is deficient. If there is any uncertainty or question about proper practice that arises during this transition period, a qualified macrobiotic counselor or medical professional should be contacted.

As mentioned earlier, introductory macrobiotic cooking classes are essential for proper orientation to the new way of eating. In addition, it is important to have a community of support consisting of other individuals or families who are eating in this way or in the general direction of more natural foods. Dishes and recipes can then be exchanged and experiences shared in the spirit of adventure and discovery.

Variables in cooking such as salt, oil, pressure, time, and liquid are always changing with the seasons and our own development and take time to master. Another factor connected with unsatisfactory cooking is the use of electricity or microwave. Some families have either recently installed expensive ranges or ovens or live in an apartment where they come furnished with the kitchen. We have found that when people, especially cancer patients, switch to gas heat they invariably get improved results, and a peaceful energy replaces the chaotic vibration of the previously prepared food. Although it may appear uneconomical in the short run to invest in another stove, the change in food quality and improved health will be well worth it in the long run. Even a small portable camping stove with one or two propane burners can be set up conveniently in a corner of the kitchen for this purpose.

All of these factors will contribute to a smoother transition and more delicious and satisfying meals.

CLASSES AND FURTHER INFORMATION

Further information on implementing a natural foods diet can be obtained from the East West Foundation, a nonprofit institution established in 1972. The East West Foundation, and its seven major affiliates or regional offices around the country, offer ongoing classes for the general public in macrobiotic cooking, Oriental medicine and philosophy, and related fields. They also provide health and dietary counseling services with trained consultants and referrals to medical doctors, registered nurses, and other professional health-care associates. Other activities include periodic weekend seminars for cancer patients and their families, conferences and research assistance for the medical profession, and mail order books and literature. There are also Macrobiotics International and East West Centers in Canada, Mexico, Latin America, Europe, the Middle East, Africa, Asia, and Australia. The whole foods and naturally processed items described in this book are available at thousands of natural foods and health food stores, as well as a growing number of supermarkets. The macrobiotic specialty items are also available by mail order from various distributors and retailers.

Contact the Boston office for further information on any of the above services or whole foods outlets in your area.

BOSTON HEADQUARTERS:
Macrobiotics International and
   the East West Foundation
17 Station St.
Brookline, MA 02147
(617) 731-0564

COLORADO
1931 Mapleton Ave.
Boulder, CO 80302
(303) 449-6754

BALTIMORE
4803 Yellowwood Rd.
Baltimore, MD 21209
(301) 367-6655

CONNECTICUT
184 East Main St.
Middletown, CT 06457
(203) 344-0090

PHILADELPHIA
606 South Ninth St.
Philadelphia, PA 19147
(215) 922-4567

ILLINOIS
1574 Asbury Ave.
Evanston, IL 60201
(312) 328-6632

CALIFORNIA
708 N. Orange Grove Ave.
Hollywood, CA 90046
(213) 651-5491

WASHINGTON, D.C.
Box 40012
Washington, DC 20016
(301) 897-8352

For those who wish to study further, the Kushi Institute, an educational institution founded in Boston in 1979 with affiliates in London, Amsterdam, and Antwerp, offers full- and part-time instruction for individuals who wish to become macrobiotic teachers and counselors. The Kushi Institute publishes a "Macrobiotic Teachers and Counselors Directory," listing graduates who are qualified to offer guidance in the macrobiotic approach to health. The Cook Referral Service is an extension of the Kushi Institute and is comprised of specially qualified graduates of the Institute's advanced cooking program. These men and women are available to assist individuals and families in learning the basics of macrobiotic food preparation and home cares in their own home.

Kushi Institute and Cook Referral Service
Box 1100
Brookline, MA 02147
(617) 731-0564

Ongoing developments in the field of cancer and diet are reported in the Kushi Foundation's periodicals, including the *East West Journal*, a monthly magazine begun in 1971 and now with an international readership of 200,000. The *EWJ* features regular articles on the macrobiotic approach to health and nutrition, as well as ecology, science, psychology, and the arts.

> *East West Journal*
> 17 Station St.
> Brookline, MA 02147
> (617) 232-1000

29.

Recipes

This chapter includes the basic recipes for the Cancer-Prevention Diet. People with cancer should be careful to follow the guidelines in the individual chapters in Part II and may need to restrict their use of oil or preparation of fruit, salad, fish, dessert, and other items. After these basic recipes are learned, those in good health may wish to consult a macrobiotic cookbook with a wider selection of recipes for supplemental food and seasonal variation as well as cooking and food preparation techniques. Several of these books are listed in the bibliography.

GRAINS

PRESSURE-COOKED BROWN RICE

1 cup organic brown rice   pinch of sea salt per cup of rice
1¼–1½ cups spring water per
    cup of rice

Gently wash and quickly place rice (short- or medium-grain) in a pressure-cooker and smooth out surface of rice so it is level. Slowly add spring water down side of pressure-cooker so surface of rice remains calm and even. Add sea salt. Place cover on pressure-cooker and bring up to pressure slowly. When pressure is up, place a flame deflector underneath and turn flame to low. Cook for 50 minutes. When rice is done, remove pressure-cooker from burner and allow to stand for about 5 minutes before reducing pressure and opening. With a bamboo rice paddle, lift rice from pot one spoonful at a time and smooth into wooden bowl. Distribute more cooked rice at bottom and less cooked rice at top evenly in bowl. The rice will have a delicious, nutty taste and impart a very peaceful feeling.

Note: Each cup of uncooked rice makes about 3 cups of cooked rice. Allow about 1 cup per person. In general, you will want to start with 3 or more cups of uncooked rice and store the remainder. Leftover rice will keep for several days. After rice cools off, place in a closed container in the refrigerator. Warm up by placing rice in a cheesecloth or piece of unbleached muslin, place in a ceramic saucepan or on top of a steamer that fits into a pot or saucepan, add ¼ to ½ inch of water, and bring to a boil. After rice has heated for a few minutes, remove from cloth and serve.

Variation: One third of an umeboshi plum may be added instead of salt for each cup of uncooked rice. Long-grain rice may occasionally be used in summer.

BOILED RICE

1 cup brown rice   pinch of sea salt
2 cups spring water

Wash rice and place in heavy pot or saucepan. Add water and salt. Cover with a lid. Bring to a boil, lower flame, and simmer for about 1 hour or until all water has been absorbed. Remove and serve.

Note: It is highly recommended that cancer patients eat pressure-cooked brown rice. It is sweeter and more energizing than boiled rice. Healthy persons should also eat primarily pressure-cooked rice. However, they may have boiled rice occasionally, especially lightly roasted rice.

SOFT BROWN RICE (Rice Kayu)

1 cup brown rice   pinch of sea salt
5 cups spring water

Wash rice and pressure-cook or boil as in either of the above recipes. However, not all of the water will be absorbed. Rice should be creamy and some of the grains should be visible after cooking. In case water boils over while pressure-cooking, turn off flame and allow to cool off. Then turn on flame again and continue to cook until done.

Note: Makes a nourishing and appetizing breakfast cereal. Especially recommended for cancer patients and others who have difficulty swallowing or holding food down.

Variation: Vegetables such as daikon or Chinese cabbage or an umeboshi plum may be added while cooking. Also a one-inch square of dried kombu is highly recommended.

GENUINE BROWN-RICE CREAM

1 cup brown rice
10 cups spring water

½ umeboshi plum or a pinch of
sea salt per cup of rice

Dry roast rice in a cast-iron or stainless-steel skillet until golden brown. Place in pot, add water and plum or salt, and bring to a boil. Cover, lower heat, and place flame deflector beneath pot. Cook until water is one half of original volume. Let cool and place in cheesecloth or unbleached muslin, tie and squeeze out the pulp. Heat the cream again, then serve. Add salt if needed. The pulp is also very good to eat and can be made into a small ball and steamed with grated lotus root or carrot.

Note: Makes a delicious breakfast cereal and is also good for those who have difficulty eating. The lives of many people who otherwise could not eat have been saved with rice cream. The love, care, and energy of the cook can be imparted to the food with his or her hands.

Variation: Garnish with scallions, chopped parsley, nori, gomashio, or roasted sunflower seeds.

FRIED RICE

4 cups cooked brown rice
1 Tablespoon dark sesame oil
1 medium onion sliced diagonally
*   or diced*

1–2 Tablespoons tamari soy
sauce

Brush skillet with sesame oil. Let heat for a minute or less but do not
let oil start to smoke. Add onion, place rice on top of vegetables. If
rice is dry, moisten with a few drops of water. Cover skillet and cook
on low flame for 10 to 15 minutes. Add tamari soy sauce and cook for
another 5 minutes. There is no need to stir. Just mix before serving.

Note: Those in good health may have fried rice several times a
week, though the amount of oil may need to be reduced depending
on the individual's condition. Cancer patients may need to restrict
their oil and may use 2 to 3 tablespoons of water to replace the oil.
Check dietary recommendations carefully.

Variation: Use scallions, parsley, or a combination of vegetables
such as carrots and onion, cabbage and mushroom, and daikon and
daikon leaves.

RICE WITH BEANS

1 cup brown rice
*¹⁄₁₀ to ¹⁄₈ cup of beans per cup of
rice*

1¼–1½ cups spring water
pinch of sea salt

Wash rice and beans. Cook beans ½ hour beforehand following basic
recipes in bean section below. Allow beans to cool; add with cooking
water to rice. Bean water counts as part of the total water in the
recipe. Pressure-cook for 45 to 50 minutes and serve as with plain
rice.

Note: Cancer patients should generally use only azuki, chickpeas,
or lentils. Those in good health may use a variety of other beans as
well. Grains and beans cooked together make for a substantial meal
and save the time and fuel needed for cooking each dish separately.

RICE AND VEGETABLES

1 cup brown rice
¼ cup dried daikon
*½ cup carrots (finely diced or
small matchsticks)*

*⅛ cup burdock (finely diced or
small matchsticks)*
*1¼–1½ cup spring water per
cup of rice*
pinch of sea salt per cup of rice

Place washed rice in pressure-cooker and mix with vegetables. Add water and salt, cover, and cook as for plain rice.

Variation: A small amount of tamari soy sauce may be added with salt before cooking. Other vegetables that go well with rice are sweet rice, green beans, green peas and carrots, etc. Soft vegetables such as onion and green leafy vegetables tend to become mushy and should be avoided for this dish. Rice and vegetables may also be cooked with sesame seeds, with walnuts, or with lotus seeds, as well as with azuki beans or black soy beans.

RICE BALLS WITH NORI SEA VEGETABLE

1 cup cooked brown rice   *½–1 umeboshi plum*
1 sheet toasted nori

Roast a thin sheet of nori by holding the shiny side over a burner about 10 to 12 inches from the flame. Rotate for 3 to 5 seconds until color changes from black to green. Fold nori in half and tear into two pieces. Fold and tear again. You should now have four pieces that are about 3 inches to a side. Add pinch of salt to a dish of water and wet your hands. Form a handful of rice into a solid ball. Press a hole in the center with your thumb and place a small piece of umeboshi inside. Then close hole and compact ball again until solid. Cover rice ball with nori, one piece at a time, until it sticks. Wet hands occasionally to prevent rice and nori from sticking to them but do not use too much water.

Note: Rice balls make a tasty, convenient lunch or snack because they can be eaten without utensils. They are great to take along when traveling and keep fresh for a few days. Use less or no umeboshi when making rice balls for children.

Variation: Rice can be made into triangles instead of balls by cupping your hands into a V-shape. Balls or triangles can be rolled in toasted sesame seeds and eaten without nori. Small pieces of salt or bran pickles, vegetables, pickled fish, or other condiments can be inserted inside instead of umeboshi. Instead of nori sheets, use roasted crushed sesame seeds, shiso leaves, pickled rice leaves, dried wakame sheets, or green leafy vegetable leaves.

MILLET

1 cup millet
2½ cups boiling water

pinch of sea salt per cup of millet

Wash millet. Lightly roast millet in dry skillet for about 5 minutes or until slightly golden. Stir gently during this time to prevent burning. Add boiling water and salt. Bring to boil, cover, lower flame, and simmer 30 to 35 minutes.

Note: Millet has a delicious nutty flavor and light, fluffy consistency.

Variation: Roast millet with a little sesame oil, or sauté onions 3 to 5 minutes on low flame, add millet and sauté another 3 to 5 minutes, add boiling water and cook as above. The sautéing methods are not recommended for most cancer patients. Millet can also be topped with a sauce to reduce its somewhat dry taste. A nourishing breakfast cereal of soft millet can be made by adding 4 cups of boiling water to the basic recipe instead of 2½ cups.

BARLEY

1 cup barley
1¼–1½ cups spring water per cup of barley

pinch of sea salt per cup of barley

Follow same method as basic pressure-cooked brown rice.

Note: Barley is very strengthening and recommended for regular use by cancer patients.

Variation: Barley may also be boiled, fried, and cooked with a variety of other grains, beans, and vegetables, and used in soups. For soft barley cereal, combine 1 cup barley, 4–5 cups water, and pinch of sea salt and boil for 1¼–1½ hours. Serve hot and garnish with scallions, chopped parsley, nori, or gomashio.

WHOLE OATS

1 cup whole oats
5–6 cups spring water

pinch of sea salt per cup of oats

Wash oats and place in pot. Add water and salt. Cover and bring to a boil. Reduce flame and simmer on a low flame for several hours or overnight until water is absorbed. Use a flame deflector to prevent burning. Makes an excellent cereal.

Note: Whole oats are very strengthening for cancer patients and are to be preferred to steel-cut oats or rolled oats.

Variation: Cooking time can be reduced by pressure-cooking following the basic brown rice recipe. For a very nourishing and peaceful dish, combine 1½ cups barley, 1 cup whole oats, and ½ cup partially cooked beans. Add 3 pinches of sea salt, about 4 cups of water, and pressure-cook as usual.

BUCKWHEAT (Kasha)

1 cup buckwheat   *pinch of sea salt*
2 cups boiling spring water

Roast buckwheat in dry skillet for 4 to 5 minutes. Put grain in pot and add boiling water and salt. Bring to boil, reduce flame, and simmer for 30 minutes or until water has been absorbed.

Note: Buckwheat is a strong, warm grain. Patients with more yin cancer may eat buckwheat frequently in this form or in noodle form as soba. Patients with more yang cancer should avoid it. See specific dietary recommendations.

Variation: Cook buckwheat with sautéed cabbage and carrots or with onion and chopped parsley. For a hearty cereal, use 4 to 5 cups of boiling water and cook as above.

SWEET RICE

1 cup sweet rice   *pinch of sea salt*
1 cup spring water

Wash rice, add water and salt, and cook in pressure-cooker following basic rice recipe.

Note: Sweet rice is more glutinous than regular rice and should be used only occasionally. It may also be added in small volume to regular rice for a sweeter taste.

MOCHI

Mochi is sweet rice served in cakes or squares. They are made by pounding cooked sweet rice with a heavy wooden pestle in a wooden bowl. Pound until grains are crushed and become very sticky. Wet pestle occasionally to prevent rice from sticking to it. Form rice into small balls or cakes, or spread on a baking sheet that has been oiled and dusted with flour and allow to dry. Cut into pieces and roast in a dry skillet, bake, or deep-fry. For occasional use and special celebrations.

RYE

1 cup rye   *pinch of sea salt*
1¼–1½ cups spring water

Cook the same as basic pressure-cooked brown rice, or boil, in which case 2 cups of water are used.

Note: Since rye is hard and requires a lot of chewing, it is usually mixed with other grains or consumed in flour form as rye bread. For a delicious, chewy dish, add 1 part rye to 3 parts brown rice. Rye may be dry roasted in a skillet for a few minutes prior to cooking to make it more digestible.

CORN

Prepare fresh corn on the cob by steaming or boiling in a saucepan for 10 minutes or until done. Instead of butter or margarine, season with a little bit of umeboshi plum.

Note: Because of hybridization and heavy pesticide use, today's corn is less strengthening than original Indian corn. Use organic and traditional open-pollinated varieties whenever possible. Corn may be prepared into dough for tortillas and many other delicious, traditional Native American dishes. Also corn is made into flour or meal for polenta, cornbread, etc. (See the August 1982 *East West Journal* for these recipes.)

WHEAT

1 cup wheat berries
1¼–1½ cups spring water

pinch of sea salt

Cook following basic pressure-cooked brown rice recipe or boiled-rice recipe. Boiled wheat will usually cook longer than rice.

Note: Wheat is difficult to digest in whole form and must be thoroughly chewed. It also requires longer cooking time. Soaking wheat berries 3 to 5 hours beforehand reduces cooking time and makes a softer, more digestible dish. For a tasty combination, combine 1 part wheat berries and 3 parts rice or other grain.

NOODLES AND BROTH

1 package soba or udon noodles
1 piece of kombu, 2–3 inches
   long
4 cups spring water

2 dried shiitake mushrooms
2–3 Tablespoons tamari soy
   sauce

Boil water. Oriental noodles already contain salt so no salt needs to be added to the water. Add noodles to water and boil. After about 10 minutes, check to see if they are done by breaking the end of one noodle. Buckwheat cooks faster than whole wheat, and thinner noodles cook faster than thicker ones. If the inside and outside are the same color, noodles are ready. Remove noodles from pot, strain and rinse with cold water to stop them from cooking and prevent clumping. To make the broth, place kombu in pot, add water and mushrooms that have been soaked, their stems cut off, and sliced. Bring to boil. Reduce flame and simmer for 3 to 5 minutes. Remove kombu and mushrooms. Add tamari soy sauce to taste for 3 to 5 minutes. Place cooked noodles into the broth to warm up. Do not boil. When hot, remove and serve immediately. Garnish with scallions, chives, or toasted nori.

Note: Soba buckwheat noodles are very strengthening. In summer they can be cooked and enjoyed cold. Udon wheat noodles are much lighter. Western-style whole-grain noodles and pasta may also be used regularly. These include whole-wheat spaghetti, shells, spirals, elbows, flat noodles, lasagna, etc. Use pinch of salt in water when cooking.

FRIED NOODLES

1 package soba or udon
1 Tablespoon sesame oil
½ cup sliced scallions

2 cups cabbage
1–2 Tablespoons tamari soy
    sauce

Cook noodles as in previous recipe, rinse under cold water, and drain. Oil skillet and put in cabbage. Place noodles on top of vegetables. Cover and cook on low flame for several minutes until noodles become warm. Add tamari soy sauce and mix noodles and vegetables well. At the very end of cooking, add scallions. Serve hot or cold.

Note: If you cannot take oil, use 2 tablespoons of water for sautéing.

Variation: Many combinations of vegetables may be used, including carrots and onions, scallions and mushrooms, cabbage and tofu.

WHOLE-WHEAT BREAD

8 cups whole-wheat flour
2 Tablespoons sesame oil
   (optional)

¼–½ teaspoon sea salt
spring water

Mix flour and salt, add oil, and sift thoroughly together by hand. Form a ball of dough by adding just enough water and knead 300 to 350 times. Oil two bread pans with sesame oil and place dough in pans. Place damp cloth over pans and let sit for 8 to 12 hours in a warm place. After dough has risen, bake at 300° for 15 minutes and then 1¼ hours longer at 350°.

Note: Flour products, including bread, are not recommended for regular use by cancer patients.

Variation: A delicious sourdough starter for bread can be made by combining 1 cup of flour and enough water to make a thick batter. Cover with damp cloth and allow to ferment for 3 to 4 days in a warm place. After starter has soured, add 1 to 1½ cups of starter to bread dough, knead, and proceed as above. For rye bread, use 3 cups rye flour to 5 cups whole-wheat flour.

RICE KAYU BREAD

2 cups brown rice   *8 cups spring water*

Pressure-cook rice in water for 1 hour or more. Take out rice and allow to cool in large bowl. While still slightly warm, add to rice:

2 teaspoons sesame oil   *enough whole-wheat flour to*
* (optional)*   * form into a ball of dough*
½ teaspoon sea salt

Add oil and salt to rice and mix well. Add enough flour to make soft ball of dough. Knead 300 to 350 times, adding flour to ball from time to time to keep from getting too sticky. Place dough in two oiled bread pans, shape into loaves, cover with damp cloth, set in warm place, and let rise 8 to 12 hours. Bake at 300° for 30 minutes and 350° for another hour, or until golden brown.

Note: This bread is better for cancer patients than whole-wheat bread, but should still be used sparingly.

SEITAN (Wheat Gluten)

3½ pounds of whole-wheat flour   *8–9 cups spring water*

Place flour in large bowl and add 8 to 9 cups of warm water. Consistency should be like oatmeal or cookie batter. Knead for 3 to 5 minutes until flour is mixed thoroughly with water. Cover with warm water and allow to sit a minimum of 5 to 10 minutes. Knead again in soaking water for 1 minute. Pour off cloudy water into jar. Place remaining gluten into a large strainer and put strainer in a large bowl or pot. Pour cold water over gluten and knead in the strainer. Repeat until the bran and starch are completely separated. Keep the starch. Alternate between cold and hot water when rinsing and kneading gluten. Always start and finish with cold water to contract the gluten.

Gluten should form a sticky mass. Separate into 5 to 6 pieces and form balls. Drop balls into 6 cups boiling water and boil for 5 minutes, or until balls rise to surface. Put balls on top of a piece of kombu, add 3 to 5 tablespoons of tamari soy sauce and 1 teaspoon grated ginger, cook 1 hour, and serve.

Note: Seitan is very versatile, tasty, and full bodied in texture. It is especially appealing for people making a transition to natural foods. Spring-wheat flour has a softer texture than winter wheat and is often preferred.

Variation: Seitan can be cut into cubes for soups and salads; used in a stew with carrots, burdock, brussels sprouts, onion, radish, or other vegetables; combined with bread crumbs, onions, mushrooms, and celery to stuff a squash; fried in larger slices for sandwiches and grainburgers.

SOUPS

BASIC VEGETABLE MISO SOUP

1 ounce dry wakame sea
  vegetable
1 cup thinly sliced onions

1 quart spring water
2–3 Tablespoons miso

Rinse wakame quickly in cold water and soak for 3 to 5 minutes and slice into ½-inch pieces. Place wakame and onions in pot and add water. Bring to a boil, cover flame, and simmer for 10 to 20 minutes or until tender. Reduce flame to very low but not boiling or bubbling. Place miso in a bowl or suribachi. Add ¼ cup of broth and puree until miso is completely dissolved in liquid. Add pureed miso to soup. Simmer for 3 to 5 minutes and serve. Garnish with scallions, parsley, ginger, or watercress.

Note: Be careful to reduce the flame while the miso is cooking in order to preserve the beneficial enzymes in miso. As a general rule, use about ½ teaspoon of miso for each cup of water in the broth. Soup shouldn't taste too salty or too bland.

Variation: Barley miso is highly recommended, especially for cancer patients and for people with other sicknesses. Hatcho (100 percent soybean) miso is strong, but not salty, and also may be used to help restore health. Other misos, such as brown rice miso, may be used occasionally. In terms of aging, select miso that has fermented one-and-a-half years or more. All types of miso may be eaten year round and slightly modified in proportion according to the season or condition of health. Vegetables may be varied often. Other basic combinations include wakame, onions, tofu; onions and squash; cabbage and carrots; daikon and daikon greens. If your health allows for oil, you may brush 1 teaspoon or less of unrefined vegetable oil, especially dark sesame oil, sauté the vegetables first, and then add to the wakame in the pot.

MISO SOUP WITH DAIKON AND WAKAME

1½ cups daikon	1 quart spring water
½ cup wakame	3 teaspoons miso

Wash and slice daikon into ½-inch slices and add to water. Cook for 5 minutes. Meanwhile, soak wakame for 3 to 5 minutes and chop into small pieces. Add wakame to pot and cook over low flame until vegetables are soft. Dilute and add miso to stock. Simmer for 3 minutes. Garnish with chopped scallion.

Note: Daikon is particularly helpful to eliminate excess mucus, fat, protein, and water from the body. Cooking time of wakame depends on how soft or hard it is.

MISO SOUP WITH MILLET

½ cup millet	1 quart spring water
1 cup sliced onions	¼ cup miso
1 cup butternut squash	1 sheet toasted nori
½ cup celery	

Wash millet and dry-roast in a skillet. In a pot, layer vegetables, starting with celery, then onions, and squash on top. Spread millet evenly on top of layered vegetables. Carefully add water to just below the level of the squash. Cook over a medium flame. Add water gradually as the millet expands. Do not stir. After millet becomes very soft, add the rest of the soup stock or water. Bring to a boil. Reduce flame.

Mix miso with small amount of soup water and puree. Add pureed miso to the soup a couple of minutes before serving. Garnish with nori and parsley.

Variation: Other grains may be substituted for millet including barley, rice, buckwheat, oats, or cracked wheat. Alternate different vegetables as well.

TAMARI SOY SAUCE BROTH

1 three-inch piece of kombu sea vegetable
2 cakes of tofu cubed
2 shiitake mushrooms
¼ cup sliced scallions
4 cups spring water
2–3 Tablespoons tamari soy sauce

Soak shiitake 10 to 20 minutes. Place kombu and shiitake in water (including soaking water) and boil for 3 to 4 minutes. Take kombu and shiitake out and save for another recipe. Add tofu and boil until tofu comes to the surface. Do not boil tofu too long or it will become too hard. Tofu in soup is best enjoyed soft. Add tamari soy sauce and simmer for 2 to 3 minutes. Garnish with scallions and nori.

Variation: This clear broth soup can be made with chopped watercress and other vegetables instead of tofu. The shiitake too is optional but very good for cancer patients.

LENTIL SOUP

1 cup lentils
2 onions diced
1 carrot diced
1 small burdock root diced
1 Tablespoon chopped parsley
1 quart spring water
¼–½ teaspoon sea salt

Wash lentils. Layer vegetables starting with onions, then carrots, burdock, and lentils on top. Add water and pinch of salt. Bring to a boil. Reduce flame to low, cover, and simmer for 45 minutes. Add chopped parsley and remaining salt. Simmer 20 more minutes and serve. Tamari soy sauce may be added for flavor.

Variation: For those who can use oil, vegetables may first be sautéed and then cooked with lentils as above.

AZUKI BEAN SOUP

1-inch square of dried kombu
1 cup azuki beans
1 medium onion sliced
½ cup sliced carrots

1 quart spring water
¼–½ teaspoon sea salt
tamari soy sauce to taste
(optional)

Soak kombu 5 minutes and slice. Wash beans, place in pot, and add water. Bring to a boil. Reduce flame and simmer for 1¼ hours or until beans are 80 percent done. Take out cooked beans or use other pot. Put onion on bottom, then carrots, then azuki beans and kombu on top. Add salt. Cook for 20 to 25 minutes more until vegetables are soft. At very end, add tamari soy sauce to taste. Garnish with scallions or parsley and serve.

Variation: Instead of carrots and onion, winter squash may be used. This is particularly recommended for kidney, spleen, pancreas, and liver troubles.

CHICKPEA SOUP

1 cup chickpeas soaked overnight
1 onion diced
1 carrot diced
1 burdock stalk quartered

1 three-inch piece kombu
4–5 cups spring water
¼–½ teaspoon sea salt

Place kombu, chickpeas, and water in pressure-cooker and cook for 1 to 1½ hours. Bring pressure down. Place beans in another pot. Add vegetables and salt. Cook for 20 to 25 minutes on medium-low flame. Garnish with scallions, parsley, or bread crumbs.

BARLEY SOUP

½ cup barley
¼ cup lentils
3 onions diced
1 celery stalk

1 carrot
5–6 cups spring water
¼–½ teaspoon sea salt

Wash barley and lentils. Layer vegetables in pot starting with celery on bottom, then onion, carrot, lentils, and barley on top. Add water just enough to cover and bring to a boil. Add sea salt just before boiling. Lower flame and simmer until barley becomes soft and milky. Check taste. You may add a drop of tamari soy sauce for flavor and garnish with nori or parsley.

Note: Barley broth is very nourishing for cancer patients. The amount of barley may be increased and other variations of vegetables may be used.

Variation: You may cook barley before using for soup, adding ½ cup of barley to 1½ cups of water. Cook 20 to 30 minutes, then follow recipe.

BROWN RICE SOUP

2 cups cooked brown rice
3 shiitake mushrooms
1 three-inch piece kombu
¼ cup dried celery

1 quart of spring water
1–2 Tablespoons tamari soy
  sauce

Boil mushrooms and kombu in water for 2 to 3 minutes. Remove and slice into thin strips or pieces. Place them back in water, add rice, and bring to a boil. Lower flame and cook for 30 to 40 minutes. Add celery and simmer for 5 minutes. Add tamari soy sauce to taste and simmer for final 5 minutes, garnish with scallion and serve.

Variation: You may also add miso for a wonderful, warming soup.

BUCKWHEAT SOUP

½ cup roasted buckwheat
1 onion diced
½ cup minced parsley

5–6 cups spring water
pinch of sea salt
tamari soy sauce to taste

Brush a small amount of sesame oil in pot. Sauté onion until translucent. Add buckwheat and water and salt. Bring to boil, cover, reduce flame, and simmer 25 to 30 minutes. Season with tamari soy sauce and simmer 10 more minutes.

Note: Not recommended for cancer patients who need to restrict oil or buckwheat intake.

Variation: Without oil, you can make a light tasting soup. For a rich, dynamic soup, add carrots, cabbage or a variety of other vegetables.

CORN SOUP

4 ears fresh corn	*5–6 cups spring water or kombu*
1 celery stalk diced	*stock*
2 onions diced	*¼ teaspoon sea salt*
	tamari soy sauce to taste

Strip kernels from corn with knife. Place celery, onions, and corn in pot. Add water and pinch of salt. Bring to a boil, lower flame, cover and simmer until celery and corn are soft. Add rest of salt and tamari soy sauce to taste if desired. Serve with chopped parsley, watercress, or scallions and nori.

SQUASH SOUP

1 large buttercup squash	*4–5 cups spring water*
1 onion diced	*½ teaspoon sea salt*

Remove skin from squash. Place diced onion in pot, add cubed squash, along with water. Add pinch of sea salt. Bring to boil, cover, and lower flame. Simmer 20 to 30 minutes or until squash is soft. Remove squash and puree in a Foley food mill. Place pureed squash in a pot; add rest of salt. Bring to a boil, lower flame, and cook for 20 minutes. Garnish with scallions or parsley.

Variation: This thick, creamy, and delicious soup may also be made with other autumn and winter squashes or pumpkins. You may add a little powdered kuzu (kudzu) after pureeing squash to make a creamy soup with a nice smooth texture.

CARP AND BURDOCK SOUP (Koi-Koku)

1 fresh carp
burdock in weight at least equal
to fish
½–1 cup used bancha tea leaves
and twigs wrapped in
cheesecloth sack

1 Tablespoon grated ginger
miso to taste
spring water and bancha
(kukicha) tea

Select a live carp and express your gratitude for taking its life. Ask fishseller to carefully remove gallbladder and yellow bitter bone (thyroid) and leave the rest of the fish intact. This includes all scales, bones, head, and fins. At home, chop entire fish into 1- to 2-inch slices. Remove eyes if you wish. Meanwhile, chop at least an equal amount of burdock (ideally 2 to 3 times the weight of fish) into thinly shaved slices or matchsticks. This quantity of burdock may take a while to prepare. When everything is chopped up, place burdock and fish in pressure-cooker. Tie old bancha (kukicha) twig leaves and stems from your teapot in cheesecloth. It should be the size of a small ball. Place this ball in pressure-cooker on top or nestled inside fish. The tea twigs will help soften the bones while cooking. Add enough liquid to cover fish and burdock, approximately ⅓ bancha tea and ⅔ spring water. Pressure-cook 1 hour. Bring down pressure, take off lid, add miso to taste (½–1 teaspoons per cup of soup), and grated ginger. Simmer for 5 minutes. Garnish with chopped scallions and serve hot.

Note: This delicious, invigorating soup is excellent for restoring strength and vitality and opening the electromagnetic channel of energy in the body. It may be eaten occasionally by all cancer patients, even those who otherwise shouldn't eat animal products. It is also good for mothers who have just given birth or who are breastfeeding. In cold weather it is particularly warming. Be careful, however, to eat only a small volume (1 cup or less) at a time. Otherwise you will become too yang and be attracted to liquids, fruits, sweets, and other strong yin. Soup will keep for a week in the refrigerator or several months in the freezer where it can be taken out from time to time as needed.

Variation: For those whose oil isn't restricted, the burdock may be sautéed for a few minutes in sesame oil at the start, prior to cooking with the fish. Soup may also be made by boiling in lidded pot for 4 to 6 hours or until all bones are soft and dissolved. As liquid evaporates, more water or bancha tea should be added. If carp is unavailable, substitute another more yin fish such as perch, red snapper, or trout. If burdock is scarce, use carrots instead, or use half burdock and half carrots.

KOMBU SEA VEGETABLE STOCK

Wipe kombu with a dried brush quickly to remove dust. Minerals are lost by wiping so, if not dusty, place immediately in pot containing cold spring water. Boil 3 to 5 minutes. Remove kombu and use in other dishes or dry out and use as a condiment or side dish. Use stock for miso, grain, bean, or vegetable soups.

SHIITAKE MUSHROOM STOCK

Soak 5 to 6 shiitakes in water for 30 minutes. Add shiitake and its soaking water to 1 to 2 quarts of spring water and bring to a boil. Boil 5 to 10 minutes. Remove shiitake and save for the soup (in which case be sure to remove stems) or use in another recipe. Kombu may also be combined with shiitake to make a stock.

FRESH VEGETABLE STOCK

Save vegetable roots, stems, tops, and leaves for a nutritious soup stock. Boil in 1 to 2 quarts of spring water for 5 to 10 minutes. Remove vegetable pieces and compost or discard.

FISH STOCK

Boil fish heads or bones for a few minutes. You may tie the fish parts in a cheesecloth sack and place in water or remove fish parts from stock by straining after boiling through a cheesecloth. Use fish stock for vegetable or grain soups, or thicken with pastry flour to make a fish sauce and season with tamari soy sauce.

Note: Not recommended for cancer patients whose fish intake is limited. Commercially available bonito flakes are not recommended. However, home-prepared freshly shaved, smoked and dried, traditional bonito is suitable.

VEGETABLES

Waterless Cooking (Nishime Style)

Use a pot with a heavy lid or one made for waterless cooking. Soak 1 or 2 long strips of kombu about 10 minutes, or until they are soft, and cut into 1-inch pieces. Place kombu in bottom of pot. Add vegetables such as carrots, daikon, turnips, burdock, lotus root, onions, dried shiitake mushrooms, and cabbage. These should be cut into 2-inch chunks and layered on top of the kombu. Add enough water to come just below the top layer of vegetables. Sprinkle several pinches of sea salt or drops of tamari soy sauce over the vegetables. Cover and set flame to high until a high steam is generated. Lower flame and cook peacefully for 15 to 30 minutes or longer depending on the kind of vegetables used. If water evaporates during cooking, add more water to the bottom of the pot. At end of cooking, turn off flame, and allow vegetables to sit for about 2 minutes. The cooked juice may be served along with the vegetables and is very delicious.

Note: This way of cooking vegetables without oil is highly recommended for cancer patients. It helps restore general strength and vitality.

Sautéing

There are two basic ways of sautéing: with oil and with water. In the first, cut the vegetables into small pieces such as matchsticks, thin slices, or shaved slices. Lightly brush skillet with dark or light sesame oil. Heat oil, but before oil begins to smoke add vegetables and a pinch of sea salt to bring out their natural sweetness. Occasionally turn over or move vegetables with chopsticks or wooden spoon to ensure even cooking. However, do not stir. Sauté for 5 minutes on medium flame, followed by 10 minutes on low flame. Gently mix from time to time to avoid burning. Season to taste with sea salt or tamari soy sauce and cook 2 to 3 minutes longer.

The second method combines water and oil. Vegetables may be

prepared either in small pieces or in large, thick pieces. Sauté as above in lightly oiled skillet for about 5 minutes. Then add enough cold water to cover the vegetables half way or just enough to cover the surface of the skillet. Add a pinch of sea salt, cover, and cook until almost tender. When 80 percent done, season with sea salt or tamari soy sauce and cook 3 to 4 minutes more. Remove cover and simmer until water evaporates.

Note: Sautéing with oil is not recommended for many cancer patients or others who need to avoid or reduce oil. However, for those in good health, sautéed vegetables may be prepared daily. For those who cannot use oil, use 1 to 2 tablespoons of water instead.

Variation: Delicious combinations include burdock and carrots; onion and carrots; cabbage, onion, and carrots; parsnips and onions; mushrooms and celery; broccoli and cauliflower; Chinese cabbage, mushrooms, and tofu; kale and seitan. Soft vegetables take only 1 to 2 minutes to sauté, while cooking time for root vegetables will take longer. Other unrefined vegetable oils may be used in this way. However, only sesame and corn oil are recommended for regular use.

Boiling

Place about ½–1 inch of cold spring water in pot, add a pinch of sea salt. Bring to a boil and add vegetables. Vegetables should be tender but crisp.

Note: In order to keep a green color, cook watercress, parsley, scallions, and other green leafy vegetables at a high flame for only 1 to 2 minutes. In order to preserve the taste, it is also better not to add salt after boiling. Tamari soy sauce may be added at end of cooking for flavor.

Variation: For an especially sweet taste, place a 3-inch piece of kombu on bottom of pot when cooking round vegetables such as carrots or daikon. Vegetables may be seasoned with tamari soy sauce or miso instead of salt. Tasty combinations of boiled vegetables include broccoli and cauliflower; cabbage, corn, and tofu; carrots, onions, and green peas.

Steaming

Place ½ inch of spring water in pot. Insert a vegetable steamer inside pot or a wooden Japanese steamer on top of pot. Place sliced vegeta-

bles in steamer and sprinkle with a pinch of sea salt. Cover and bring
water to boil. Steam until tender but slightly crisp. Greens will take
only 1 to 2 minutes, other vegetables 5 to 7 minutes depending on
type, size, and thickness.

Note: Lightly steamed greens can be eaten every day. These include leafy tops of turnip, daikon, and carrot; watercress; kale; mustard greens; Chinese cabbage; parsley.

Variation: If you don't have a steamer, place ½ inch of water in
bottom of pot. Add vegetables and pinch of sea salt. Bring to a boil,
lower flame to medium, and steam until tender. Save vegetable water
for soup stock or sauces.

Other Cooking Styles

Vegetables may be prepared in a variety of other styles including
baking, broiling, and tempuraing (deep frying). However, these are
not generally recommended for cancer patients. For those in good
health who wish to try these methods, seek proper instruction and
guidance or consult another cookbook such as *Macrobiotic Cooking
for Everyone* by Edward and Wendy Esko.

AZUKI, KOMBU, AND SQUASH

1 cup azuki beans   *1 hard winter squash*
2 3-inch strips of kombu

Wash and soak azuki beans with kombu. Remove kombu after soaking
and chop into 1-inch-square pieces. Place kombu at bottom of pot and
add chopped hard winter squash such as acorn, butternut, or hokkaido. Add azukis on top of squash. Cover with water and cook over a
low flame until beans and squash are soft. Sprinkle lightly with sea
salt. Cover and let cook for 10 to 15 minutes. Turn off flame and let
sit for several minutes before serving.

Note: This dish is helpful in regulating blood sugar levels, especially in those who are hypoglycemic, diabetic, or have pancreatic
or liver disorders. It is naturally sweet and delicious and will reduce
the craving for sweets. May be prepared 1 to 2 times per week.

Variation: You may cook azuki beans 50 to 70 percent, then add
on top of squash, and proceed as above.

DRIED DAIKON WITH KOMBU AND TAMARI

2 six-inch strips of kombu   *tamari soy sauce to taste*
½ cup dried daikon (long white
radish)

Soak kombu and slice lengthwise into ¼-inch strips and place in bottom of heavy pot with a heavy lid. Soak daikon until soft. If daikon is very dark in color wash first. Place dried daikon on top of kombu in pot. Add enough kombu and daikon soaking water and spring water if needed to just cover top of daikon. Cover pot, bring to boil, lower flame, add tamari soy sauce, and simmer 30 to 40 minutes until kombu is tender. Cook away excess liquid.

Note: This dish helps to dissolve fat deposits throughout the body.

Variation: Fresh daikon has more power than dried. Slice fresh daikon and cook as above until very tender. If daikon is unavailable, red radish may be used, though the effect is not so strong.

BOILED SALAD

1 cup sliced Chinese cabbage   *½ cup sliced celery*
½ cup sliced onion   *1 bunch watercress*
½ cup thinly sliced carrots

When making a boiled salad, boil each vegetable separately. All vegetables, however, may be boiled in the same water. Cook the mildest tasting vegetables first, so that each will retain its distinctive flavor. Place 1 inch of water and a pinch of sea salt in a pot and bring to a boil. Drop Chinese cabbage slices into water and boil 1 to 2 minutes. All vegetables should be slightly crisp, but not raw. To remove vegetables from water, pour into a strainer that has been placed inside a bowl so as to retain the cooking water. Put the drained-off water back into the pot and reboil. Next boil the sliced onion. Drain as above, retaining water and returning to boil. Next boil sliced carrots followed by sliced celery. Last, drop watercress into boiling water for just a few seconds. In order for vegetables to keep their bright color, each vegetable should be allowed to cool off. Sometimes you can run under cold water while in the strainer, but it is not ideal. Mix vegeta-

bles together after boiling. A dressing of 1 umeboshi plum or 1 teaspoon of umeboshi paste may be added to ½ cup of water (vegetable
stock from boiling may be used) and pureed in a bowl or suribachi for
seasoning.

Note: A refreshing way to prepare vegetables in place of raw
salad. Especially recommended for cancer patients who cannot have
uncooked foods. This method just takes out the raw taste and preserves the crispy freshness.

PRESSED SALAD

Wash and slice desired vegetables into very thin pieces, such as ½
cabbage (may be shredded), 1 cucumber, 1 stalk celery, 2 red
radishes, 1 onion. Place vegetables in a pickle press or large bowl and
sprinkle with ½ teaspoon sea salt and mix. Apply pressure to the
press. If you use a bowl in place of the press, place a small plate on
top of the vegetables and place a stone or weight on top of the plate.
Leave it for at least 30 to 45 minutes. You may leave it up to 3 to 4
days but the longer you press the vegetables the more they resemble
light pickles.

Note: This is a method to remove excess liquid from raw vegetables. For cancer patients, a boiled salad is preferable.

Variation: A press is not necessary when using soft vegetables.
Just mix with salt and serve after 30 minutes.

PRESSED SALT PICKLES

2 large daikon and their leaves   *heavy ceramic or wooden crock*
¼–½ cup sea salt   *or keg*

Wash daikon and their leaves with enough cold water 2 to 3 times,
making sure all dirt is removed, especially from the leaves. Set aside
and let dry for about 24 hours. Slice the daikon into small rounds.
Sprinkle sea salt on the bottom of the crock. Next layer some of the
daikon leaves, followed by a layer of daikon rounds. Then sprinkle
with sea salt again. Repeat this until the daikon is used or the crock is
filled. Place a lid or plate that will fit inside the crock on top of the
daikon, daikon leaves, and salt. Place a heavy rock or brick on top of

the lid or plate. Cover with a thin layer of cheesecloth to keep out dust. Soon water will begin to be squeezed out and rise to the surface of the plate. When this happens, replace heavy weight with a lighter one. Store in a dark, cool place for 1 to 2 weeks or longer. If water is not entirely squeezed out, add more salt. And make sure water is always covered or it will spoil. When ready, remove a portion, wash under cold water, slice and serve.

Note: Pickles are a naturally fermented food and aid in digestion. A small volume may be eaten daily. However, commercial pickles such as dill pickles that have been made with vinegar and spices should be strictly avoided.

Variation: Pickles may also be made from Chinese cabbage, carrots, cauliflower, and other vegetables in this manner.

TAMARI SOY SAUCE PICKLES

Mix equal parts spring water and tamari soy sauce in a bowl or glass jar. Slice vegetables such as turnips or rutabaga and place in this liquid. Soak for 4 hours to 2 weeks, depending on the strength desired.

RICE BRAN PICKLES (Nuka)

Long Time (Ready in 3 to 5 months)
10–12 cups of nuka (rice bran) or wheat bran
1½–2 cups of sea salt
3–5 cups spring water

Short Time (Ready in 1 to 2 weeks)
10–12 cups nuka
⅛–¼ cup sea salt
3–5 cups spring water

Roast nuka or wheat bran in a dry skillet until it gives off a nutty aroma. Allow to cool. Combine roasted nuka or wheat bran with salt and mix well. Place a layer of bran mixture on the bottom of a wooden keg or ceramic crock. A single vegetable such as daikon, turnips, rutabaga, onion, or Chinese cabbage may be used. Slice vegetables into 2- to 3-inch pieces and layer on top of the nuka. If more than one type of vegetable is used, layer one on top of another. Then sprinkle a layer of nuka on top of the vegetables. Repeat this layering until the nuka mixture is used up or until the crock is filled. Always make sure that the nuka mixture is the top layer. Place a wooden disk or plate to fit inside the crock, on top of the vegetables and nuka. Place a heavy weight, such as a rock or brick, on top of the plate. Soon water will begin to be squeezed out and rise to the surface of the plate. When this happens, replace heavy weight with a lighter one. Cover with a thin layer of cheesecloth and store in a cool room. To serve, take out pickled vegetables as needed and rinse under cold water to remove excess bran and salt. The same nuka paste may be used for several years. Just keep adding vegetables and a little more bran and salt.

BEANS AND BEAN PRODUCTS

AZUKI BEANS

1 cup azuki beans
2½ cups spring water per cup of
beans

¼ teaspoon sea salt per cup of
beans

Wash beans and place in pressure-cooker. Add water, cover, and bring to pressure. Reduce flame to medium-low and cook 45 minutes. Remove pressure-cooker from burner and rinse cold water over it to bring pressure down quickly. Open, add salt, cook uncovered until liquid evaporates.

Note: Most other types of beans can be pressure-cooked in this way. Chickpeas and yellow soybeans should first be soaked. Black soybeans should not be pressure-cooked because they clog up the gauge.

Variation: Beans may also be boiled by putting in a pot, adding 3½ to 4 cups of water per cup of beans, and cooking for about 1 hour and 45 minutes. When 80 percent cooked, add salt and cook for another 15 to 20 minutes until liquid is evaporated. To reduce cooking time, add flavor, and make beans more digestible, lay a 3-inch piece of kombu under beans at the beginning. A small volume of vegetables may also be cooked along with beans, such as chopped squash, onions, or carrots.

LENTILS

1 cup lentils   ¼ teaspoon sea salt
2½ cups spring water

Wash lentils and place in pot. Add water, cover, and bring to a boil. Reduce flame to medium-low. After 30 minutes, add salt and cook another 15 to 20 minutes. Remove cover and allow liquid to cook off.

Variation: Chopped onions and celery go well with lentils and may be cooked together.

CHICKPEAS

1 cup chickpeas   ½ teaspoon sea salt
3 cups spring water

Wash beans and soak overnight. Place beans and soaking water in pressure-cooker. Add more water if necessary. Bring to pressure, turn down flame to medium-low, and cook 1 to 1½ hours. Take off burner and allow pressure to come down. Remove lid, add salt, and return to burner. Cook uncovered for another 45 to 60 minutes.

Variation: Diced onion and carrots may be added to beans during last hour of cooking.

COLORFUL SOYBEAN CASSEROLE

2 cups yellow soybeans   1 carrot sliced
2 3-inch pieces of kombu   1 burdock sliced
1 shiitake mushroom   1 stalk of celery sliced
5 large pieces of dried lotus root   soaking water
6 dried tofu   1½ Tablespoons tamari soy sauce
1 dried daikon shredded   1 teaspoon kuzu

Soak soybeans in cold water overnight in 2½ cups of water per cup of soybeans. Next day, place beans and soaking water in pressure-cooker and bring to pressure. Soak kombu, shiitake, lotus root, and dried tofu for 10 minutes. After beans have cooked 70 to 80 percent (approximately 15 minutes) reduce pressure, open, and layer kombu, shiitake, lotus root, and dried tofu on top. Bring back to pressure and cook 10 more minutes. Reduce pressure, open, skim off hulls from beans and take out vegetables and put on separate plates. Meanwhile, cut up carrot, burdock, celery, and dried daikon. Slice up cooked kombu and put in bottom of a large saucepan in a little water. On top of kombu add soft vegetables such as celery, shiitake, daikon, and tofu; then root vegetables including carrots, burdock, and lotus root; and finally soybeans and any original water remaining in pressure-cooker. Add 1½ tablespoons of tamari soy sauce, cover, cook 30 minutes. Add 1 teaspoon of kuzu to make creamy and a little grated ginger for flavoring. Soybeans should be very tender and sweet.

Note: This dish is extremely nourishing and highly recommended for cancer patients. However, those with yin cancer should be careful not to use more than one shiitake mushroom. Those with a yang cancer or healthy persons may use 5 to 6 shiitake.

Variation: Depending on availability, some vegetables may be omitted or added. Also, seitan makes this dish especially delicious.

BLACK SOYBEANS

2 cups black soybeans *spring water*
1 teaspoon sea salt *tamari soy sauce*

Wash beans quickly and soak overnight in cold water, adding ¼ to ½ teaspoon of sea salt per cup of beans. The salt will prevent the skins from peeling. In the morning, place beans and soaking water in pot. If necessary, add additional water to cover surface of beans. Bring to a boil, reduce heat, and simmer uncovered. When a dark foam rises to the surface, skim and discard. Continue in this way until no more foam rises. Cover beans and cook for 2½ to 3 hours. Add water to cover surface of beans if necessary. Toward end of cooking, uncover and add a little tamari soy sauce to give the skins a shiny, black color. Cook away excess liquid. Shake pot up and down to coat beans with remaining juice, and serve.

Note: This dish is particularly beneficial for the sexual organs and to relieve an overly yang condition caused by excess meat or fish. Avoid pressure-cooking black beans since they may clog the valve.

MISO

Miso (fermented soybean paste) is highly recommended for daily use. Cancer patients and others with illness, weakness, or fatigue should use barley miso that has aged for 3 years. Hatcho miso (100% soybean) and brown rice miso may be used occasionally. Avoid misos that have aged less than 1½ years. Store-bought miso should be made with organic or all-natural ingredients. Miso sold in bulk is usually preferable to miso sold in sealed plastic, which has been pasteurized, thereby reducing the beneficial enzymes and bacteria that aid digestion. Instant miso mixes are not recommended for daily use if regular miso is available. Instant miso is all right for traveling, and if circumstances permit should be cooked for a few minutes in water rather than seaped like a tea bag. Miso can be made at home with a grain called koji, which contains a special bacteria that enables the soybeans to ferment. Koji is available in some natural foods stores or can be made at home with a koji starter available from American Type Culture Collection, 12301 Park Lawn Drive, Rockville, Maryland 20852. (Request koji culture, aspergilus oryzae, Ahlburg Cohn, Code No. 14805.) Miso is used primarily in making miso soup (see soup section). However, it can also be used in cooking with vegetables, as a seasoning in place of salt, and in spreads, dips, dressings, pickles, relishes, and condiments. For complete miso recipes, see *How to Cook with Miso* by Aveline Kushi (Japan Publications, 1978).

HOMEMADE TOFU

3 cups organic yellow soybeans   *6 quarts spring water*
4½ teaspoons natural nigari

Soak beans overnight, strain, and grind in an electric blender. Place ground beans in pot with 6 quarts of water and bring to a boil. Reduce flame to low and simmer for 5 minutes, stirring constantly to avoid burning. Sprinkle cold water on beans to stop bubbling. Gently boil again and sprinkle with cold water. Repeat a third time. Place a cotton cloth or several layers of cheesecloth in a strainer and pour this liquid into a bowl. This is soy milk. Fold corners of the cloth to form a sack or place cloth in a strainer and squeeze out remaining liquid. Pulp in sack is called okara and may be saved for other recipes. In a suribachi or blender, grind the nigari, which is a special salt made from sea water and available in many natural foods stores. Sprinkle powdered nigari over soy milk in a bowl. With a wooden spoon carefully make a large X-shaped cut with two deep strokes in this mixture and allow to sit 10 to 15 minutes. During this time it will begin to curdle. The next step calls for a wooden or stainless-steel tofu box (available in many natural foods stores) or a bamboo steamer. Line box or steamer with cheesecloth and gently spoon in soy milk. Cover top with layer of cheesecloth and place lid on top of box or steamer so it rests on cheesecloth and curdling tofu. Place small stone or weight on lid and let stand for about 1 hour or until tofu cake is formed. Then gently place tofu in a dish of cold water for 30 minutes to solidify. Keep tofu covered in water and refrigerate until used. Tofu will keep several days fresh in the refrigerator. However, it is best to change water daily.

Note: Raw tofu is somewhat difficult to digest, so it is preferably eaten cooked. Tofu bought at the store should be made from organically grown soybeans and natural nigari. Refined solidifiers are sometimes used instead of natural nigari and should be avoided when possible. Cancer patients on an oil-restricted diet should avoid tofu mayonnaise, tofu dips, and other tofu products that contain oil, vinegar, or spices.

Variation: Tofu is very versatile, picks up the taste of the foods it is combined with, and has a variety of textures depending upon how it is cooked. It may be sliced, cubed, diced, pressed, or mashed and boiled in soups, sautéed with vegetables or grains, or baked in casseroles. It may also be used in dips, sauces, dressings, and desserts. The okara or pulp can be added to soups or cooked with vegetables.

TEMPEH (Soy Meat)

Tempeh is a traditional fermented soyfood originating in Indonesia. In the last decade it has become increasingly popular in the Far East and West and is now available in many natural foods stores. Tempeh is crisp, delicious, and nourishing and may be steamed, boiled, baked, or sautéed. It is enjoyed with a wide variety of grains, vegetables, and noodles and may be used in soups, salads, or sandwiches. Tempeh should always be cooked before eating. Tempeh may also be made at home. A special culture is available in many natural foods stores or may be ordered from The Farm, 156 Drakes Lane, Summertown, Tennessee 38483. For recipes and further information on tempeh making, see *The Book of Tempeh* by William Shurtleff and Akiko Aoyagi (Harper & Row, 1980).

CABBAGE-ROLL TEMPEH

Several outer layers of cabbage   *2 strips kombu*
   leaves   *2 onions*
8 ounces tempeh

Soak kombu one hour or more. Steam cabbage until soft. Cut the tempeh into 2-inch rectangles and steam or boil. Place on cabbage leaves and roll up. Slice soaked kombu and onions thinly. Layer kombu and onions on bottom of pot. Add water and cabbage rolls. Add sea salt to taste if desired. Cook until very soft.

   Note: Avoid cooking with salt or tamari soy sauce when serving tempeh to children. Tempeh is very energizing and salt could make them overactive.

NATTO

Natto is a fermented soy product that aids digestion and strengthens the intestines. It looks like baked beans connected by long slippery strands and has a unique odor. Natto is available in macrobiotic specialty stores or can be made at home (see recipe in *Introducing Macrobiotic Cooking* by Wendy Esko, Japan Publications, 1978). Natto is usually eaten with a little tamari soy sauce, mixed with rice, or served on top of buckwheat noodles.

SEA VEGETABLES

HIJIKI AND ARAME

2 cups soaked hijiki or arame   *3–4 Tablespoons tamari soy*
1 medium onion sliced   *sauce*
1 carrot sliced in matchsticks
spring water

Wash hijiki quickly under cold water. Place in bowl, cover with water, and soak 5 to 10 minutes. Drain water and save. Slice hijiki in 1- to 2-inch pieces. Place hijiki on top of other vegetables in pot. Add enough soaking water to cover top of hijiki. Bring to a boil, cover, reduce flame to low. Add one tablespoon of tamari soy sauce. Cook on low flame for 45 to 60 minutes. Season with additional tamari soy sauce to taste and simmer for 20 more minutes until liquid evaporates. Mix vegetables only at end and serve.

Note: Hijiki is thicker and coarser in texture than arame. Arame is milder, softer, has less of a briny taste, takes less time to cook, and is usually the sea vegetable preferred by those new to macrobiotic cooking.

Variation: Both hijiki and arame can be cooked with lotus root, daikon, and other vegetables; combined with grains or tofu; added to a salad; or put into a pie crust and baked as a roll. For those who can use oil, a strong, rich dish can be created by adding a little oil at the beginning of cooking.

WAKAME

2 cups soaked wakame   *soaking water*
1 medium onion sliced   *2 teaspoons tamari soy sauce*

Rinse wakame quickly under cold water and soak 3 to 5 minutes. Slice into 1-inch pieces. Put onion in pot and wakame on top. Add soaking water to cover vegetables. Bring to boil, lower flame, and simmer for 30 minutes or until wakame is soft. Add tamari soy sauce to taste and simmer 10 to 15 more minutes.

Note: Wakame is the chief vegetable added to miso soup. It also makes a tasty side dish or can be used as an alternative in most recipes calling for kombu.

KOMBU

1 12-inch strip kombu   *1 Tablespoon tamari soy sauce*
1 onion halved, then quartered   *spring water*
1 carrot cut in triangular pieces

Soak kombu 3 to 5 minutes, slice in half, and then slice diagonally into 1-inch pieces. Place in pot and add vegetables and enough soaking water to cover vegetables halfway. Add one tablespoon of tamari soy sauce. Bring to a boil. Reduce the flame to low and simmer for 30 minutes. Add additional tamari soy sauce to taste if desired, and cook for 5 to 10 more minutes.

Note: Kombu is delicious as a side dish or can be used as a stock for soups. Adding a 3-inch piece of kombu beneath beans will speed up cooking, add flavor, and make beans more digestible. When cooking with kombu, oil is usually not used.

NORI

Nori comes in thin sheets and can be used for wrapping rice balls (see recipe in grain section). It is also used to make sushi and makes an attractive garnish for soups, noodles, and salads. Toast lightly by holding nori, shiny side up, 10 to 12 inches from flame and rotate about 3 to 5 seconds until the nori changes from black to green.

DULSE

Dulse may be eaten dry as a snack or dry-roasted and ground into a powder in a suribachi to make a condiment. Dulse can also be used to season soups at the very end of cooking, salad, and main dishes.

AGAR-AGAR

This whitish sea vegetable forms into a gelatin when cooked and is used to make vegetable aspics and delicious fruit desserts. See recipe for kanten in dessert section.

SAUCES, DRESSINGS, AND SPREADS

KUZU SAUCE

1½ cups vegetable stock or water   1 Tablespoon kuzu

Dilute kuzu (a white starch, also known as kudzu) in small volume of cold water and add to pot containing stock or water. Bring to a boil, lower flame, and simmer 10 to 15 minutes. Stir constantly. Add tamari soy sauce to taste. Serve over vegetables, tofu, noodles, grains, or beans.

Variation: Arrowroot powder may be used instead of kuzu. Avoid thickeners such as corn starch.

BECHAMEL SAUCE

*½ cup whole-wheat pastry flour
  or brown-rice flour
3 cups spring water or kombu
  stock or vegetable soup stock*

*1 medium onion diced
1 teaspoon sesame oil
1 Tablespoon tamari soy sauce*

Sauté onion in lightly oiled skillet until transparent. Stir in flour and sauté 2 to 3 minutes until each piece of onion is coated. Gradually add water or stock and stir continually to prevent lumping. Bring to a boil, lower flame, and simmer 2 to 3 minutes. Add tamari soy sauce to taste and cook 10 to 12 minutes more until thick and brown. Serve over millet, buckwheat, or seitan.

Note: This savory sauce can be mucus-producing and should only be used occasionally by those in good health. Cancer patients should avoid it altogether.

UMEBOSHI DRESSING

*2 umeboshi plums
½ teaspoon sesame oil*

*½ cup spring water
¼–½ teaspoon grated onion*

Puree umeboshi and onion in suribachi. Add slightly heated oil and mix. Add water and mix to smooth consistency. Serve on salad.

Note: Cancer patients can make this dressing without oil by adding a little bit more water.

Variation: Umeboshi paste may be used instead of plums. Use 1 teaspoon of paste per plum. Also chives and scallions may be substituted for onions and the mixture used as a dip for crackers or chips.

TOFU DRESSING

8 ounces of tofu
½ teaspoon pureed umeboshi
   plum

¼ onion grated or diced
2 teaspoons spring water
chopped scallions or parsley

Puree umeboshi, onion, and water in suribachi. Add tofu and puree until creamy. Add water to increase creaminess if desired. Garnish with scallions or parsley. Serve with salad.

TAHINI DRESSING

2 umeboshi plums
2 Tablespoons tahini

½ small onion grated or diced
½–¾ cup spring water

Puree umeboshi, onion, and tahini in suribachi. Add water and puree until creamy. Serve with salad.

Note: Tahini is high in oil and generally not recommended for cancer patients.

MISO–TAHINI SPREAD

6 Tablespoons tahini

1 Tablespoon barley or rice miso

Dry-roast tahini in a skillet over medium-low flame until golden brown. Stir constantly to prevent burning. In suribachi stir tahini with miso. Add chopped scallions for variation. Delicious with bread or crackers.

Note: This spread is high in oil and should be avoided by most cancer patients.

CONDIMENTS

TAMARI SOY SAUCE

Tamari soy sauce is the name given by George Ohsawa to traditional, naturally made soy sauce to distinguish it from the commercial, chemically processed soy sauce found in many Oriental restaurants and supermarkets. Tamari soy sauce is also called natural shoyu. In natural foods stores there is now also available a wheatless soy sauce, known as genuine or real tamari. It is stronger in flavor. Tamari soy sauce, however, is recommended for regular use and should be used primarily in cooking and not added to rice or vegetables at the table.

GOMASHIO (Sesame Salt)

Dry roast 1 part sea salt. Wash and dry roast 10 to 14 parts sesame seeds. Add seeds to sea salt and grind in a suribachi until about two thirds of the seeds are crushed. Used to season grains, noodles, vegetables, salad, or soup at the table.

Note: For more yin cancer, prepare with 10 to 12 parts sesame to 1 part salt. For more yang cancer, use 14 to 16 parts sesame to 1 part salt. For cancer caused by a combination of both, prepare with 12 parts seeds to 1 part salt. Use about 1 teaspoon per day.

ROASTED SEA VEGETABLE POWDER

Use either wakame, kombu, dulse, or kelp. Roast sea vegetable in oven until nearly charred (approximately 10 to 15 minutes at 350°) and crush in a suribachi.

Note: For more yin cancer, this powder can be used more frequently in larger amounts (up to 1 teaspoon per day). For more yang cancer, slightly less volume is advisable (about ½ teaspoon per day). For cancers caused by a combination of both, an in-between volume is recommended.

UMEBOSHI PLUMS

Umeboshi are special plums (imported from Japan and now also grown in this country) that have been dried and pickled with sea salt and aged from one to three years. They usually come with shiso (beefsteak) leaves, which contribute to their distinctive red color. Umeboshi may be eaten by themselves or used to enhance grains and vegetables. They may also be pureed for making a tart and tangy dressing, sauce, or tea. The umeboshi contains a harmonious balance of more yin factors, such as the natural sourness of the plum, and more yang factors created by the salt, pressure, and aging used in their preparation. Umeboshi are excellent for strengthening the intestines and may be used regularly by persons with all types of cancer. Some natural foods stores also sell umeboshi paste without the pits. The paste is not as strong or balanced, and cancer patients are advised to use the whole plums.

TEKKA (Root Vegetable Condiment)

¼ cup sesame oil
⅓ cup finely minced burdock
⅓ cup finely minced carrot

⅓ cup finely minced lotus root
½ teaspoon grated ginger
⅔ cup hatcho miso

Prepare vegetables and mince as finely as possible. Heat oil in a skillet and sautée vegetables. Add miso. Reduce flame to low and cook 3 to 4 hours. Stir frequently until liquid evaporates and a dry, black mixture is left.

Note: Tekka is very strengthening for the blood but should be used sparingly because of its strong contractive nature. For more yin cancer, it can be used daily (about ½ teaspoon). For more yang cancer or cancer caused by a combination of yin and yang, use small volume only on occasion.

TAMARI-NORI CONDIMENT

Place dried nori or several sheets of fresh nori in ½ to 1 cup of spring water and simmer until most of the water cooks down to a thick paste. Add tamari soy sauce several minutes before end of cooking for a light to moderate taste.

Note: This special condiment helps the body recover its ability to discharge toxins. It may be eaten by persons with all types of cancer. For more yang cancer, use a slightly smaller volume (approximately ½ teaspoon per day). For more yin cancer, use up to 1 teaspoon daily. Those with cancers caused by a combination of both may eat an in-between volume.

SHIO-KOMBU CONDIMENT

1 cup sliced kombu   *½ cup tamari soy sauce*
½ cup spring water

Soak kombu until soft and chop into 1-inch-square pieces. Add sliced kombu to water and tamari soy sauce. Bring to a boil and simmer until the liquid evaporates. Cool off and place in a covered jar to keep for several days.

Note: This condiment is very high in minerals and aids in the discharge of toxins. Cancer patients may eat several pieces daily. If it is too salty, reduce the tamari.

SAUERKRAUT

A small amount of sauerkraut made from organic cabbage and sea salt may be used as a condiment occasionally.

VINEGAR

Brown rice vinegar, sweet brown rice vinegar, and umeboshi vinegar may be used moderately. Avoid red wine or apple cider vinegars.

GINGER

Fresh grated gingerroot may be used occasionally in a small volume as a garnish or flavoring in vegetable dishes, soups, pickled vegetables, and especially with fish or seafoods.

HORSERADISH

May be used occasionally by those in good health to aid digestion, especially for fish and seafood.

DESSERTS AND SNACKS

COOKED APPLES

Wash apples and peel unless organically grown, in which case skins may be eaten. Slice and place in a pot with a small amount of water to keep from burning (about ¼–½ cup). Add pinch of sea salt and simmer for 10 minutes, or until soft.

Note: Those with yin cancer should avoid desserts completely. Those with yang cancer may have a small volume of cooked fruit on occasion if craved.

Variation: Puree in a Foley food mill to make applesauce. Other fruits may be cooked in this way.

ROASTED SEEDS

Dry roast sesame, sunflower, pumpkin, or squash seeds by placing several cups of seeds in a skillet. Turn on flame to medium-low and gently stir with wooden roasting paddle or spoon for 10 to 15 minutes. When done, seeds should be darker in color, crisp, and give off a fragrant aroma. Seeds may be lightly seasoned with tamari soy sauce while roasting.

Note: Cancer patients may occasionally have roasted seeds in small volume.

KANTEN (Gelatin)

3 apples sliced　　　　　　　*pinch of sea salt*
2 cups spring water　　　　　*agar-agar flakes*
2 cups apple juice

Wash and slice fruit and place in pot with liquid. Add agar-agar flakes in amount according to directions on package (varies from several teaspoons to several tablespoons). Stir well and bring to boil. Reduce flame to low and simmer 2 to 3 minutes. Place in shallow dish or mold and put in refrigerator to harden.

Note: This delicious natural gelatin is not recommended for some cancer patients because of the high fruit and fruit juice content.

Variation: Kanten may also be made with other temperate-climate fruits including strawberries, blueberries, peaches, or melons. Nuts and raisins may be added to the fruit. Vegetable aspics may be made in this same way with vegetable soup stock instead of fruit juice, and vegetable pieces instead of fruit. Azuki beans and raisins are a delicious combination.

AMASAKE (Sweet Rice Beverage)

4 cups sweet brown rice   *8 cups spring water*
½ cup koji

Wash rice, drain, and soak in 8 cups of water overnight. Place rice in pressure-cooker and bring to pressure. Reduce flame and cook for 45 minutes. Turn off heat and allow to sit in pressure-cooker for 45 minutes. When cool enough, mix koji into rice by hand and allow to ferment 4 to 8 hours. During fermentation, place mixture in a glass bowl, cover with wet cloth or towel, and place near oven, radiator, or other warm place. During fermentation period, stir the mixture occasionally to melt the koji. After fermenting, place ingredients in a pot and bring to boil. When bubbles appear, turn off flame. Allow to cool. Refrigerate in a glass bowl or jar.

Note: Amasake may be served hot or cold as a nourishing beverage or used as a natural sweetener for making cookies, cakes, pies, or other desserts. As a beverage, first blend the amasake and place in a saucepan with a pinch of sea salt and spring water in volume to desired consistency. Bring to a boil and serve hot or allow to cool off.

Note: Cancer patients may have amasake occasionally as a beverage, especially to satisfy craving for a sweet taste.

RICE PUDDING

3½ cups cooked brown rice   *¼ teaspoon cinnamon*
1½ cups apple juice   *½ cup almonds*
¼ teaspoon sea salt   *¾ cup spring water*
⅓–½ cup spring water   *3–4 Tablespoons tahini*

Boil almonds and tahini in ¾ cup water and puree in a blender. Place mixture and other ingredients in pressure-cooker for 45 minutes.

After pressure has come down, take out and place mixture in a baking dish or covered casserole, and bake at 350° for 45 to 60 minutes.

Note: A tasty dessert for those in good health but best avoided by cancer patients.

BEVERAGES

BANCHA OR KUKICHA TEA

Dry roast twigs in skillet for 2 to 3 minutes. Stir constantly and shake pan to prevent burning. Store in air-tight jar. To make tea, add 2 tablespoons of roasted twigs to 1½ quarts of spring water and bring to a boil. Lower flame and simmer for several minutes. Place bamboo tea strainer in cup and pour out tea. Twigs in strainer may be returned to teapot.

Note: This tea is the main beverage in macrobiotic cooking. It may be eaten at the end of every meal and in between meals. However, everyone should watch their liquid consumption and drink only when thirsty.

BROWN RICE TEA

Dry roast uncooked brown rice over medium flame for 10 minutes or until a fragrant aroma develops. Stir and shake pan occasionally to prevent burning. Add 2 to 3 tablespoons of roasted rice to 1½ quarts of spring water. Bring to a boil, reduce flame, and simmer 10 to 15 minutes.

Variation: Teas may be made from other whole grains in this way.

ROASTED BARLEY TEA

Prepare same way as roasted brown rice tea above. This tea is especially good for melting animal fat from the body. Roasted barley tea also makes a very nice summer drink and may also aid in the reduction of fever.

GRAIN COFFEE

Roast separately each of the following: 3 cups of uncooked brown rice, 2½ cups of wheat, 1½ cups of azuki beans, 2 cups of chickpeas, 1 cup chicory root. Roast ingredients until dark brown, then mix together and grind into a fine powder in a grain mill. This mixture is known as yannoh. For a coffeelike drink, use 1 tablespoon per cup of water. Bring to a boil, lower flame, and simmer for 5 to 10 minutes.

Note: There are also a variety of grain coffees available in natural foods stores. Avoid any that contain dates, figs, molasses, or honey. Others may be used occasionally as an alternative to bancha tea at the meal.

MU TEA

Mu tea is a medicinal tea made with a variety of herbs, including ginseng. Mu #9 is excellent for strengthening the female sex organs and for stomach troubles and may also be used therapeutically by men. Mu tea is sold prepackaged in most natural foods stores. Stir package in 1 quart of water and simmer for 10 minutes. Except for medicinal purposes, macrobiotic cooking does not recommend ginseng, which is extremely yang, and fragrant and aromatic herbs, which are too yin, for ordinary daily consumption.

30.

Menus

The following weekly menu is a sample of the kinds of meals that might be prepared by an individual or family in relatively good health. It is set for the end of the summer and early autumn, so seasonal adjustments would be recommended for other times of the year.

	Breakfast	Lunch	Dinner
SUNDAY	Vegetable Miso Soup Soft Brown Rice with Kombu and Shiitake Mushroom Bancha Tea	Udon and Broth Steamed Brussel Sprouts Garden Salad Bancha Tea	Brown Rice Tamari Broth Sou, Colorful Soybean Casserole Steamed Mustard Greens Hijiki with Onion Cooked Peaches Bancha Tea
MONDAY	Tamari Broth Soup Soft Barley with Shiitake Mushroom Bancha Tea	Seitan with Bechamel Sauce Boiled Peas and Mushrooms Grain Coffee	Brown and Sweet Rice Azuki Beans with Kombu and Winter Squash Corn Soup Arame with Carrots, Burdock, and Onions Bancha Tea

	Breakfast	Lunch	Dinner
TUESDAY	Miso Soup with Millet Whole Oatmeal Bancha Tea	Corn on the Cob with Umeboshi Paste Pressed Salad Arame Bancha Tea	Brown Rice Lentil Soup Boiled Kale, Broccoli and Carrots Watermelon Bancha Tea
WEDNESDAY	Soft Brown Rice with Winter Squash Rice Kayu Bread Bancha Tea	Fried Rice with Scallions and Chinese Cabbage Navy Beans with Kombu Bancha Tea	Whole-Wheat Lasagna with Tofu Filling Boiled String Beans and Onions Steamed Watercress Bancha Tea
THURSDAY	Miso with Daikon and Wakame Soft Millet Bancha Tea	Whole Oats with Barley and Chickpeas Steamed Kale Fresh Cantaloupe Grain Coffee	Brown Rice Squash Soup Boiled Mustard Greens Cabbage Roll Tempeh Arame with Dried Daikon Bancha Tea
FRIDAY	Barley Miso Soup Steamed Rye Bread Bancha Tea	Fried Soba Boiled Celery Natto Bancha Tea	Baked Scrod with Ginger Sauce Millet Boiled Carrots and Onions Steamed Parsley Blueberry Pie Roasted Barley Tea
SATURDAY	Tamari Broth Soup Whole Oatmeal Bancha Tea	Rice Ball with Nori Boiled Salad Bancha Tea	Kasha Brown Rice Soup with Vegetables Kidney Beans with Kombu Steamed Cabbage Bancha Tea

MENUS FOR CANCER PATIENTS

The following suggested meal plans are for people with cancer. They
do not include pickles, condiments, and special side dishes or special
beverages which should also be prepared. Check the dietary recommendations for each particular illness.

*More Yin Cancer (Mouth, Esophagus, Upper Stomach,
Breast, Skin, Leukemia, Lymphomas, Hodgkin's Disease,
and Tumors in the Outer Region of the Brain)*

	Breakfast	Lunch	Dinner
SUNDAY	Vegetable Miso Soup Soft Brown Rice Bancha Tea	Brown Rice Cabbage-Roll Tempeh Arame Bancha Tea	Brown Rice Miso Soup Nishime Style Carrots, Onion Lotus Root, an Burdock Steamed Kale Bancha Tea
MONDAY	Miso Soup Soft Barley Bancha Tea	Brown Rice with Wheat Berries Steamed Tofu with Miso Dressing Boiled Watercress Salad Bancha Tea	Brown Rice and Rye Miso Soup with Chickpeas Steamed Caulifloι and Broccoli Boiled Wakame a Onions Bancha Tea
TUESDAY	Vegetable Miso Soup Whole Oatmeal Steamed Rice Kayu Bread Bancha Tea	Sweet Rice Sautéed Burdock and Carrots Grain Coffee	Brown Rice Buckwheat Soup Azuki, Kombu, ar Squash Boiled Chinese Cabbage Bancha Tea

	Breakfast	Lunch	Dinner
WEDNESDAY	Miso Soup with Millet Soft Brown Rice Bancha Tea	Brown Rice Seitan Stew Hiziki Boiled Daikon Bancha Tea	Brown Rice with Barley Miso Soup with Azuki Beans Colorful Soybean Casserole Steamed Mustard Greens Bancha Tea
THURSDAY	Miso Soup with Daikon and Wakame Soft Buckwheat Bancha Tea	Millet with Vegetables Natto Boiled Salad Bancha Tea	Brown Rice Tamari Broth Soup Lentils with Onions and Celery Steamed Parsnips and Parsley Amasake
FRIDAY	Miso Soup with Barley Steamed Rye Bread Bancha Tea	Rice Ball with Nori Steamed Kale Grain Coffee	Brown Rice Carp and Burdock Soup Boiled Salad with Daikon, Cabbage, Onions, Carrots, and Watercress Bancha Tea
SATURDAY	Vegetable Miso Soup Brown-Rice Cream Bancha Tea	Whole Oats and Barley Azuki Beans Steamed Watercress Bancha Tea	Brown Rice Miso Soup with Squash Dried Daikon with Kombu Boiled Sauerkraut and Scallions Grain Coffee

More Yang Cancer (Colon, Rectum, Prostate, Ovary, Bone, Pancreas, and Tumors in the Inner Regions of the Brain)

	Breakfast	Lunch	Dinner
SUNDAY	Miso Soup with Corn Soft Brown Rice Bancha Tea	Udon Noodles and Broth Steamed Brussels Sprouts Garden Salad with Umeboshi Dressing Bancha Tea	Brown Rice Miso Soup with Chickpeas Steamed Mustar Greens Hijiki with Carr Bancha Tea
MONDAY	Soft Barley with Kombu and Shiitake Mushroom Steamed Rice Kayu Bread Bancha Tea	Millet Boiled Seitan, Peas, Corn, and Carrots Grain Coffee	Brown and Swee Rice Vegetable Miso Soup Azuki Beans wit Kombu and Winter Squasl Steamed Kale Bancha Tea
TUESDAY	Miso Soup with Millet Whole Oatmeal Bancha Tea	Brown Rice Cabbage-Roll Tempeh Arame Pressed Salad Bancha Tea	Brown Rice Miso Soup with Broccoli and Cauliflower Boiled Chinese Cabbage and Carrot Greens Cooked Apples Bancha Tea
WEDNESDAY	Vegetable Miso Soup Soft Brown Rice Bancha Tea	Fried Rice with Scallions and Chinese Cabbage Azuki Beans with Kombu Bancha Tea	Brown Rice Miso Soup with Squash Nishime Style Onions, Carro Burdock, Lotu Root, and Kon Steamed Watercr Bancha Tea

	Breakfast	*Lunch*	*Dinner*
THURSDAY	Miso Soup with Daikon and Wakame Soft Millet Bancha Tea	Whole Oats with Barley, Chickpeas, and Kombu Boiled Cabbage Grain Coffee	Brown Rice Miso Soup with String Beans and Carrots Steamed Leeks and Parsley Arame Bancha Tea
FRIDAY	Soft Barley with Kombu Steamed Rye Bread Grain Coffee	Corn on the Cob with Umeboshi Sauce Natto Dried Daikon with Arame Bancha Tea	Brown Rice and Whole-Wheat Berries Miso Soup with Onions and Wakame Steamed Tofu and Kale Bancha Tea
SATURDAY	Vegetable Miso Soup Brown-Rice Cream with Kombu and Shiitake Mushroom Bancha Tea	Rice Ball with Nori Boiled Salad Amasake	Brown Rice Azuki Bean Soup Nishime Style Daikon, Cabbage, Burdock Steamed Daikon Tops Strawberry Kanten with Kuzu Grain Coffee

Cancer from a Combination of Yin and Yang
(Lung, Bladder, Kidney, Lower Stomach, Cervix, Endometrium, Melanoma, Spleen, Liver, Tongue)

	Breakfast	Lunch	Dinner
SUNDAY	Vegetable Miso Soup Soft Brown Rice Bancha Tea	Buckwheat Noodles and Broth Steamed Brussels Sprouts and Kale Bancha Tea	Brown Rice Miso Soup with Chickpeas Steamed Broccoli Hijiki with Dried Daikon Bancha Tea
MONDAY	Tamari Broth Soup Soft Barley Bancha Tea	Brown Rice Boiled Seitan, Peas, Carrots, and Shiitake Mushroom Grain Coffee	Brown and Sweet Rice Miso Soup with Cauliflower Azuki Beans with Kombu and Winter Squash Steamed Kale Bancha Tea
TUESDAY	Miso Soup with Millet Whole Oatmeal Bancha Tea	Brown Rice Cabbage-Roll Tempeh Arame Boiled Salad Bancha Tea	Brown Rice Miso Soup with Daikon Colorful Soybean Casserole Steamed Carrot Greens and Chinese Cabbage Grain Coffee
WEDNESDAY	Vegetable Miso Soup Steamed Rye Bread Bancha Tea	Fried Rice with Scallions and Chinese Cabbage Azuki Beans with Kombu Bancha Tea	Brown Rice Miso Soup with String Beans and Onions Nishime Style Onions, Carrots, Lotus Root, and Kombu Steamed Watercress Bancha Tea

	Breakfast	Lunch	Dinner
THURSDAY	Miso Soup with Daikon and Wakame Soft Millet	Whole Oats with Barley and Chickpeas Boiled Broccoli and Grain Coffee	Brown Rice Miso Soup with Squash Sautéed Burdock Steamed Leeks and Parsley Amasake
FRIDAY	Soft Barley Steamed Rice Kayu Bread Bancha Tea	Corn on the Cob with Umeboshi Sauce Dried Daikon with Kombu Bancha Tea	Brown Rice with Whole-Wheat Berries Miso Soup with Cauliflower and Kale Steamed Tofu Bancha Tea
SATURDAY	Vegetable Miso Soup Brown-Rice Cream Bancha Tea	Rice Ball with Nori Boiled Salad Bancha Tea	Brown Rice Tamari Broth Soup Nishime Style Daikon, Burdock, Cabbage Steamed Daikon Greens Strawberry Kanten with Kuzu Grain Coffee

31.

Kitchen Utensils

Pressure-Cooker

A pressure-cooker is an essential item in preparing the Cancer-Prevention Diet, especially in preparing brown rice and other whole grains. Stainless steel is recommended.

Cooking Pots

Stainless steel and cast iron are recommended, although Pyrex, stoneware, or unchipped enamelware may also be used. Avoid aluminum or teflon-coated pots.

Metal Flame Deflectors

These are especially helpful when cooking rice and other grains as they help distribute heat more evenly and prevent burning. Avoid asbestos pads.

Suribachi (Grinding Bowl)

A suribachi is a ceramic bowl with grooves set into its surface. It is used with a wooden pestle and is needed in preparing condiments, pureed foods, salad dressings, and other items. A six-inch size is generally fine for regular use.

Flat Grater

A small enamel or steel hand-style grater that will grate finely is recommended.

Pickle Press

Several pickle presses or heavy crocks with a plate and weight should be available for regular use in the preparation of pickles and pressed salads.

Steamer Basket

The small stainless steamers are suitable. Bamboo steamers are also fine for regular use.

Wire Mesh Strainer

A large strainer is useful for washing grains, beans, sea vegetables, some vegetables, and draining noodles. A small, fine mesh strainer is good for washing smaller items such as millet or sesame seeds.

Vegetable Knife

A sharp, high-quality Oriental knife with a wide rectangular blade allows for the more even, attractive, and quick cutting of vegetables. Stainless steel and carbon steel varieties are recommended.

Cutting Board

It is important to cut vegetables on a clean, flat surface. Wooden cutting boards are ideal for this purpose. They should be wiped clean after each use. A separate board should be used for the preparation of dishes containing animal foods.

Foley Hand Food Mill

This utensil is useful for pureeing, especially when preparing baby foods or dishes requiring a creamy texture.

Glass Jars

Large glass jars are useful for storing grains, seeds, nuts, beans, or dried foods. Wood or ceramic containers, which allow air to circulate, are better but may be difficult to locate.

Tamari Dispenser

This small glass bottle with a spout is very helpful in controlling the quantity of tamari soy sauce used in cooking.

Tea Strainer

Small, inexpensive bamboo strainers are ideal, but small mesh strainers may also be used.

Vegetable Brush

A natural-bristle vegetable brush is recommended for cleaning vegetables.

Utensils

Wooden utensils such as spoons, rice paddles, and cooking chopsticks are recommended since they will not scratch pots and pans or leave a metallic taste in your foods.

Bamboo Mats

Small bamboo mats may be used in covering food. They are designed to allow heat to escape and air to enter so that food does not spoil quickly if unrefrigerated.

Electrical Appliances

Avoid all electrical appliances as far as possible when preparing foods or cooking. Electricity produces a chaotic vibration that is transmitted to the energy of the food. Instead of toasting bread, steam or bake it. Instead of using an electric blender, use a suribachi to puree sauces and dressings. Occasionally, however, an automatic blender may be used to grind the soybeans for making tofu or when cooking for a party or large numbers of people. Use common sense.

32.

Baby Food
Suggestions

Our diet should change in accordance with the development of our teeth. The ideal food for the human infant is mother's milk, and all of the baby's nourishment should come from this source for the first 6 months. At about that age, the quantity of breastmilk can gradually be decreased over the next six months while soft foods, containing practically no salt, are introduced and proportionately increased. Mother's milk should usually be stopped around the time the first molars appear (12 to 14 months) and the baby's diet by then consist entirely of soft mashed foods.

Harder foods should be introduced around the time the first molars appear and gradually increase in percentage over the next year. By the age of 20 to 24 months, softly mashed foods should be replaced entirely by harder foods and comprise the mainstay of the diet.

At the beginning of the third year, a child can receive one third to one fourth the amount of salt used by an adult depending upon its health. A child's intake of salt should continue to be less than an adult's until about the seventh or eighth year.

At age four, the standard diet may be introduced, along with mild sea salt, miso, and other seasonings, including ginger. Until this age, infants ideally should not have any animal food, including fish, except in special cases where the child is weak, slightly anemic, or lacks energy. Then give about one tablespoon of white-meat fish or seafood that has been well boiled with vegetables and mashed. At age four, if desired, a small amount of white-meat fish or seafood may be included from time to time for enjoyment. Different tastes appeal to us at different periods of our development. A natural sweet taste particularly nourishes babies and children.

The following dietary recommendations may be followed for healthy infants as well as those with serious sicknesses, including childhood leukemia, lymphoma, or brain or kidney tumors.

Whole Grain Cereal can be introduced after 8 months to 1 year as the baby's main food. The cereal should be in the form of a soft whole grain porridge consisting of 4 parts brown rice (short-grain), 3 parts sweet brown rice, and 1 part barley. The porridge is preferably cooked with a piece of kombu, although this sea vegetable does not always have to be eaten. Millet and oats can be included in this cereal from time to time. However, buckwheat, wheat, and rye are usually not given.

The porridge may be prepared by pressure-cooking or boiling. To pressure-cook, soak cereals for 2 to 3 hours and pressure-cook with 5 times more water for 1 hour or longer until soft and creamy in consistency. To boil, soak cereals for 2 to 3 hours and boil with 10 times more water until one half the original volume of water is left. Use a slow flame after the rice comes to a boil. If rice boils over, turn off flame and start it again when rice stops boiling over.

If the cereal is introduced to a baby less than 5 months old, the porridge is best digested if mashed well, preferably in a suribachi or with a mortar and pestle. If the baby is less than 1 year old, rice syrup or barley malt may be added to maintain a sweet taste similar to the mother's milk.

The proportion of water to grains depends upon the age of the baby and usually ranges from ten to one, to seven to one, to three to one. Younger babies require a softer cereal and thus more water.

The porridge can also be given the baby as a replacement for mother's milk if the mother cannot breastfeed.

Be careful to avoid giving babies porridges or ready-to-eat creamy grain cereals made from flour products.

Soup can be introduced after 5 months, especially broth. The contents may include vegetables that have been well mashed until creamy in form. No salt, miso, or tamari soy sauce should be added before 10 months old. Thereafter, a slightly salty taste may be used for flavoring. However, in such special cases as the baby's stool is green or the baby experiences digestive troubles, a salty taste may need to be used, only in small volume and for a short period.

Vegetables can be introduced after 5 to 7 months, usually when teeth come in and grains have been given for 1 month. When introducing vegetables to children, start by giving sweet vegetables such as carrots, cabbage, squash, onions, daikon, Chinese cabbage. These may be boiled or steamed and should be well cooked and thoroughly mashed. Because it is usually difficult for children to eat greens, parents should make a special effort to see that they are eaten. Sweet greens such as kale and broccoli are generally preferred over slightly bitter-tasting ones such as watercress and mustard greens. Very mild seasoning may be added to vegetables after 10 months to encourage the appetite.

Beans can be introduced after 8 months, but only small amounts of azuki beans, lentils, or chickpeas, cooked well with kombu and mashed thoroughly, are recommended. Other beans such as kidney beans, soybeans, and navy beans can also be used occasionally provided they are well cooked until very soft and mashed thoroughly. Beans may be seasoned with a tiny amount of sea salt or tamari soy sauce or sweetened with squash, barley malt, or rice syrup.

Sea vegetables can be introduced as a separate side dish after the child is from 1½ to 2 years old, although grains are preferably cooked with kombu, and vegetables and beans may also be cooked with sea vegetables even if they are not always eaten.

Fruit should be given to babies or infants occasionally. Temperate-climate fruit, in season, can be introduced in small volume, about one tablespoon, in cooked and mashed form, after 1½ and 2 years of age. However, in some special cases, cooked apples or apple juice may be used temporarily as an adjustment for some conditions.

Pickles that are traditionally made, quick and light in aging and seasoning can be introduced after the child is 2 to 3 years old.

Beverages may include spring or well water, boiled or cooled, bancha twig tea, cereal grain tea, apple juice (warmed or hot), and amasake (which has been boiled with 2 times as much water and cooled).

For further information on infant or childhood nutrition or health, please refer to my forthcoming book, *Macrobiotic Pregnancy* (Japan Publications, 1983) or contact a qualified macrobiotic counselor or medical professional.

33.

Home Cares

The following home remedies are based on traditional macrobiotic Oriental medicine and folk medicine, modified and adjusted for more practical use in modern society. Similar remedies have been used for thousands of years to help alleviate various imbalances caused by faulty diet or unhealthy lifestyle activities. They should be followed only after complete understanding of their uses. If there is any doubt as to whether these remedies should be used, please seek out an experienced macrobiotic counselor or medical professional for proper guidance.

Bancha Stem Tea

Used for strengthening the metabolism in all sicknesses. Use 1 tablespoon of tea to 1 quart of water, bring to a boil, reduce flame, and simmer 4 to 5 minutes.

Brown-Rice Cream

Used in cases when a person in a weakened condition needs to be nourished and energized or when the digestive system is impaired. Dry roast brown rice evenly until all the grains turn a yellowish color. To 1 part rice, add a tiny amount of sea salt and 3 to 6 parts water, and pressure-cook for at least 2 hours. Squeeze out the creamy part of the cooked rice gruel through a cheesecloth sanitized in boiling water. Eat with a small volume of condiment such as umeboshi plum, gomashio, tekka, kelp or other sea vegetable powder.

Brown-Rice Plaster

When the swelling of a boil or infection is not opened by the taro plaster, the rice plaster can be used to help reduce the fever around the infected area. Hand grind 70 percent cooked brown rice, 30 percent raw leafy vegetables, and a few crushed sheets of raw nori in a suribachi—the more grinding the better. (If the mixture is very sticky, add water.) Apply the paste to the affected area. If the plaster begins to burn, remove it, since it is no longer effective. To remove, rinse with warm water to remove direct paste.

Buckwheat Plaster

Purpose: Draws retained water and excess fluid from swollen areas of the body.

Preparation: Mix buckwheat flour with enough hot water to form a hard, stiff dough, and then combine thoroughly with 5 to 10 percent fresh grated ginger. Apply in a ½-inch layer to the affected area; tie in place with a bandage or piece of cotton linen.

Special Consideration for Cancer Cases: A buckwheat plaster should be applied in cases where a patient develops a swollen abdomen due to retention of fluid. If this fluid is surgically removed, the patient may temporarily feel better but on some occasions may suddenly become much worse after several days, so it is better to avoid such a drastic procedure.

This plaster can be applied anywhere on the body. In cases where a breast has been removed, for example, the surrounding lymph nodes, the neck, or in some cases, the arm, often become swollen after several months. To relieve this condition, apply ginger compresses to the swollen area for about five minutes, then apply a buckwheat plaster, and place a salt pack (see instructions below) on top of the plaster to maintain a warm temperature. Replace the buckwheat plaster every four hours. After removing the plaster, you may notice that fluid is coming out through the skin or that the swelling is starting to go down. A buckwheat plaster will usually eliminate the swelling after only several applications or at most after two or three days.

Burdock Tea

Used for strengthening vitality. To 1 portion of fresh burdock shavings, add 10 times the amount of water. Bring to a boil, reduce flame, and simmer for 10 minutes.

Carrot–Daikon Drink

To help eliminate excessive fats and dissolve hardening accumulation in the intestines. Grate 1 tablespoon each of raw daikon and carrot. Cook in 2 cups of spring water for 5 to 8 minutes with a pinch of sea salt or 7 to 10 drops of tamari soy sauce.

Daikon Radish Drink

Drink No. 1: Serves to reduce a fever by inducing sweating. Mix half a cup of grated, fresh daikon with 1 tablespoon of tamari soy sauce and ¼ teaspoon of grated ginger. Pour hot bancha tea or hot water over this mixture, stir, and drink while hot.

Drink No. 2: Induces urination. Use a piece of cheesecloth to squeeze the juice from the grated daikon. Mix 2 tablespoons of this juice with 6 tablespoons of hot water to which a pinch of sea salt or 1 teaspoon of tamari soy sauce has been added. Boil this mixture and drink only once a day. Do not use this preparation more than three consecutive days without proper supervision and never use it without first boiling.

Drink No. 3: Helps dissolve fat and mucus. In a tea cup place 1 tablespoon of fresh grated daikon and 1 teaspoon of tamari soy sauce. Pour hot bancha tea over mixture and drink. It is most effective when taken just before sleeping. Do not use this drink longer than 5 days unless otherwise advised by an experience macrobiotic counselor.

Dandelion Root Tea

Used to strengthen the lungs and large intestine function and increase vitality. One teaspoon of root to 1 cup of water. Bring to a boil, reduce flame, and simmer 10 minutes.

Dentie

Helps to prevent tooth problems, promotes a healthy condition in the mouth, and stops bleeding anywhere in the body by contracting expanded blood capillaries. Bake an eggplant, particularly the calix or cap, until black. Crush into a powder and mix with 30 to 50 percent roasted sea salt. Use daily as a tooth powder or apply to any bleeding area—even inside the nostrils in case of nosebleed—by inserting squeezed, wet tissue dipped in dentie into the nostril.

Dried Daikon Leaves

Used to warm the body and to treat various disorders of the skin and female sex organs. Also helpful in drawing odors and excessive oils from the body. Dry fresh daikon leaves in the shade, away from direct sunlight, until they turn brown and brittle. (If daikon leaves are unavailable, turnip greens may be substituted.) Boil 4 to 5 bunches of the leaves in 4 to 5 quarts of water until the water turns brown. Stir in a handful of sea salt and use in one of the following ways: 1) Dip cotton linen into the hot liquid and wring lightly. Apply to the affected area repeatedly, until the skin becomes completely red. 2) Women experiencing problems in their sexual organs should sit in a hot bath to which the daikon-leaves liquid described above has been added along with one handful of sea salt. The water should come to waist level with the upper portion of the body covered with a towel. Remain in the water until the whole body becomes warm and sweating begins. This generally takes about 10 minutes. Repeat as needed, up to 10 days. Following this bath, douche with warm bancha tea, ½ teaspoon of sea salt, and juice of half a lemon or similar volume of brown rice vinegar.

Ginger Compress

Purpose: Stimulates blood and body fluid circulation, helps loosen and dissolve stagnated toxic matter, cysts, tumors, etc.

Preparation: Place a handful of grated ginger in a cheesecloth and squeeze out the ginger juice into a pot containing 1 gallon of very hot water. Do not boil the water or you will lose the power of the ginger. Dip a cotton hand-towel into the ginger water, wring it out tightly and apply, very hot but not uncomfortably hot, to the area of the body to be treated. A second, dry towel can be placed on top to reduce heat loss. Apply a fresh hot towel every 2 to 3 minutes until the skin becomes red.

Special Considerations for Cancer Cases: The ginger compress should be prepared in the usual manner. However, it should be applied for only a short time (about 5 minutes maximum) to activate circulation in the affected area and should be immediately followed by a taro potato or potato plaster. If a ginger compress is applied repeatedly over an extended time, it may accelerate the growth of the cancer, particularly if it is a more yin variety. The ginger compress should be considered only as a preparation for the taro plaster (see instructions below) in cancer cases, not as an independent treatment, and applied for several minutes only. Please seek more specific recommendations from a qualified macrobiotic adviser.

Ginger Sesame Oil

Activates the function of the blood capillaries, circulation, and nerve reactions. Also relieves aches and pains. Mix the juice of grated, fresh ginger with an equal amount of sesame oil. Dip cotton linen into this mixture and rub briskly into the skin of the affected area. This is also helpful for headache, dandruff, and hair growth.

Grated Daikon

A digestive aid, especially for fatty, oily, heavy foods and for animal food. Grate fresh daikon (red radish or turnip may be used if daikon is not available). Sprinkle with tamari soy sauce and eat about 1 tablespoon. You may also add a pinch of grated ginger.

Green Magma Tea

Young barley grass powder available in many natural foods stores. Good for reducing and melting fats, cysts, and tumors arising from animal foods. Take 1 to 2 teaspoons and pour hot water over and drink. Consult an experienced macrobiotic counselor for length of time to use.

Kombu Tea

Good for strengthening the blood. Use 1 three-inch strip of kombu to 1 quart of water. Bring to a boil, reduce flame, and simmer for 10 minutes. Another method is to dry kombu in a 350° oven for 10 to 15 minutes, or until crisp. Grate ½ to 1 teaspoon of kombu into a cup and add hot water.

Kuzu Drink

Strengthens digestion, increases vitality, and relieves general fatigue. Dissolve a heaping teaspoon of kuzu powder in 2 teaspoons of water, then add to 1 cup of cold water. Bring the mixture to a boil, reduce the heat to the simmering point, and stir constantly until the liquid becomes a transparent gelatin. Stir in 1 teaspoon of tamari soy sauce and drink while hot. Kuzu is also known as kudzu.

Lotus Root Plaster

Draws stagnated mucus from the sinuses, nose, throat, and bronchi. Mix grated, fresh lotus root with 10 to 15 percent pastry flour and 5 to 10 percent grated, fresh ginger. Spread a half-inch layer onto cotton linen and apply the lotus root directly to the skin. Keep on for several hours or overnight and repeat daily for several days. A ginger compress can be applied before this application to stimulate circulation and to loosen mucus in the area being treated.

Lotus Root Tea

Helps relieve coughing and dissolves excess mucus in the body. Grate ½ cup of fresh lotus root, squeeze the juice into a pot, and add a small amount of water. Cook for 5 to 8 minutes, add a pinch of sea salt or tamari soy sauce, and drink hot.

Mustard Plaster

Stimulates blood and body fluid circulation and loosens stagnation. Add hot water to dry mustard powder and stir well. Spread this mixture onto a paper towel and sandwich it between two thick cotton towels. Apply this "sandwich" to the skin area and leave on until the skin becomes red and hot and then remove. After removing, wipe off remaining mustard plaster from the skin with towels.

Nachi Green Tea

Helps dissolve and discharge animal fats and reduce high cholesterol levels. Place ½ teaspoon of tea into the serving kettle. Pour 1 cup of hot water over the tea and steep for 3 to 5 minutes. Strain and drink 1 cup per day.

Salt Bancha Tea

Used to loosen stagnation in the nasal cavity or to cleanse the vaginal region. Add enough salt to warm bancha tea (about body temperature) to make it just a little less salty than sea water. Use the liquid to wash deep inside the nasal cavity through the nostrils or as a douche. Salt bancha tea can also be used as a wash for problems with the eyes, sore throat, and fatigue.

Salt Pack

Used to warm any part of the body. For the relief of diarrhea, for example, apply the pack to the abdominal region. Roast salt in a dry pan until hot and then wrap in thick cotton linen pillowcase or towel and tie with string or cord like a package. Apply to the troubled area and change when the pack begins to cool.

Salt Water

Cold salt water will contract the skin in the case of burns while warm salt water can be used to clean the rectum, colon, and vagina. When the skin is damaged by fire, immediately soak the burned area in cold salt water until irritation disappears. Then apply vegetable oil to seal the wound from the air. For constipation or mucus or fat accumulation in the rectum, colon, and vaginal regions, use warm water (body temperature) as an enema or douche.

Sesame Oil

Used to relieve stagnated bowels or to eliminate retained water. Take 1 to 2 tablespoons of raw sesame oil with ¼ teaspoon of ginger and tamari soy sauce on an empty stomach to induce the discharge of stagnated bowels. To eliminate water retention in the eyes, put a drop or two of pure sesame oil (preferably dark sesame oil) in the eyes with an eyedropper, ideally before sleeping. Continue up to a week, until the eyes improve. Before using the sesame oil for this purpose, boil and then strain it through a sanitized cheesecloth to remove impurities, and let cool.

Shiitake Mushroom Tea

Used to relax an overly tense, stressful condition and helps to dissolve excessive animal fats. Soak a dried black shiitake mushroom cut in quarters. Cook in 2 cups of water for 20 minutes with a pinch of sea salt or 1 teaspoon of tamari soy sauce. Drink only ½ cup at a time.

Tamari Bancha Tea

Neutralizes an acidic blood condition, promotes blood circulation, and relieves fatigue. Pour 1 cup of hot bancha twig tea over 1 to 2 teaspoons of tamari soy sauce. Stir and drink hot.

Tofu Plaster

This treatment is more effective than an ice pack to draw out a fever. Squeeze the water from the tofu, mash it, and then add 10 to 20 percent pastry flour and 5 to 10 percent grated ginger. Mix the ingredients and apply directly to the skin. Change every 2 to 3 hours, or sooner if plaster becomes hot.

Taro Potato (Albi) Plaster

Purpose: Often used after a ginger compress to collect stagnated toxic matter and draw it out of the body.

Preparation: Peel off taro potato skin and grate the white interior. Mix with 5 to 10 percent grated fresh ginger. Spread this mixture in a ⅔ to 1-inch-thick layer onto a fresh cotton linen and apply the taro side directly to the skin. Change every 4 hours.

Taro potato can usually be obtained in most major cities in the United States and Canada from Chinese, Armenian, or Puerto Rican grocery stores or natural foods stores. The skin of this vegetable is brown and covered with "hair." The taro potato is grown in Hawaii as well as in the Orient. Smaller taro potatoes are the most effective for use in this plaster. If taro is not available, a preparation using regular white potato can be substituted. While not as effective as taro, it will still produce a beneficial result. Mix 50 to 60 percent grated white potato with 40 to 50 percent grated or mashed green leafy vegetables, mixing them together in a suribachi. Add enough wheat flour to make a paste and add 5 to 10 percent grated ginger. Apply as above.

Special Considerations for Cancer Patients: The taro plaster has the effect of drawing cancerous toxins out of the body and is particularly effective in removing carbon and other minerals often contained in tumors. If, when the plaster is removed, the light-colored mixture has become dark or brown, or if the skin where the plaster was applied also takes on a dark color, this change indicates that excessive carbon and other elements are being discharged through the skin. This treatment will gradually reduce the size of the tumor if applied repeatedly once or twice daily.

If the patient feels chilly from the coolness of the plaster, a hot ginger compress applied for 5 minutes while changing plasters will help relieve this. If chill persists, roast sea salt in a skillet, wrap it in a towel, and place it on top of the plaster. Be careful not to let the patient become too hot from this salt application.

Ume Extract

A concentrated form of umeboshi plums, available in some natural foods stores. Good for neutralizing an acid or nauseous condition and diarrhea in the stomach. Pour hot water or bancha tea over ¼ to ⅓ teaspoon of ume extract.

Umeboshi Plum

Baked umeboshi plum or powdered baked whole umeboshi plum neutralizes an acidic condition and relieves intestinal problems, including those caused by microorganisms. Take ½ to 1 umeboshi plum (baked is stronger than unbaked) with 1 cup bancha tea. If you bake and crush into a powder, add a teaspoon to 1 cup of hot water.

Ume-Sho-Bancha

Strengthens the blood and the circulation through the regulation of digestion. Pour 1 cup of bancha tea over the meat of ½ to 1 umeboshi plum and 1 teaspoon of tamari soy sauce. Stir and drink hot. Also helps relieve headaches in the front part of the head.

Ume-Sho-Bancha with Ginger

Helps to increase blood circulation. Same as above, but add ¼ teaspoon of grated ginger juice and pour 1 cup of hot bancha tea over. Stir and drink.

Ume-Sho-Kuzu Drink

Strengthens digestion, revitalizes energy, and regulates the intestinal condition. Prepare the kuzu drink according to the instructions for Kuzu Drink and add the meat of ½ to 1 umeboshi plum. One-eighth teaspoon of fresh grated ginger may also be added.

Glossary

Acid phosphatase test Lab test measuring the amount of an enzyme produced in the prostate and released into the blood. High levels indicate possible multiple myeloma or metastatic prostate cancer.

Acupressure Shiatsu massage, a healing art based on stimulating the flow of energy through the meridians of the body.

Acupuncture Far Eastern medical art based on inserting needles in various parts of the body to relieve pain and release blocked energy.

Alkaline phosphatase test Lab test measuring an enzyme in the blood and bone. High levels signify possible liver and pancreatic cancer or other serious condition.

Amasake A sweetener or refreshing drink made from sweet brown rice and koji starter that is allowed to ferment into a thick liquid.

Angiogram A medical procedure in which a radiosensitive dye or other material is injected into the arteries to diagnose cancer or other serious conditions in the inner organs, brain, heart, or limbs.

Arame A thin, wiry black sea vegetable similar to hijiki.

Arrowroot A starch flour processed from the root of an American plant. It is used as a thickening agent for making sauces, stews, gravies, or desserts.

Azuki bean A small, dark red bean originally from Japan but also now grown in the United States.

Bancha tea The stems and leaves from mature Japanese tea bushes, also known as kukicha. Bancha aids in digestion and is high in calcium. It contains no chemical dyes.

Benign tumor A tumor that does not spread to other regions but remains confined to its original location.

430

Bioassay A medical test in which living organisms are used, such as a carcinogenesis test.

Biopsy Extraction of a sample of living tissue or fluid for microscopic examination and diagnosis.

Bok choy A leafy green vegetable.

Bone scan Medical procedure in which radioisotopes are introduced into the bone marrow for detection of bone cancer or metastasis.

Brown rice Whole, unpolished rice. Comes in three main varieties: short-, medium-, and long-grain. Brown rice contains an ideal balance of minerals, protein, and carbohydrates.

Buckwheat A staple food in the Soviet Union and many European countries. This cereal food is eaten widely in the form of kasha, whole groats, and soba noodles.

Burdock A wild, hardy plant that grows throughout the United States. The long, dark root is valued in cooking for its strengthening qualities.

Cancer A disease of the whole body in which mucus and toxins accumulated over years of imbalanced eating are localized as tumors or a degenerating blood or lymph condition.

Carcinogen Any substance that augments cancer in humans or animals.

Carcinoma Cancer in an epithelial tissue, further differentiated into types such as squamous-cell, basal-cell, or adenocarcinoma.

Case-control study A medical study in which exposure data (such as food intake) are collected for individuals (cases) with a specific type of cancer and compared with similar data for a suitable noncancer group (controls).

CAT scan Computer-Assisted Transaxial device that takes cross-sectional x-rays of the brain and torso.

Catheter A hollow tube for discharging fluids from a body cavity.

CBC Complete Blood Count, a computerized lab test that analyzes the constituents of the blood. The normal range for erythroctes (red-blood cells) is 4.5 to 5 million per cubic millimeter; WBC (White-Blood Count), 5,000 to 10,000; granulocytes, 2,000 to 4,000; differential count (ratio of mature to immature cells), 100; blasts (abnormal cells in marrow), less than 5 percent; hematocrit (percentage of red-blood cells), 42 to 46 percent in men and 38 to 42 percent in women; hemoglobin, 13 to 16 grams per 100 milliliters; reticulocytes (young red-blood cells), 0.5 to 1.5 percent of red-blood cells.

CEA assay Lab test measuring the presence of Carcinoembryonic antigen in the blood. High levels indicate possible cancer in the digestive system, lung cancer, and other diseases.

Chemotherapy Treatment of cancer with chemicals or drugs.

Cholesterol A constituent of all animal fats and oils, which in excess can give rise to heart disease, cancer, and other illnesses.

Condition   An individual's day-to-day or year-to-year state of health in contrast to constitution or characteristics acquired at birth.

Constitution   An individual's characteristics determined before birth by the health and vitality of the parents, grandparents, and ancestors, especially by the food eaten by the mother during pregnancy.

Couscous   Partially refined, cracked wheat.

Cyst   A sac containing fluid, mucus, or other material; a possible precancerous sign

Daikon   A long, white radish. Besides making a delicious side dish, daikon is a specific aid in dissolving fat and mucus deposits that have accumulated as a result of past animal food intake. Grated daikon aids in the digestion of oily foods. If unavailable, red radish may be substituted.

Dentie   A black tooth powder made from sea salt and charred eggplant.

Disaccharide   Double sugar such as sucrose (cane sugar) and lactose (milk sugar), which enters the bloodstream rapidly and can lead to imbalance.

Discharge   The body's elimination of mucus, toxins, and other accumulations through normal or abnormal mechanisms ranging from urination and bowel movement to coughing and sneezing to cysts and tumors.

Do-in   A form of Oriental self-massage based on harmonizing the energy flowing through the meridians.

Dulse   A reddish-purple sea vegetable. Used in soups, salads, and vegetable dishes. Very high in iron.

Electromagnetic energy   Natural energy from the environment that flows through all things. Includes atmospheric and celestial forces and the energy generated by the Earth's rotation and orbit.

Endoscope   An instrument for viewing the interior of a body cavity.

Epidemiology   The study of the occurrence and distribution of disease among human populations.

Estrogen   A female hormone that regulates ovarian activity and that may be taken synthetically to control the birth cycle, menopause, or the development of breast, prostate, or other sex-related cancers.

Fiber   The part of vegetable foods that is not broken down in the digestive process and facilitates the elimination of wastes through the intestine. Especially found in whole grains and legumes and to a lesser extent in vegetables and fruits.

Foley food mill   A special steel food mill operated by a hand crank to make purees, sauces, dips, etc.

Gallium scan A total body scan in which radioactive gallium-67 is introduced into the veins. Used particularly to detect the spread of cancer to the lymph nodes.

Genmai miso Miso made from fermented brown rice, soybeans, and sea salt. Also referred to as Brown Rice Miso.

GI series A diagnostic study of the gastrointestinal tract. Usually divided into upper and lower series. The upper observes abnormalities in the esophagus, stomach, and small intestine. The lower (also known as a barium enema) focuses on the large intestine.

Ginger A spicy, pungent, golden-colored root used in cooking and for medicinal purposes.

Ginger compress A compress made from grated gingerroot and water. Applied hot to an affected area of the body, it serves to stimulate circulation and dissolve stagnation.

Gluten The sticky substance that remains after the bran has been kneaded and rinsed from whole wheat flour. Used to make seitan.

Gomashio Sesame salt. A condiment made from roasted, ground sesame seeds and sea salt.

Hatcho miso A fermented soybean paste made from soybeans and sea salt and aged for two years. Used in making condiments, soup stocks, and seasoning for vegetable dishes.

Hijiki A dark, brown sea vegetable, which, when dried, turns black. It has a wiry consistency and may be strong tasting. Hijiki is imported from Japan but also grows off the coast of Maine.

Hokkaido pumpkin A round, dark-green or orange squash that is very sweet and harvested in the fall. Originally from New England, it was introduced to Japan and named after the island of Hokkaido.

Hysterectomy Total or partial surgical removal of the uterus.

Intravenous pylegram (IVP) A fluoroscopic x-ray exam of the urinary system.

Iriko Small dried fish.

Jinenjo A light brown Japanese mountain potato which grows to be several feet long and two to three inches wide.

Kanten A jelled dessert made from agar-agar.

Kasha Buckwheat groats.

Kayu Cereal grain porridge that has been cooked with approximately 5 to 10 times as much water as grain for a long period of time until it is soft and creamy.

Kelp A large family of sea vegetables that grow mainly in northern latitudes. Available packaged whole, granulated, or powdered.

Kinpira A sautéed burdock or burdock and carrot dish that is seasoned with tamari soy sauce.

Koji A grain inoculated with bacteria and used in making fermented foods such as miso, tamari, amasake, natto, and sake.

Kokkoh Baby food porridge made from brown rice, sweet rice, barley, and kombu.

Kombu A wide, thick, dark-green sea vegetable that grows in deep ocean water. Used in making soup stocks, condiments, candy, and cooked with vegetables and beans.

Kukicha Bancha tea. Older stems and leaves of a tea bush grown in Japan.

Kuzu A white starch made from the root of a wild plant. Used in making soups, gravies, desserts, and for medicinal purposes. Also known as kudzu. If unavailable, arrowroot may be substituted.

Laboratory studies Medical tests in which food constituents or chemicals are analyzed for molecular structure, short-term effects on bacteria, yeast, or other biological systems, or long-term effects on animals.

Laparotomy Major abdominal surgery in which a biopsy may be taken of the inner organs.

Lotus root The root of water lily, which is brown-skinned with a hollow, chambered, off-white inside. Especially good for respiratory organs.

Malignant tumor A tumor with the ability to invade adjacent tissue or spread to distant body sites; life-threatening.

Mammogram X-ray of the breast.

Mastectomy Surgical removal of the breast.

Meridian Channel or pathway of electromagnetic energy in the body. Oriental medicine, massage, and the martial arts are based on understanding the flow of energy through the meridians.

Metastasis The spread of cancer from a primary to a secondary site through the blood or lymph systems.

Millet A small, yellow grain, originally native to China, other parts of Asia, and Africa. It can be used regularly in soups, vegetable dishes, and in cereal form.

Miso Fermented soybean paste, used in soups, spreads, and for seasonings.

Mochi A rice cake or dumpling made from cooked, pounded sweet rice.

Monosaccharide Simple sugar such as glucose, fructose, and galactose. Both mono- and disaccharides enter the bloodstream quickly and can elevate blood sugar levels and cause hypoglycemic reactions.

Moxibustion Oriental medical technique of burning mugwort or other herb on the skin to release blocked energy and promote circulation.

Mucus   Viscid liquid secreted by mucous glands and produced from eating foods high in fat and sugar, as well as flour products.

Mugi miso   Soybean paste made from fermented barley, soybeans, sea salt, and water.

Mu tea   A tea made from a variety of herbs that have the medicinal properties of warming the body and strengthening the female organs.

Natto   Soybeans that have been cooked and mixed with beneficial enzymes and allowed to ferment 24 hours.

Natural foods   Whole foods that are unprocessed and untreated with artificial additives or preservatives.

Nigari   Hard crystallized salt made from liquid droppings of dampened sea salt. Used in making tofu.

Nori   Thin sheets of dried sea vegetable. Black or dark purple when dried, they turn green when roasted over a flame. Used as a garnish, wrapped around rice balls, in making sushi, or cooked with tamari soy sauce and used as a condiment.

Okara   Coarse soybean pulp left over when making tofu. Can be put into soups.

Organic foods   Foods grown without the use of artificial chemical fertilizers, herbicides, and pesticides.

Palm healing   Healing method utilizing the palms of the hands to focus electromagnetic energy on various parts of the body.

Pap test   Medical test in which cell samples are taken from the cervix to detect possible cancer.

Physiognomy   The art of judging a person's health from the features of the face or the form of the body.

Polysaccharides   Complex sugars that gradually become absorbed during the digestive process. They include starch and cellulose found in large quantities in whole grains and vegetables.

Polyunsaturated fats   Essential fatty acids found in high concentration in grains, beans, seeds, and in smaller quantities in animal foods, especially fish.

Refined oil   Cooking oil that has been chemically processed to alter or remove color, taste, and odor.

Sarcoma   Cancer of bone, muscle, or connective tissue. Differentiated by site such as osteosarcoma, fibrosarcoma, etc.

Saturated fat   Animal fat primarily, which contributes to the formation of cholesterol and hardening of the arteries.

Sea salt Salt obtained from the ocean and either sun-baked or kiln-baked. Unlike refined table salt, it is high in trace minerals and contains no chemicals, sugar, or iodine.

Seitan Wheat gluten cooked in tamari soy sauce, kombu, and water.'

Shiatsu Traditional Oriental massage based on harmonizing the electromagnetic energy in the body and releasing blockages along the meridians.

Shiitake A medicinal, dried mushroom imported from Japan and now also grown in the United States. Scientific name is *Lentinus edodes*.

Shio kombu Salty kombu. Pieces of kombu cooked for a long time in tamari soy sauce and used in small amounts as a condiment.

Shio nori Pieces of nori cooked for a long time in tamari soy sauce and water and used as a condiment.

Shiso Pickled beefsteak plant leaves.

Shoyu Naturally processed tamari soy sauce.

Soba Noodles made from buckwheat flour or in combination with whole-wheat flour.

Somen Very thin, white or whole-wheat Japanese noodles.

Suribachi A serrated, glazed clay bowl. Used with a pestle, called a surikogi, for grinding and pureeing foods.

Sushi Rice rolled with vegetables, fish, or pickles wrapped in nori and sliced in rounds.

Tai chi A martial art developed in China based on fluid circular movements.

Taro A potato that has a thick, hairy skin. Used in making taro potato plaster to draw toxins from the body. Also called albi.

Tamari soy sauce Traditional, naturally made soy sauce as distinguished from refined, chemically processed soy sauce. Original tamari is made during the process of making miso. The water that comes to the top of the miso and poured off is called tamari.

Tekka Condiment made from hatcho miso, sesame oil, burdock, lotus root, carrot, and gingerroot.

Tempeh A traditional Indonesian soyfood made from split soybeans, water, and a special bacteria, which is allowed to ferment for almost a day. Available prepackaged in some natural foods stores or can be made at home.

Tofu Soybean curd made from soybeans and nigari. High in protein, used in soups, vegetable dishes, dressings, etc.

Tomogram A cross-sectional view of an organ obtained by taking two x-rays in a single plane.

Toxin A poisonous product of animal or vegetable origin, which produces formation of antibodies.

Tumor A swelling or growth of abnormal cells or tissues. May be benign or malignant.

Udon Japanese noodles made from wheat, whole wheat, or whole-wheat and unbleached white flour.

Ultrasound Diagnostic procedure using high-frequency sound echoes to produce an image of the body tissue.

Umeboshi A salty, pickled plum originally from Japan but now also made in the United States.

Unrefined oil Vegetable oil that has been prepressed and/or solvent-extracted to retain the color, aroma, flavor, and nutrients of the natural substance.

Wakame A long, thin green sea vegetable used in making soups, salads, and vegetable dishes.

Whole foods Foods in their entire natural form that have not been refined or processed, such as brown rice, whole-wheat berries, etc.

Yang One of the two complementary and antagonistic forces that combine to produce all phenomena. Yang refers to the relative tendency of contraction, centripetality, fusion, heat, light, density, etc.

Yin The antagonistic, complementary force to yang. Yin is the relative tendency of expansion, growth, centrifugality, diffusion, cold, darkness, etc.

Recommended Reading

Aihara, Cornellia, *The Do of Cooking*, Chico, Calif.: George Ohsawa Macrobiotic Foundation, 1972.

Dietary Goals for the United States, Washington, D.C.: Select Committee on Nutrition and Human Needs, U.S. Senate, 1977.

Diet, Nutrition, and Cancer, Washington, D.C.: National Academy of Sciences, 1982.

Dufty, William, *Sugar Blues*, New York: Warner, 1975.

East West Foundation, *Cancer and Heart Disease: The Macrobiotic Approach to Degenerative Disorders*, New York: Japan Publications, 1982.

Esko, Edward and Wendy, *Macrobiotic Cooking for Everyone*, New York: Japan Publications, 1980.

Esko, Wendy, *Introducing Macrobiotic Cooking*, New York: Japan Publications, 1978.

Fukuoaka, Masanobu, *The One-Straw Revolution*, Emmaus, Pa.: Rodale Press, 1978.

Healthy People: The Surgeon General's Report on Health Promotion and Disease Prevention, Washington, D.C.: Government Printing Office, 1979.

Hippocrates, *Hippocratic Writings*, edited by G.E.R. Lloyd, translated by J. Chadwick and W.N. Mann, New York: Penguin Books, 1978.

I Ching or Book of Changes, translated by Richard Wilhelm and Cary F. Baynes, Princeton: Bollingen Foundation, 1950.

Jacobson, Michael, *The Changing American Diet*, Washington, D.C.: Center for Science in the Public Interest, 1978.

Kohler, Jean and Mary Alice, *Healing Miracles from Macrobiotics*, West Nyack, N.Y.: Parker, 1979.

Kushi, Aveline, *How to Cook with Miso,* New York: Japan Publications 1978.

Kushi, Michio, *The Book of Do-In: Exercise for Physical and Spiritual Development,* New York: Japan Publications, 1979.

——————*The Book of Macrobiotics,* New York: Japan Publications, 1977.

——————*The Era of Humanity,* Brookline, Mass.: East West Journal, 1980.

——————*How to See Your Health: The Book of Oriental Diagnosis,* New York: Japan Publications, 1980.

——————*Natural Healing Through Macrobiotics,* New York: Japan Publications, 1978.

Mendelsohn, Robert S., M.D., *Confessions of a Medical Heretic,* Chicago: Contemporary Books, 1979.

——————*Male Practice,* Chicago: Contemporary Books, 1980.

Ohsawa, George, *Cancer and the Philosophy of the Far East,* Oroville, Calif.: George Ohsawa Macrobiotic Foundation, 1971 edition.

——————*You Are All Sanpaku,* edited by William Dufty, New York: University Books, 1965.

——————*Zen Macrobiotics,* Los Angeles: Ohsawa Foundation, 1965.

Price, Weston A., D.D.S., *Nutrition and Physical Degeneration,* Santa Monica, Calif.: Price-Pottenger Nutritional Foundation, 1945.

Sattilaro, Anthony, M.D. with Tom Monte, *Recalled by Life: The Story of My Recovery from Cancer,* Boston: Houghton-Mifflin, 1982.

Yamamoto, Shizuko, *Barefoot Shiatsu,* New York: Japan Publications, 1979.

The Yellow Emperor's Classic of Internal Medicine, translated by Ilza Veith, Berkeley: University of California Press, 1949.

Periodicals

East West Journal, Brookline, Mass.

Macrobiotic Review, Baltimore, Md.

Nutrition Action, Washington, D.C.

"The People's Doctor" by Robert S. Mendelsohn, M.D. and Marian Tompson, Evanston, Ill.

Index

441

12, 29–30, 101, 150–51, 193, 196, 240–42, 243, 305, 328
agricultural basis of, 242–43
annual deaths from, 3
beneficial nature of, 24
causes of, 20–23, 52–54, 75
contributing factors to, 52–54
cure vs. control of, 79
development of, 35–41
dietary prevention of, 42–49, 305
dietary relief of, 69–77, 81
environmental factors in, 25, 52–54, 73–76
history of, 5–10
holistic approach to, 23, 75
increase in, 3, 5, 12, 193, 194
and lifestyle, 26–27, 28, 73–76
national rates of, 31
origin of the word for, 5
protective factors against, 52–54, 104
seasonal incidence of, 88–89
and society, 19, 96–97
and spiritual awareness, 74–76, 113–14
treatment vs. no treatment of, 8, 79
two basic types of, 66
wartime decline of, 12–13, 155, 192–93
as a whole vs. local disease, 21–25, 35–41, 69–70, 96, 100, 105–06, 150, 192
yin/yang diagnosis of, 67–68, 69
Cancer (earlier journal), 6, 151, 243
Cancer (later journal), 195, 244, 257, 293, 306, 317
Cancer Research
case-control studies in, 152, 155
epidemiological studies in, 154, 171, 215, 267, 317, 329
laboratory studies in, 100, 125, 151, 214, 227, 292, 306
Cancer Treatment Reports, 267
Caraka Samhita, 9, 82
Carbohydrates, 33, 40, 112, 225
Carcinogens, 99–100
discovery of, 22, 99
fear of, 99–100
theory of, 105–07
Carroll, K.K., 152, 154

Carrot juice, 243
Case histories. *See* Personal experiences
CAT scan, 144
Cataracts, 39, 157
Catholicism, 10, 75–76, 275–76
CEA test, 206, 235, 287
Cellular level, cancer at the mechanism of, vii, 20, 28, 35, 104–07
modern medical approach to, 20–22, 24–25, 70
rise of interest in, 11
Cervical cancer. *See* Female cancers
Cervical dysplasia, 165
Cheese. *See also* Dairy food
effects on body of, 37, 295
guidelines for use of, 45, 348
rising use of, 30, 32, 181, 288
substitute for, 55
Chemicals, 45, 52–54, 103, 257, 228–29
Chemotherapy
benefits of, 80
limits of, 78, 90, 94, 146
personal experiences of, 144, 205, 262–63, 273, 274–75, 286, 312
recovering from the effects of, 76, 90, 94, 120, 274–75
theory of, 105–07
Chewing, proper
importance of, 48
metabolism of, 71, 316
patients' practice of, 132, 180, 196, 335
Cheyne, George, 150
Chihara, G., 125
Childhood cancers
dietary recommendations for, 417–19
China
cancer rates in, 222, 241, 244, 245, 306, 318
traditional teachings of, 9, 16, 58, 82, 317
Chinese Journal of Preventive Medicine, 306
Cholesterol
disease promoted by, 40, 258, 280, 295
metabolism of, 224–25
reduction of, by whole foods, 55, 189, 195, 227–28, 298, 425

RECIPE INDEX

Notes on the Authors

Michio Kushi, leader of the international macrobiotic, natural health movement, has guided thousands of people with cancer toward physical, psychological, and spiritual health and lectured on Oriental medicine and philosophy to medical professionals across North and South America, Europe, and the Far East. He has inspired macrobiotic research projects at the Harvard School of Public Health, Shattuck Hospital in Boston, and other hospitals, medical schools, and prisons around the country. He is the president of the Kushi Foundation, Kushi Institute, and East West Foundation in Boston with 500 affiliate centers worldwide. Since 1977 he has presided over the East West Foundation's annual Conference on Cancer and Other Degenerative Diseases. He has also spoken at numerous international seminars, governmental conferences, universities, medical schools, civic organizations, and the United Nations.

Born in Kokawa, Wakayama-ken, Japan in 1926, Michio Kushi devoted his early years to the study of international law at Tokyo University. Following World War II, he became interested in world peace through world government and met Yukikazu Sakurazawa (known in the West as George Ohsawa), who had revised and reintroduced the principles of Oriental medicine and philosophy under the name *macrobiotics*. Inspired by Ohsawa's teaching, he began his lifelong study of the application of traditional understanding to solving the problems of the modern world.

In 1949 Michio Kushi came to the United States to pursue graduate studies at Columbia University. Since that time he has resided in this country and lectured on medicine, philosophy, and culture and given personal counseling to individuals and families. In 1972 he founded the East West Foundation, a nonprofit cultural and educational organization, with headquarters in Boston, to help develop and spread the macrobiotic way of life through seminars, publications, research, and other means. He is also the founder of Erewhon, a leading distributor of natural and macrobiotic foods in North America; the *East West Journal*, a monthly magazine unifying traditional Oriental philosophy and medicine with Western science; and the *Order of the Universe*, a journal of philosophy and science. In 1978 he founded the Kushi Institute, an educational organization for the training of macrobiotic teachers, counselors, and cooks, with affiliates in London, Amsterdam, and Antwerp. As a further means toward addressing problems of world health and world peace, he established the Macrobiotic Congresses of North America and Western Europe, which meet annually and draw delegates from many states and nations.

Michio Kushi has published a dozen books including *The Book of Macrobiotics, How to See Your Health: Book of Oriental Diagnosis,* and *The Macrobiotic Way of Natural Healing.* He currently resides in Brookline, Massachusetts, with his wife Aveline, five children, and their families.

Alex Jack has been involved in the natural foods and holistic health movements as an author, journalist, and speaker. For seven years he worked on the staff of the *East West Journal*, serving as editor from 1979 to 1982. During this time he coordinated investigative reporting on diet, nutrition, cancer, heart disease, and other degenerative illnesses as well as writing on topics such as natural healing in the Bible and the *Divine Comedy*. In 1980, as a guest of the Buddhist Association of China, he organized a macrobiotic banquet featuring brown rice and miso from the United States at the Zen temple in Peking for Buddhist, Taoist, Islamic, and Christian leaders.

Alex Jack was born in Chicago in 1945 and grew up in Evanston, Illinois and Scarsdale, New York. His interest in the Far East developed at age eleven when he accompanied his father, a Unitarian minister, to an international peace conference in Japan. During the mid-1960's, he served as a civil rights organizer in Mississippi, helped set up an arts festival with atomic bomb survivors in Hiroshima, and reported on the war in Southeast Asia for a syndicate of university, small-town, and peace publications. He adopted a natural foods diet while studying philosophy and religion at Banaras Hindu University in India in 1965.

Alex Jack received a degree in philosophy from Oberlin College in 1967 and went on to graduate work in theology in the Boston area. His books include *The Adamantine Sherlock Holmes* and *The New Age Dictionary*. He has lectured at the East West Foundation, the New England Acupuncture Center, and other organizations. He lives in Brookline, Massachusetts.